Practical Issues in Geriatrics

Series Editor

Stefania Maggi
Aging Branch
CNR-Neuroscience Institute
Padua, Italy

This practically oriented series presents state of the art knowledge on the principal diseases encountered in older persons and addresses all aspects of management, including current multidisciplinary diagnostic and therapeutic approaches. It is intended as an educational tool that will enhance the everyday clinical practice of both young geriatricians and residents and also assist other specialists who deal with aged patients. Each volume is designed to provide comprehensive information on the topic that it covers, and whenever appropriate the text is complemented by additional material of high educational and practical value, including informative video-clips, standardized diagnostic flow charts and descriptive clinical cases. Practical Issues in Geriatrics will be of value to the scientific and professional community worldwide, improving understanding of the many clinical and social issues in Geriatrics and assisting in the delivery of optimal clinical care.

More information about this series at http://www.springer.com/series/15090

Nicola Veronese • Charlotte Beaudart
Shaun Sabico

Editors

Sarcopenia

Research and Clinical Implications

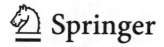 Springer

Editors
Nicola Veronese
Department of Internal Medicine
University of Palermo
Palermo
Italy

Shaun Sabico
Chair for Biomarkers of Chronic Diseases
Biochemistry Department
College of Science
King Saud University
Riyadh
Saudi Arabia

Charlotte Beaudart
WHO Collaborating Center for Public
Health Aspects of Musculo-skeletal Health
and Ageing, Division of Public Health
Epidemiology and Health Economics
University of Liège
Liège
Belgium

ISSN 2509-6060 ISSN 2509-6079 (electronic)
Practical Issues in Geriatrics
ISBN 978-3-030-80040-6 ISBN 978-3-030-80038-3 (eBook)
https://doi.org/10.1007/978-3-030-80038-3

This Springer imprint is published by the registered company Springer Nature Switzerland AG
The registered company address is: Gewerbestrasse 11, 6330 Cham, Switzerland

Preface

From a single concept to a consistently hot topic in major medical congresses and scholastic journals, sarcopenia has undoubtedly become one of modern medicine's most active areas of research within the geriatric field in such a short span of time. At its most basic definition, sarcopenia just means muscle, or flesh (sarx) loss (penia). But because it is a syndrome, sarcopenia is compounded with both physiologic and pathologic components that are multifactorial in nature, making it a genuine medical challenge. Fortunately, landmark investigations on sarcopenia have started to accumulate at warp speed to shed some much-needed light on this condition. Interdisciplinary collaborations of major clinical organizations took advantage of this momentum, to set the foundational platform for which sarcopenia guidelines can evolve, eventually culminating in the recognition and birth of sarcopenia as a distinct disease entity. The present book intends to update the global academic and medical community on major and emerging aspects of sarcopenia, from epidemiology to molecular mechanisms, from screening to future drugs, and from nutrition to the complex interactions between the skeletal and muscular tissues. This herculean objective has been accomplished not by us, but by the well-respected international field experts, who graciously accepted to contribute high-quality chapters and make this book a repository of cutting-edge knowledge on sarcopenia. It is the hope of the editors that through this book, its intended audience will not only become adept on what's latest in sarcopenia, but will also be able to identify several gaps that are yet to be filled for the continuous understanding of this disease in the right direction. Perhaps the biggest accomplishment this book can attain is to attract the new generation of geriatricians who will continue the expansion and advancement of the field that is arguably, still, at its infancy. We are confident that we have successfully assembled an up-to-date book on sarcopenia with wide coverage of the most recent literature, to serve as a reference not only for early career scientists and physicians but also for experts, in their quest to further improve the field's knowledge and ultimately serve our biggest benefactors, the elderly population.

Palermo, Italy   Nicola Veronese
Liège, Belgium   Charlotte Beaudart
Riyadh, Saudi Arabia   Shaun Sabico

Contents

Epidemiology of Sarcopenia

1

Fiona Ecarnot ⓘ, Domenico Rogoli, and Stefania Maggi

1.1   Introduction

The term sarcopenia derives from the Greek "sarx" meaning flesh and "pcnia" meaning loss or poverty. It was first introduced by Rosenberg [1] in 1997 to describe the age-related loss of skeletal muscle mass and function, after seminal publications by Evans and Campbell regarding the declining functional status observed in older individuals with changes in body composition [2–4]. Initially, it was thought that only muscle wasting occurred in elderly individuals, but sarcopenia is now recognized as a complex concept that involves not only loss of muscle mass but also decreased muscle strength, and a resulting decline in functional capacity. Functional parameters came to be included in the definition because they have consistently been shown to be a stronger predictor of outcomes than muscle mass alone [5]. Indeed, sarcopenia is a progressive and generalized skeletal disorder that is not necessarily synonymous with leanness. It may also be present in overweight and obese individuals, a condition now termed "sarcopenic obesity" (*see* Chap. 14). A distinction may also be made between primary, or age-related sarcopenia, and secondary sarcopenia, which is more disease-related.

F. Ecarnot (✉)
Department of Cardiology, University Hospital Besancon, Besancon, France

EA3920, University of Burgundy Franche-Comté, Besancon, France
e-mail: Fiona.ecarnot@univ-fcomte.fr

D. Rogoli · S. Maggi
CNR, Aging Branch-NI, Padua, Italy
e-mail: stefania.maggi@in.cnr.it

© Springer Nature Switzerland AG 2021   1
N. Veronese et al. (eds.), *Sarcopenia*, Practical Issues in Geriatrics,
https://doi.org/10.1007/978-3-030-80038-3_1

1.2   Definitions

Over the years since its first description, there has been a steady increase in research and publications about sarcopenia, and a number of groups and societies have published operational definitions of sarcopenia for use in clinical practice and in research settings. Following a meeting of a group of geriatricians and scientists from academia and industry in 2009, the International Working Group on Sarcopenia published a definition of sarcopenia, namely the "age-associated loss of skeletal muscle mass and function" [6]. In 2010, the European Working Group on Sarcopenia in Older People (EWGSOP) developed a clinical definition together with consensus diagnostic criteria for age-related sarcopenia, which recommended that both low muscle mass and low muscle function (i.e., strength or performance) be considered [7]. The EWGSOP further defined stages of severity, with a gradual scale from pre-sarcopenia to sarcopenia to severe sarcopenia. The EWGSOP consensus was updated in 2019 to reflect the growing body of evidence that has emerged since its first publication [8]. In parallel, professional societies in Asia also worked to prepare consensus definitions on sarcopenia, due to the fact that the cultural, lifestyle, and anthropometric differences call for specific considerations when diagnosing sarcopenia in people of Asian descent. In this regard, the Asian Working Group on Sarcopenia published a diagnostic algorithm for sarcopenia using cut-offs and reference levels derived from Asian populations [9], which was updated in 2019, revising some of the component criteria and cut-offs [10]. In 2011, the Society on Sarcopenia, Cachexia and Wasting Disorders Trialist Workshop convened a consensus conference, which concluded that "sarcopenia, i.e., reduced muscle mass, with limited mobility should be considered an important clinical entity" [11]. Their definition was based on walk speed on the 6-min walk test and lean appendicular mass corrected for height. Finally, the Foundation for the National Institutes of Health (FNIH) Sarcopenia Project also developed an operational definition of sarcopenia based on data from 9 sources totalling over 26,000 individuals to identify clinically relevant and independently validated thresholds that could be used to identify participants for clinical trials, and individuals with significant functional limitation [12].

The abundance of research in the field of sarcopenia culminated in the recognition of sarcopenia as a distinct disease, with its inclusion in the International Classification of Diseases tenth Revision (ICD-10) in 2016 (under the ICD code M62.84) [13, 14]. This important step meant that the condition could be cited on medical records, death certificates, and other data sources, which can help harmonize practices, compare data, and promote research. The recognition of sarcopenia as a disease entity also provides additional stimulus for pharmaceutical companies to invest in research and development in this area, by allowing for billing and reimbursement possibilities.

The various definitions of sarcopenia developed by professional societies, as well as other combinations of criteria used in the literature to define sarcopenia, will be discussed in greater detail in Chap. 3. Suffice to say, however, that there are wide variations across all these definitions in the components included, the methods used to measure these components, and the cut-off values used to distinguish pathological states. For the measurement of muscle mass, dual-energy X-ray absorptiometry (DXA) is a widely available, noninvasive method for determining muscle quantity (i.e., total body lean tissue mass or appendicular skeletal muscle mass) and is considered by many as the gold standard. However, inconsistencies may exist across measurements performed with different machines, rendering comparison difficult [15]. Other methods used to assess muscle mass include bioelectrical impedance analysis (BIA), computed tomography (CT), or magnetic resonance imaging (MRI), as well as simple anthropometric measures. Muscle strength can be measured easily and inexpensively by assessing hand-grip strength with a calibrated handheld dynamometer. For patients in whom disability of any type precludes measurement of hand-grip strength, leg strength can be used as a proxy, for example, via the chair stand test, timed chair stand test, or the timed up-and-go test. Other measures of mobility, such as gait speed, or walk test performance are also widely used. The heterogeneity of definitions, criteria, measurement methods, and cut-off values makes it extremely difficult to compare estimates of sarcopenia prevalence between studies. Estimates are also affected by the populations used to define the normal range reference values and the setting in which those cut-offs are applied (e.g., community-dwelling adults, versus nursing home residents, versus acute hospital care) [16]. This underlines the need for a consensual definition, to enable comparison of the burden of disease worldwide, as the lack of agreement between definitions hampers the integration of sarcopenia into clinical practice.

1.3   Prevalence of Sarcopenia

The prevalence of sarcopenia is notoriously difficult to compare across studies, in view of this heterogeneity of definitions and measurement possibilities. Nevertheless, recent years have seen a striking increase in the number of publications investigating sarcopenia prevalence, risk factors, and outcomes. Many of these are now using established definitions, thus allowing for some comparison of rates across studies as the body of evidence grows. Table 1.1 displays a selection of prevalence estimates from recent publications in various populations. It can be seen that there are wide variations in reported rates between studies, and even within studies, when different criteria are used to define sarcopenia. The burgeoning volume of publications on the prevalence of sarcopenia has led to ever more precise estimates, and reports providing pooled estimates from systematic reviews and/or meta-analysis. For example, in a systematic review and meta-analysis, Mayhew et al. examined 109 studies using 8 different sarcopenia definitions (including the EWGSOP, AWGS, FNIH, and IWGS definitions), with a total of 227 individual prevalence estimates in community-dwelling older adults (>60 years) without specific health conditions [24]. Overall, estimated prevalence ranged from 9.9 to 40.4% and was lowest with the EWGSOP/AWGS (12.9%, 95% CI: 9.9, 15.9%), IWGS (9.9%, 95% CI: 3.2, 16.6%), and FNIH (18.6%, 95% CI: 11.8, 25.5%) definitions [24]. In another systematic review and meta-analysis, Shafiee et al. included 35 population-based studies reporting the prevalence of sarcopenia in healthy adults aged ≥60 years from different regions of

Table 1.1 Selected data from the literature on prevalence of sarcopenia in different populations

Author, year (Reference)	Study population	Age	Findings
Purcell, 2020 [17]	12,592 community-dwelling subjects from the Canadian Longitudinal Study on Aging (6314 men (50.1%), 6278 women (49.9%))	All 65 y or older	Across different definitions, prevalence (all ages combined) ranged from: − 0.2% (EWGSOP2) to 5.2% (IWGS) in men − 0.2% (EWGSOP2) to 7.2% (IWGS) in women
Martone, 2020 [18]	11,253 community-dwelling subjects from the Italian Longevity Check-up 7+ project (4897 men (44%), 6356 women (56%))	Mean 55.6 ± 14.8 y Range 18–98 y	8.6% had probable sarcopenia according to the EWGSOP2 definition. Prevalence increased with age to reach 54.2% in women and 42.4% in men older than 80 y
Ligthart-Melis, 2020 [19]	Meta-analysis of 15 studies totalling 4014 hospitalized patients	Mean ranged from 62 to 86 y across studies	Pooled estimates: − 37% (95% CI 26–48) overall − 44% (95% CI 29–58) in the medical subgroup − 22% (95% CI 19–25) in the surgical subgroup − 25% (95% CI 9–40) in the mixed medical/surgical subgroup
Pang, 2020 [20]	542 community-dwelling Singaporeans (57.9% women)	Mean 58.5 ± 18.8 Range 21–90 y	Prevalence estimates according to definition: AWGS 2014: − 6.7% overall, 6.9% in men, 6.4% in women AWGS 2019: − 13.6% overall, 13% in men, 14.2% in women EWGSOP2: − 7.1% overall, 9.2% in men, 5.3% in women
Wearing, 2020 [21]	219 community-dwelling Swiss subjects	82.6 ± 5.2 (men), 84.1 ± 5.7 (women)	Using the cut-off for hand-grip strength from EWGSOP2, prevalence of probable sarcopenia was 26.3% in women and 28% in men
Nguyen, 2020 [22]	600 outpatients attending the National Geriatric Hospital in Hanoi, Vietnam (60.8% females)	70 ± 8 y	Prevalence estimates according to definition: AWGS 2019: − 54.7% overall FNIH: − 40.5% overall Rates were significantly higher in men than in women in both definitions

Table 1.1 (continued)

Author, year (Reference)	Study population	Age	Findings
Makizako, 2019 [23]	7974 community-dwelling Japanese subjects from 9 studies (3723 men, 4367 women)	All 60 y or older	Using AWGS criteria: In individual studies: − 4.7–25.7% overall prevalence − 4.9–25.0% in men − 4.5–26.1% in women Pooled prevalence estimates: − 9.9% (95% CI 6.2–15.4) overall − 9.8% (95% CI 6.2–15.2) in men − 10.1% (95% CI 6.4–15.5) in women
Mayhew, 2018 [24]	Meta-analysis of 109 articles totalling 58 cohorts from 26 countries; all community-dwelling adults without specific diseases	Minimum 55 y	Pooled prevalence estimates according to definition: EWGSOP/AWGS: − 58,283 participants from 83 studies: 12.9% (95% CI 9.9–15.9) IWGS: − 10,381 participants from 12 studies: 9.9% (95% CI 3.2–16.6) FNIH: − 6467 participants from 16 studies: 18.6% (95% CI 11.8–25.5)
Churilov, 2018 [16]	Meta-analysis of 6 studies of post-acute inpatient rehabilitation (of which 5 post hip fracture)	Mean ranged from 79.7 ± 7.4 to 84.6 ± 6.6 y	Prevalence ranged from 28 to 69% across studies Pooled prevalence: 56% (95% CI 46–65%)
Shafiee, 2017 [25]	Meta-analysis of 35 articles totalling 58,404 community-dwelling individuals (55.9% men, 44.1% women)	All ≥60 y	Articles included used EWGSOP, AWGS, and/or IWGS definitions. Overall prevalence 10% (95% CI 8–12%) in men and 10% (95% CI 8–13%) in women Across individual studies, rates ranged from 0.35% to 36.6% according to the study and definition used
Kim, 2016 [26]	1464 community-dwelling Japanese subjects (246 men, 1218 women)	74.3 ± 5.17 y (men) 79.9 ± 4.43 y (women)	Using DXA measured definitions: − 2.5–28.0% in men − 2.3–11.7% in women Using BIA-measured definitions: − 7.1–98.0% in men − 19.8–88.0% in women

(continued)

Table 1.1 (continued)

Author, year (Reference)	Study population	Age	Findings
Sousa, 2015 [27]	608 hospitalized adults from medical and surgical wards, conscious and not cognitively impaired; critically ill patients excluded	Median 57 y Range 18–90 y 31.7% ≥65 y 4.6% >80 y	25.3% sarcopenic using the EWGSOP definition. Depending on age and criteria used to define sarcopenia, estimated prevalence ranged from 5% to 41.1% in men and from 4.9% to 38.3% in women
Cruz-Jentoft, 2014 [28]	18 studies of prevalence: 15 in community-dwellers, 2 in long-term institutions, 1 in acute hospital care	Mean (when given) ranged from 59.2 to 85.8 y	Prevalence: – 1–29% in community-dwellers (up to 30% in women) – 14–33% in long-term institutions (up to 68% in men) – 10% in the study of acute hospital care
Volpato, 2014 [29]	730 community-dwelling Italian individuals from the InCHIANTI study	All ≥65 y Mean 83.8 ± 5.92 in sarcopenic vs. 76.3 ± 4.96 in non-sarcopenic individuals	Using the EWGSOP definition, 16.7% were pre-sarcopenic and 7.5% were sarcopenic
Lee, 2013 [30]	386 elderly community-dwellers from the I-Lan Longitudinal Ageing Study, Taiwan (57.8% men)	74.4 ± 6.1 y (men) 72.8 ± 4.9 y (women)	Using relative skeletal mass index: EWGSOP: – 7.8% overall, 10.8% in men, 3.7% in women IWGS: – 4.1% overall, 5.8% in men, 1.8% in women. Using percentage skeletal muscle index: EWGSOP: – 16.6% overall, 14.9% in men, 19.0% in women IWGS: – 11.1% overall, 10.8% in men, 11.7% in women.
Pongchaiyakul, 2013 [31]	832 Thai subjects (435 urban, 397 rural dwellers)	49.34 ± 17.26 y (men) 50.45 ± 15.54 y (women)	35.33% (95% CI, 29.91–40.41) in men 34.74% (95% CI, 30.56–39.10) in women
Janssen, 2006 [32]	5036 noninstitutionalized elderly men and women from the Cardiovascular Health Study	>65 y	Moderate sarcopenia: – 70.7% in men – 41.9% in women Severe sarcopenia: – 17.1% in men – 10.7% in women

Table 1.1 (continued)

Author, year (Reference)	Study population	Age	Findings
Rolland, 2003 [33]	1458 non-institutionalized women recruited from electoral lists; final sample for analysis comprised 1311 women	All >70 y Mean 80.3 ± 3.8 y	Prevalence 9.5% (95% CI 7.9–11.1%)
Lauretani, 2003 [34]	1030 persons (469 men, 561 women) from the InCHIANTI epidemiological study	Range 20–102 y	Men: – 20% at 65 years – 70% at 85 years Women: – 5% at 65 years – 15% at 85 years
Baumgartner, 1998 [35]	808 elderly Hispanic and non-Hispanic white men and women from the New Mexico Elder Health Study (47.3% women)	73.6 ± 5.8 y (men) 73.7 ± 6.1 (women)	<70 y: – 13.5–16.9% (men) – 23.1–24.1% (women) 70–74 y: – 18.3–19.8% (men) – 33.3–35.1% (women) 75–80 y: – 26.7–36.4% (men) – 35.3–35.9% (women) >80 y: – 52.6–57.6% (men) – - 43.2–60.0% (women)

y ycars, *CI* confidence interval, *EWGSOP* European Working Group on Sarcopenia in Older People, *EWGSOP2* 2019 revised European consensus on definition and diagnosis of sarcopenia, *IWGS* International Working Group on Sarcopenia, *AWGS* Asian Working Group on Sarcopenia, *FNIH* Foundation for the National Institutes of Health, *DXA* dual-energy X-ray absorptiometry, *BIA* bioelectrical impedance analysis

the world, using the EWGSOP, IWGS, and AWGS definitions [25]. They reported an overall prevalence of 10% in both men and women, although estimates ranged from 0.35 to 36.6% across studies, depending on the definition used. There was significant heterogeneity between men and women in Shafiee's meta-analysis [25]. Furthermore, analysis by region showed that individuals in non-Asian countries were more likely to have sarcopenia than those from Asian countries, in both genders (11% vs. 10% in men, 13% vs. 9% in women) [25].

Even though it is almost impossible to pinpoint an actual rate of prevalence of sarcopenia, projections indicate that the rate is rising and looks set to continue increasing in the future, as worldwide population ageing adds growing numbers of older people to the pool of potentially sarcopenic individuals. In a study using the various diagnostic cut-offs proposed by the EWGSOP for lean mass, muscle strength, and gait speed, Ethgen et al. applied interpolated age- and gender-specific estimates of sarcopenia prevalence to the Eurostat population projections for Europe up to 2045 [36]. From a previous publication comparing prevalence rates at different cut-offs [37], Ethgen et al. chose first the definition yielding the lowest prevalence estimates, applied it to projected population estimates for Europe, and found that it would correspond to a 72.4% increase in overall prevalence of sarcopenia in the elderly, rising from 11.1% in 2016 to 12.9% in 2045. Applying the definition yielding the highest prevalence estimates, overall prevalence rates were projected to increase from 20.2% in 2016 to 22.3% in 2045 [36]. These projections portend a substantial burden of sarcopenia in coming decades, which will have important repercussions for society in terms of healthcare delivery and costs.

1.4   Risk Factors

Numerous risk factors for sarcopenia have been reported in the literature, some of which are non-modifiable, such as age and gender; others are modifiable and exert their influence across the life course. Among the non-modifiable risk factors, the most consistent body of evidence supports an increasing risk of sarcopenia with older age [5, 18, 22, 27, 29, 38]. Indeed, muscle mass begins to decline around the fifth decade of life, with an annual decline rate of 1–2% [39–41], accelerating in the sixth and subsequent decades to reach a loss of around 15% per decade beyond the age of 70 [42, 43]. Regarding gender, conflicting results have been reported regarding the difference in risk in men and women, but consensus seems to be emerging in favor of an increased risk of sarcopenia in men. Landi et al. reported a 13-fold increased risk in male nursing home residents (odds ratio (OR) 13.39; 95% CI 3.51–50.63) [44], while Nguyen et al. reported a twofold increase in risk of sarcopenia among male outpatients at a geriatric hospital (OR 2.03, 95% CI 1.29–3.21) [22]. Despite the existence of differences in baseline strength between the sexes, with men having greater baseline strength than women, it has been reported that muscle strength declines to a greater degree in men, thus potentially contributing to their higher risk of sarcopenia [45–47].

Concerning modifiable risk factors, nutrition and lifestyle behaviors (notably exercise) appear to be associated with muscle mass and strength in older age [48, 49]. Older people experience a natural decline in energy requirements [50], which may be accompanied by declining appetite, impaired taste or smell, and changes in gastrointestinal motility and digestion [51]. If also compounded by functional impairment reducing the ability to prepare food, or social isolation, which may reduce the desire to eat or enjoyment of mealtimes, all these features come together in a vicious circle that may lead to loss of weight and muscle mass and strength, putting older individuals at risk of malnutrition and in turn, sarcopenia and/or frailty [48, 49]. The contribution of adequate nutrition to healthy aging has long been established [52], and there have been a number of studies examining the effects of various dietary components and patterns on sarcopenia and its constituent elements. However, apart from the obvious need to ensure that all older adults have adequate nutrition both in terms of quantity and quality, the potential of individual dietary patterns to affect outcome remains unclear. Indeed, there have been conflicting findings regarding the association between protein intake and muscle strength, for example, although observational evidence tends to suggest that both strength and function are improved with increased protein intake [48]. In the same way, it is difficult to distinguish the effects of individual nutrients, such as antioxidants and omega-3 fatty acids, although overall, the best evidence supports the benefits of the Mediterranean dietary pattern in terms of functional status and incident disability [48].

The effect of exercise in reducing the negative impact of sarcopenia has been demonstrated by several studies [53–55]. In a systematic umbrella review, Beckwee et al. investigated the efficacy of different exercise interventions to counter sarcopenia in older adults [53]. They found high-quality evidence in favor of a positive and significant effect of resistance training on muscle mass, muscle strength, and physical performance from a total of 14 systematic reviews, of which 7 performed meta-analysis. Based on the evidence from their review, these authors suggest that benefits in terms of muscle mass, muscle strength, and gait speed can be expected with high-intensity resistance training, which they recommend for at least 6–12 weeks, in order to achieve these levels of improvement [53]. Similarly, Lai et al. compared the effects of exercise interventions on lean body mass, muscle strength, and physical performance in a network meta-analysis and found that resistance training (of a minimum 6 weeks duration) was the most effective intervention in improving muscle strength in older individuals [54].

Other risk factors have been less extensively investigated. Nonetheless, a meta-analysis of 12 studies totalling 22,515 participants found smoking to be an independent risk factor for sarcopenia (OR 1.20 (95% CI 1.06–1.35) in men and 1.21 (95% CI 0.92–1.59) in women) [56]. The same group also performed a meta-analysis of 13 studies including 13,155 participants to investigate the effect of alcohol on sarcopenia, but their findings did not support the hypothesis that alcohol consumption could be a risk factor for sarcopenia [57].

Other factors that have been shown to be associated with sarcopenia include age-related loss of motor-neuron end plates [58], loss of anabolic hormones and insulin resistance [42, 59], diabetes [60], obesity/waist circumference [46], level of education [29], and dependency [27, 44].

1.5   The Health Economic Burden of Sarcopenia

Sarcopenia is associated with an increased risk of falls and fractures [61, 62], frailty [63], disability [64], and cognitive impairment [65]. Low grip strength has been shown to be associated with increased morbidity and mortality [66, 67], and a meta-analysis of 11 studies investigating the impact of EWGSOP-defined sarcopenia on mortality found a more than threefold increase in the risk of mortality among sarcopenic subjects (pooled OR 3.596 (95% CI 2.96–4.37)) [68]. These deleterious outcomes can in turn translate into extended recovery time, longer length of hospital stay, and increased medical costs [68, 69].

In community-dwelling adults in the Netherlands, Mijnarends et al. reported that the mean healthcare costs of individuals with sarcopenia were significantly higher than those of non-sarcopenic subjects (€ 4325, 95% CI € 3198–€5471 vs. €1533,

95% CI €1153–€1912, respectively), mainly driven by the living situation (i.e., residential care) [70]. In the hospital setting, two studies from Portugal investigated the costs of hospitalization associated with sarcopenia. Sousa et al. assessed the hospitalization costs in 656 medical and surgical patients (24.2% sarcopenic) using diagnosis-related group codes at discharge [71]. They found that sarcopenic patients were generally older and had a longer length of stay, resulting in a median (interquartile) cost of € 3151 (€ 4175) per sarcopenic patient, compared to non-sarcopenic patients (median (IQR) € 2170 (€ 2515), $p < 0.001$) [71]. After adjustment for confounders, the economic impact of sarcopenia on hospitalization cost, i.e., the incremental cost per patient, in the overall sample was estimated at € 1117 (95% CI €644–1588), and sarcopenia was estimated to increase hospitalization costs by 39.2% in those with no comorbidities and by 54.3% in those with comorbidities [71]. In the second Portuguese study, Antunes et al. assessed hospitalization costs among 201 hospitalized older adults in a general hospital [72]. After adjustment, both sarcopenia (OR = 5.70, 95% CI 1.57–20.71) and low muscle strength alone (OR = 2.40, 95% CI 1.12–5.15) were associated with increased hospital costs. From a societal perspective, Janssen et al. evaluated the costs of sarcopenia in a representative sample of US adults aged 60 years and older, from the NHANES III and National Medical Care Utilization and Expenditures Survey (NMCUES) datasets [73]. They estimated that the direct healthcare cost attributable to sarcopenia in the USA in 2000 was $18.5 billion ($10.8 billion in men, $7.7 billion in women), representing 1.5% of total healthcare expenditure, with sensitivity analyses indicating that the cost could be as low as $11.8 billion and as high as $26.2 billion. They further estimated that a 10% reduction in the prevalence of sarcopenia would result in savings of $1.1 billion (dollar value in the year 2000) per year in US healthcare costs [73]. A more recent study from the USA updates this information and shows that costs are already on the rise; Goates et al. performed a retrospective economic burden study among 4011 adults aged 40 years and over from the NHANES dataset [74], of whom 15.1% were sarcopenic. They reported an annual total cost of hospitalization for individuals with sarcopenia of $40.4 billion, with an average estimated marginal cost increase in annual hospital spending of $2315 per sarcopenic individual, compared to those with normal muscle mass and function. In addition, they reported that individuals with sarcopenia had an almost twofold increase in the risk of hospitalization (OR 1.94, $p < 0.001$) and more hospital stays on average, compared to those without sarcopenia [74]. There is wide heterogeneity among studies on the economic burden of sarcopenia, with different approaches used to estimate costs, different time horizons for measurements, and different definitions of sarcopenia. With populating ageing continuing its onward march around the world, there is a compelling need to continue providing up-to-date estimates of sarcopenia-associated healthcare costs, particularly using standardized definitions and cost analysis parameters, not least to prepare for the substantial burden that this will represent on healthcare systems in the coming decades. The alarming estimates of the burden that sarcopenia represents on healthcare also underscores the need to focus preventive measures on preserving muscle mass, strength, and function as long as possible into older age.

1.6 Conclusion

Sarcopenia is characterized by an age-related loss of muscle mass, muscle strength, and/or physical function. It is associated with a high risk of morbidity and mortality, poor clinical outcomes, and increased events, such as falls, fractures, and hospitalizations. It represents a significant burden on healthcare systems worldwide, which looks set to increase in the coming decades. A strong research agenda is warranted to expand our knowledge of the etiological factors involved in the development of sarcopenia, and which could be leveraged to prevent or slow the onset of sarcopenia, or its progression to more severe forms. Systematic screening of older individuals is warranted to detect those with lower muscle strength, with a view to initiating early interventions to retard sarcopenia. Resistance training, of a minimum 6 weeks duration, has been shown to be most effective in achieving improvements in muscle strength in older adults. The benefit of adequate nutrition in contributing to healthy ageing has also been well established. Other interventions to promote healthy ageing and preserve muscle mass, strength and function into older age are warranted, to counter the effects of ageing and maintain functional capacity as long as possible. The considerable economic burden of sarcopenia on healthcare costs justifies the implementation of preventive measures, perhaps over the life course and almost certainly warranted from midlife onwards, in order to stem the tide of negative consequences that flows from the presence of sarcopenia.

References

1. Rosenberg IH. Sarcopenia: origins and clinical relevance. J Nutr. 1997;127:990S–1S. https://doi.org/10.1093/jn/127.5.990S.
2. Evans WJ, Campbell WW. Sarcopenia and age-related changes in body composition and functional capacity. J Nutr. 1993;123:465–8. https://doi.org/10.1093/jn/123.suppl_2.465.
3. Evans WJ. What is sarcopenia? J Gerontol A Biol Sci Med Sci. 1995;50 Spec No:5–8. https://doi.org/10.1093/gerona/50a.special_issue.5.
4. Evans WJ. Skeletal muscle loss: cachexia, sarcopenia, and inactivity. Am J Clin Nutr. 2010;91:1123S–7S. https://doi.org/10.3945/ajcn.2010.28608A.
5. Cruz-Jentoft AJ, Sayer AA. Sarcopenia. Lancet. 2019;393:2636–46. https://doi.org/10.1016/S0140-6736(19)31138-9.
6. Fielding RA, Vellas B, Evans WJ, Bhasin S, Morley JE, Newman AB, Abellan van Kan G, Andrieu S, Bauer J, Breuille D, Cederholm T, Chandler J, De Meynard C, Donini L, Harris T, Kannt A, Keime Guibert F, Onder G, Papanicolaou D, Rolland Y, Rooks D, Sieber C, Souhami E, Verlaan S, Zamboni M. Sarcopenia: an undiagnosed condition in older adults. Current consensus definition: prevalence, etiology, and consequences. International Working Group on Sarcopenia. J Am Med Dir Assoc. 2011;12:249–56. https://doi.org/10.1016/j.jamda.2011.01.003.
7. Cruz-Jentoft AJ, Baeyens JP, Bauer JM, Boirie Y, Cederholm T, Landi F, Martin FC, Michel JP, Rolland Y, Schneider SM, Topinkova E, Vandewoude M, Zamboni M, European Working Group on Sarcopenia in Older P. Sarcopenia: European consensus on definition and diagnosis: report of the European Working Group on Sarcopenia in older people. Age Ageing. 2010;39:412–23. https://doi.org/10.1093/ageing/afq034.
8. Cruz-Jentoft AJ, Bahat G, Bauer J, Boirie Y, Bruyere O, Cederholm T, Cooper C, Landi F, Rolland Y, Sayer AA, Schneider SM, Sieber CC, Topinkova E, Vandewoude M, Visser M,

Zamboni M, Writing Group for the European Working Group on Sarcopenia in Older P, the Extended Group for E. Sarcopenia: revised European consensus on definition and diagnosis. Age Ageing. 2019;48:16–31. https://doi.org/10.1093/ageing/afy169.

9. Chen LK, Liu LK, Woo J, Assantachai P, Auyeung TW, Bahyah KS, Chou MY, Chen LY, Hsu PS, Krairit O, Lee JS, Lee WJ, Lee Y, Liang CK, Limpawattana P, Lin CS, Peng LN, Satake S, Suzuki T, Won CW, Wu CH, Wu SN, Zhang T, Zeng P, Akishita M, Arai H. Sarcopenia in Asia: consensus report of the Asian Working Group for Sarcopenia. J Am Med Dir Assoc. 2014;15:95–101. https://doi.org/10.1016/j.jamda.2013.11.025.

10. Chen LK, Woo J, Assantachai P, Auyeung TW, Chou MY, Iijima K, Jang HC, Kang L, Kim M, Kim S, Kojima T, Kuzuya M, Lee JSW, Lee SY, Lee WJ, Lee Y, Liang CK, Lim JY, Lim WS, Peng LN, Sugimoto K, Tanaka T, Won CW, Yamada M, Zhang T, Akishita M, Arai H. Asian Working Group for Sarcopenia: 2019 consensus update on sarcopenia diagnosis and treatment. J Am Med Dir Assoc. 2020;21:300–307.e2. https://doi.org/10.1016/j.jamda.2019.12.012.

11. Morley JE, Abbatecola AM, Argiles JM, Baracos V, Bauer J, Bhasin S, Cederholm T, Coats AJ, Cummings SR, Evans WJ, Fearon K, Ferrucci L, Fielding RA, Guralnik JM, Harris TB, Inui A, Kalantar-Zadeh K, Kirwan BA, Mantovani G, Muscaritoli M, Newman AB, Rossi-Fanelli F, Rosano GM, Roubenoff R, Schambelan M, Sokol GH, Storer TW, Vellas B, von Haehling S, Yeh SS, Anker SD, Society on Sarcopenia C, Wasting Disorders Trialist W. Sarcopenia with limited mobility: an international consensus. J Am Med Dir Assoc. 2011;12:403–9. https://doi.org/10.1016/j.jamda.2011.04.014.

12. Studenski SA, Peters KW, Alley DE, Cawthon PM, McLean RR, Harris TB, Ferrucci L, Guralnik JM, Fragala MS, Kenny AM, Kiel DP, Kritchevsky SB, Shardell MD, Dam TT, Vassileva MT. The FNIH sarcopenia project: rationale, study description, conference recommendations, and final estimates. J Gerontol A Biol Sci Med Sci. 2014;69:547–58. https://doi.org/10.1093/gerona/glu010.

13. Anker SD, Morley JE, von Haehling S. Welcome to the ICD-10 code for sarcopenia. J Cachexia Sarcopenia Muscle. 2016;7:512–4. https://doi.org/10.1002/jcsm.12147.

14. Cao L, Morley JE. Sarcopenia is recognized as an independent condition by an international classification of disease, tenth revision, clinical modification (ICD-10-CM) code. J Am Med Dir Assoc. 2016;17:675–7. https://doi.org/10.1016/j.jamda.2016.06.001.

15. Buckinx F, Landi F, Cesari M, Fielding RA, Visser M, Engelke K, Maggi S, Dennison E, Al-Daghri NM, Allepaerts S, Bauer J, Bautmans I, Brandi ML, Bruyere O, Cederholm T, Cerreta F, Cherubini A, Cooper C, Cruz-Jentoft A, McCloskey E, Dawson-Hughes B, Kaufman JM, Laslop A, Petermans J, Reginster JY, Rizzoli R, Robinson S, Rolland Y, Rueda R, Vellas B, Kanis JA. Pitfalls in the measurement of muscle mass: a need for a reference standard. J Cachexia Sarcopenia Muscle. 2018;9:269–78. https://doi.org/10.1002/jcsm.12268.

16. Churilov I, Churilov L, MacIsaac RJ, Ekinci EI. Systematic review and meta-analysis of prevalence of sarcopenia in post acute inpatient rehabilitation. Osteoporos Int. 2018;29:805–12. https://doi.org/10.1007/s00198-018-4381-4.

17. Purcell SA, MacKenzie M, Barbosa-Silva TG, Dionne IJ, Ghosh S, Olobatuyi OV, Siervo M, Ye M, Prado CM. Sarcopenia prevalence using different definitions in older community-dwelling Canadians. J Nutr Health Aging. 2020;24:783–90. https://doi.org/10.1007/s12603-020-1427-z.

18. Martone AM, Marzetti E, Salini S, Zazzara MB, Santoro L, Tosato M, Picca A, Calvani R, Landi F. Sarcopenia identified according to the EWGSOP2 definition in community-living people: prevalence and clinical features. J Am Med Dir Assoc. 2020;21:1470–4. https://doi.org/10.1016/j.jamda.2020.03.007.

19. Ligthart-Melis GC, Luiking YC, Kakourou A, Cederholm T, Maier AB, de van der Schueren MAE. Frailty, sarcopenia, and malnutrition frequently (co-)occur in hospitalized older adults: a systematic review and meta-analysis. J Am Med Dir Assoc. 2020;21:1216–28. https://doi.org/10.1016/j.jamda.2020.03.006.

20. Pang BWJ, Wee SL, Lau LK, Jabbar KA, Seah WT, Ng DHM, Ling Tan QL, Chen KK, Jagadish MU, Ng TP. Prevalence and associated factors of sarcopenia in Singaporean

adults-the Yishun study. J Am Med Dir Assoc. 2021;22(4):885.e1–10. https://doi.org/10.1016/j.jamda.2020.05.029.

21. Wearing J, Konings P, de Bie RA, Stokes M, de Bruin ED. Prevalence of probable sarcopenia in community-dwelling older Swiss people—a cross-sectional study. BMC Geriatr. 2020;20:307. https://doi.org/10.1186/s12877-020-01718-1.

22. Nguyen TN, Nguyen TN, Nguyen AT, Nguyen TX, Nguyen HTT, Nguyen TTH, Pham T, Vu HTT. Prevalence of sarcopenia and its associated factors in patients attending geriatric clinics in Vietnam: a cross-sectional study. BMJ Open. 2020;10:e037630. https://doi.org/10.1136/bmjopen-2020-037630.

23. Makizako H, Nakai Y, Tomioka K, Taniguchi Y. Prevalence of sarcopenia defined using the Asia Working Group for Sarcopenia criteria in Japanese community-dwelling older adults: a systematic review and meta-analysis. Phys Ther Res. 2019;22:53–7. https://doi.org/10.1298/ptr.R0005.

24. Mayhew AJ, Amog K, Phillips S, Parise G, McNicholas PD, de Souza RJ, Thabane L, Raina P. The prevalence of sarcopenia in community-dwelling older adults, an exploration of differences between studies and within definitions: a systematic review and meta-analyses. Age Ageing. 2019;48:48–56. https://doi.org/10.1093/ageing/afy106.

25. Shafiee G, Keshtkar A, Soltani A, Ahadi Z, Larijani B, Heshmat R. Prevalence of sarcopenia in the world: a systematic review and meta- analysis of general population studies. J Diabetes Metab Disord. 2017;16:21. https://doi.org/10.1186/s40200-017-0302-x.

26. Kim H, Hirano H, Edahiro A, Ohara Y, Watanabe Y, Kojima N, Kim M, Hosoi E, Yoshida Y, Yoshida H, Shinkai S. Sarcopenia: prevalence and associated factors based on different suggested definitions in community-dwelling older adults. Geriatr Gerontol Int. 2016;16(Suppl 1):110–22. https://doi.org/10.1111/ggi.12723.

27. Sousa AS, Guerra RS, Fonseca I, Pichel F, Amaral TF. Sarcopenia among hospitalized patients—a cross-sectional study. Clin Nutr. 2015;34:1239–44. https://doi.org/10.1016/j.clnu.2014.12.015.

28. Cruz-Jentoft AJ, Landi F, Schneider SM, Zuniga C, Arai H, Boirie Y, Chen LK, Fielding RA, Martin FC, Michel JP, Sieber C, Stout JR, Studenski SA, Vellas B, Woo J, Zamboni M, Cederholm T. Prevalence of and interventions for sarcopenia in ageing adults: a systematic review. Report of the International Sarcopenia Initiative (EWGSOP and IWGS). Age Ageing. 2014;43:748–59. https://doi.org/10.1093/ageing/afu115.

29. Volpato S, Bianchi L, Cherubini A, Landi F, Maggio M, Savino E, Bandinelli S, Ceda GP, Guralnik JM, Zuliani G, Ferrucci L. Prevalence and clinical correlates of sarcopenia in community-dwelling older people: application of the EWGSOP definition and diagnostic algorithm. J Gerontol A Biol Sci Med Sci. 2014;69:438–46. https://doi.org/10.1093/gerona/glt149.

30. Lee WJ, Liu LK, Peng LN, Lin MH, Chen LK, Group IR. Comparisons of sarcopenia defined by IWGS and EWGSOP criteria among older people: results from the I-Lan longitudinal aging study. J Am Med Dir Assoc. 2013;14(528):e521–7. https://doi.org/10.1016/j.jamda.2013.03.019.

31. Pongchaiyakul C, Limpawattana P, Kotruchin P, Rajatanavin R. Prevalence of sarcopenia and associated factors among Thai population. J Bone Miner Metab. 2013;31:346–50. https://doi.org/10.1007/s00774-013-0422-4.

32. Janssen I. Influence of sarcopenia on the development of physical disability: the cardiovascular health study. J Am Geriatr Soc. 2006;54:56–62. https://doi.org/10.1111/j.1532-5415.2005.00540.x.

33. Rolland Y, Lauwers-Cances V, Cournot M, Nourhashemi F, Reynish W, Riviere D, Vellas B, Grandjean H. Sarcopenia, calf circumference, and physical function of elderly women: a cross-sectional study. J Am Geriatr Soc. 2003;51:1120–4. https://doi.org/10.1046/j.1532-5415.2003.51362.x.

34. Lauretani F, Russo CR, Bandinelli S, Bartali B, Cavazzini C, Di Iorio A, Corsi AM, Rantanen T, Guralnik JM, Ferrucci L. Age-associated changes in skeletal muscles and their effect on mobility: an operational diagnosis of sarcopenia. J Appl Physiol (1985). 2003;95:1851–60. https://doi.org/10.1152/japplphysiol.00246.2003.

35. Baumgartner RN, Koehler KM, Gallagher D, Romero L, Heymsfield SB, Ross RR, Garry PJ, Lindeman RD. Epidemiology of sarcopenia among the elderly in New Mexico. Am J Epidemiol. 1998;147:755–63. https://doi.org/10.1093/oxfordjournals.aje.a009520.
36. Ethgen O, Beaudart C, Buckinx F, Bruyere O, Reginster JY. The future prevalence of sarcopenia in Europe: a claim for public health action. Calcif Tissue Int. 2017;100:229–34. https://doi.org/10.1007/s00223-016-0220-9.
37. Beaudart C, Reginster JY, Slomian J, Buckinx F, Locquet M, Bruyere O. Prevalence of sarcopenia: the impact of different diagnostic cut-off limits. J Musculoskelet Neuronal Interact. 2014;14:425–31.
38. Iannuzzi-Sucich M, Prestwood KM, Kenny AM. Prevalence of sarcopenia and predictors of skeletal muscle mass in healthy, older men and women. J Gerontol A Biol Sci Med Sci. 2002;57:M772–7. https://doi.org/10.1093/gerona/57.12.m772.
39. von Haehling S, Morley JE, Anker SD. An overview of sarcopenia: facts and numbers on prevalence and clinical impact. J Cachexia Sarcopenia Muscle. 2010;1:129–33. https://doi.org/10.1007/s13539-010-0014-2.
40. Abellan van Kan G. Epidemiology and consequences of sarcopenia. J Nutr Health Aging. 2009;13:708–12. https://doi.org/10.1007/s12603-009-0201-z.
41. Doherty TJ. Invited review: aging and sarcopenia. J Appl Physiol (1985). 2003;95:1717–27. https://doi.org/10.1152/japplphysiol.00347.2003.
42. Kim TN, Choi KM. Sarcopenia: definition, epidemiology, and pathophysiology. J Bone Metab. 2013;20:1–10. https://doi.org/10.11005/jbm.2013.20.1.1.
43. Grimby G, Saltin B. The ageing muscle. Clin Physiol. 1983;3:209–18. https://doi.org/10.1111/j.1475-097x.1983.tb00704.x.
44. Landi F, Liperoti R, Fusco D, Mastropaolo S, Quattrociocchi D, Proia A, Russo A, Bernabei R, Onder G. Prevalence and risk factors of sarcopenia among nursing home older residents. J Gerontol A Biol Sci Med Sci. 2012;67:48–55. https://doi.org/10.1093/gerona/glr035.
45. Fuggle N, Shaw S, Dennison E, Cooper C. Sarcopenia. Best Pract Res Clin Rheumatol. 2017;31:218–42. https://doi.org/10.1016/j.berh.2017.11.007.
46. Shaw SC, Dennison EM, Cooper C. Epidemiology of sarcopenia: determinants throughout the lifecourse. Calcif Tissue Int. 2017;101:229–47. https://doi.org/10.1007/s00223-017-0277-0.
47. Goodpaster BH, Park SW, Harris TB, Kritchevsky SB, Nevitt M, Schwartz AV, Simonsick EM, Tylavsky FA, Visser M, Newman AB. The loss of skeletal muscle strength, mass, and quality in older adults: the health, aging and body composition study. J Gerontol A Biol Sci Med Sci. 2006;61:1059–64. https://doi.org/10.1093/gerona/61.10.1059.
48. Robinson SM, Reginster JY, Rizzoli R, Shaw SC, Kanis JA, Bautmans I, Bischoff-Ferrari H, Bruyere O, Cesari M, Dawson-Hughes B, Fielding RA, Kaufman JM, Landi F, Malafarina V, Rolland Y, van Loon LJ, Vellas B, Visser M, Cooper C, ESCEO working group. Does nutrition play a role in the prevention and management of sarcopenia? Clin Nutr. 2018;37:1121–32. https://doi.org/10.1016/j.clnu.2017.08.016.
49. Welch AA. Nutritional influences on age-related skeletal muscle loss. Proc Nutr Soc. 2014;73:16–33. https://doi.org/10.1017/S0029665113003698.
50. Wakimoto P, Block G. Dietary intake, dietary patterns, and changes with age: an epidemiological perspective. J Gerontol A Biol Sci Med Sci. 2001;56 Spec No 2:65–80. https://doi.org/10.1093/gerona/56.suppl_2.65.
51. Malafarina V, Uriz-Otano F, Gil-Guerrero L, Iniesta R. The anorexia of ageing: physiopathology, prevalence, associated comorbidity and mortality. A systematic review. Maturitas. 2013;74:293–302. https://doi.org/10.1016/j.maturitas.2013.01.016.
52. Kadoch MA. The power of nutrition as medicine. Prev Med. 2012;55:80. https://doi.org/10.1016/j.ypmed.2012.04.013.
53. Beckwee D, Delaere A, Aelbrecht S, Baert V, Beaudart C, Bruyere O, de Saint-Hubert M, Bautmans I. Exercise interventions for the prevention and treatment of sarcopenia. A systematic umbrella review. J Nutr Health Aging. 2019;23:494–502. https://doi.org/10.1007/s12603-019-1196-8.

54. Lai CC, Tu YK, Wang TG, Huang YT, Chien KL. Effects of resistance training, endurance training and whole-body vibration on lean body mass, muscle strength and physical performance in older people: a systematic review and network meta-analysis. Age Ageing. 2018;47:367–73. https://doi.org/10.1093/ageing/afy009.

55. Law TD, Clark LA, Clark BC. Resistance exercise to prevent and manage sarcopenia and dynapenia. Annu Rev Gerontol Geriatr. 2016;36:205–28. https://doi.org/10.1891/0198-8794.36.205.

56. Steffl M, Bohannon RW, Petr M, Kohlikova E, Holmerova I. Relation between cigarette smoking and sarcopenia: meta-analysis. Physiol Res. 2015;64:419–26. https://doi.org/10.33549/physiolres.932802.

57. Steffl M, Bohannon RW, Petr M, Kohlikova E, Holmerova I. Alcohol consumption as a risk factor for sarcopenia—a meta-analysis. BMC Geriatr. 2016;16:99. https://doi.org/10.1186/s12877-016-0270-x.

58. Drey M, Krieger B, Sieber CC, Bauer JM, Hettwer S, Bertsch T, Group DS. Motoneuron loss is associated with sarcopenia. J Am Med Dir Assoc. 2014;15:435–9. https://doi.org/10.1016/j.jamda.2014.02.002.

59. Morley JE, Anker SD, von Haehling S. Prevalence, incidence, and clinical impact of sarcopenia: facts, numbers, and epidemiology-update 2014. J Cachexia Sarcopenia Muscle. 2014;5:253–9. https://doi.org/10.1007/s13539-014-0161-y.

60. Kim TN, Park MS, Yang SJ, Yoo HJ, Kang HJ, Song W, Seo JA, Kim SG, Kim NH, Baik SH, Choi DS, Choi KM. Prevalence and determinant factors of sarcopenia in patients with type 2 diabetes: the Korean Sarcopenic Obesity Study (KSOS). Diabetes Care. 2010;33:1497–9. https://doi.org/10.2337/dc09-2310.

61. Schaap LA, van Schoor NM, Lips P, Visser M. Associations of sarcopenia definitions, and their components, with the incidence of recurrent falling and fractures: the longitudinal aging study Amsterdam. J Gerontol A Biol Sci Med Sci. 2018;73:1199–204. https://doi.org/10.1093/gerona/glx245.

62. Zhang Y, Hao Q, Ge M, Dong B. Association of sarcopenia and fractures in community-dwelling older adults: a systematic review and meta-analysis of cohort studies. Osteoporos Int. 2018;29:1253–62. https://doi.org/10.1007/s00198-018-4429-5.

63. Syddall H, Cooper C, Martin F, Briggs R, Aihie Sayer A. Is grip strength a useful single marker of frailty? Age Ageing. 2003;32:650–6. https://doi.org/10.1093/ageing/afg111.

64. Xu W, Chen T, Cai Y, Hu Y, Fan L, Wu C. Sarcopenia in community-dwelling oldest old is associated with disability and poor physical function. J Nutr Health Aging. 2020;24:339–45. https://doi.org/10.1007/s12603-020-1325-4.

65. Peng TC, Chen WL, Wu LW, Chang YW, Kao TW. Sarcopenia and cognitive impairment: a systematic review and meta-analysis. Clin Nutr. 2020;39:2695–701. https://doi.org/10.1016/j.clnu.2019.12.014.

66. Cooper R, Kuh D, Cooper C, Gale CR, Lawlor DA, Matthews F, Hardy R, Falcon THAS. Objective measures of physical capability and subsequent health: a systematic review. Age Ageing. 2011;40:14–23. https://doi.org/10.1093/ageing/afq117.

67. Cooper R, Kuh D, Hardy R, Mortality Review G, Falcon THAS. Objectively measured physical capability levels and mortality: systematic review and meta-analysis. BMJ. 2010;341:c4467. https://doi.org/10.1136/bmj.c4467.

68. Beaudart C, Zaaria M, Pasleau F, Reginster JY, Bruyere O. Health outcomes of sarcopenia: a systematic review and meta-analysis. PLoS One. 2017;12:e0169548. https://doi.org/10.1371/journal.pone.0169548.

69. Norman K, Otten L. Financial impact of sarcopenia or low muscle mass—a short review. Clin Nutr. 2019;38:1489–95. https://doi.org/10.1016/j.clnu.2018.09.026.

70. Mijnarends DM, Schols JMGA, Halfens RJG, Meijers JMM, Luiking YC, Verlaan S, Evers SMAA. Burden-of-illness of Dutch community-dwelling older adults with sarcopenia: health related outcomes and costs. Eur Geriatr Med. 2016;7:276–84. https://doi.org/10.1016/j.eurger.2015.12.011.

71. Sousa AS, Guerra RS, Fonseca I, Pichel F, Ferreira S, Amaral TF. Financial impact of sarcopenia on hospitalization costs. Eur J Clin Nutr. 2016;70:1046–51. https://doi.org/10.1038/ejcn.2016.73.
72. Antunes AC, Araujo DA, Verissimo MT, Amaral TF. Sarcopenia and hospitalisation costs in older adults: a cross-sectional study. Nutr Diet. 2017;74:46–50. https://doi.org/10.1111/1747-0080.12287.
73. Janssen I, Shepard DS, Katzmarzyk PT, Roubenoff R. The healthcare costs of sarcopenia in the United States. J Am Geriatr Soc. 2004;52:80–5. https://doi.org/10.1111/j.1532-5415.2004.52014.x.
74. Goates S, Du K, Arensberg MB, Gaillard T, Guralnik J, Pereira SL. Economic impact of hospitalizations in US adults with sarcopenia. J Frailty Aging. 2019;8:93–9. https://doi.org/10.14283/jfa.2019.10.

Definitions of Sarcopenia Across the World

2

Domenico Azzolino, Shaea Alkahtani, and Matteo Cesari

2.1 Introduction

The musculoskeletal system is pivotal for physical functionssing. Advancing age is associated with several changes in body composition. The most evident of these changes (both phenotypically and functionally speaking) is probably the progressive loss of muscle mass and strength. In fact, after the age of 40, a progressive decline both in muscle mass (about 1–2% per year) and strength (about 1.5% per year, but even up to 3% per year after the sixth decade of life) is observed [1].

In 1988, during a meeting in Albuquerque (New Mexico, USA), Rosenberg explained that no change occurring with aging was more significant and clinically relevant than the progressive decline of the skeletal muscle. To give adequate recognition to this major feature of the aging process, he proposed using the term "sarcopenia" or" sarcomalacia." Since then, sarcopenia, from the Ancient Greek σάρξ (sárx, "flesh") and πενίᾱ (peníā, "poverty"), has been widely accepted and increasingly adopted [2].

The first studies on sarcopenia were focused mainly on the quantitative aspect of the skeletal muscle decline (i.e., the loss of muscle mass). Subsequently, evidence started to point out the prominent role of muscle quality (i.e., muscle strength) in the clinical characterization of the phenomenon. In particular, it became evident that muscle mass alone (at least as measured with the instruments available at that time)

D. Azzolino · M. Cesari (✉)
Department of Clinical Sciences and Community Health, University of Milan, Milan, Italy

Geriatric Unit, IRCCS Istituti Clinici Scientifici Maugeri, Milan, Italy
e-mail: domenico.azzolino@unimi.it

S. Alkahtani
Department of Exercise Physiology, King Saud University, Riyadh, Saudi Arabia
e-mail: shalkahtani@ksu.edu.sa

© Springer Nature Switzerland AG 2021
N. Veronese et al. (eds.), *Sarcopenia*, Practical Issues in Geriatrics,
https://doi.org/10.1007/978-3-030-80038-3_2

had a lower predictive capacity than muscle functioning for adverse clinical outcomes [3]. In this context, the term "dynapenia" was also proposed to capture the muscle strength abnormality [4].

It is also noteworthy the theoretical evolution of the sarcopenia concept over the years. If, at the beginning, sarcopenia was primarily considered as a geriatric syndrome [4], a specific International Classification of Diseases (ICD-10) code was applied to it in 2016, allowing to view it today as a formal disease [5]. This legitimation has substantially boosted the interest around it, and several molecules are in the pipeline of pharmaceutical industries for potentially treating sarcopenia in the next future [6, 7].

Over the past decade, several consensus definitions have been released by expert groups worldwide to (1) find an agreement on the definition, assessment, and diagnosis of sarcopenia and (2) stimulate research on this age-related condition globally impacting on our aging societies. Unfortunately, this field is still very debated and controversial. Several operational definitions have been proposed, frequently differing in the quality of the defining criteria and the cut-points setting the thresholds distinguishing normality from abnormality. Furthermore, it has been pointed out that body composition is substantially influenced by ethnicity. Therefore, the designing of diagnostic algorithms may need adaptations to the local context where these are applied. In this context, it is well-known how the scientific literature is strongly biased by the vast majority of evidence coming from high-income regions, in particular the United States and Europe. It is thus fully justified and meritorious the effort of many for adapting the concept of sarcopenia designed by task forces and expert groups to the reality of regions and countries which, despite being highly populated, are still not adequately represented in the literature [8]. In this chapter, we will present and discuss the main definitions and operationalizations of sarcopenia across the world.

2.2   Sarcopenia: Different Definitions Across the World

The first operational definition of sarcopenia was provided by Baumgartner and colleagues [9]. Low muscle mass was defined as the reduced amount (i.e., less than two standard deviations) of appendicular lean mass standardized by height in square meters. It is evident how the condition of interest was considered in a monodimensional way, exclusively looking at the skeletal muscle mass. Furthermore, the definition of the critical cut-points was based on the characteristics of the participants enrolled in the New Mexico Elder Health Survey 1993–1995.

A milestone in the field was subsequently set in 2010 when the European Working Group on Sarcopenia in Older People (EWGSOP) [10] released a well-known and highly cited consensus document. The recommendations have been recently revised and updated (in the so-called EWGSOP2 document) [11]. The first EWGSOP definition considered sarcopenia as the simultaneous presence of low muscle mass and poor muscle function (i.e., muscle weakness or physical performance impairment). In other words, the EWGSOP introduced the dimension of muscle function into the definition of sarcopenia. The choice was mainly motivated by the fact that muscle strength had consistently been a better predictor of adverse health-related outcomes than muscle mass alone. Muscle strength is not dependent only on muscle mass, and the relationship between these two components is not linear. Furthermore, it could not be ignored that muscle weakness is more likely to be reported as a complaint by the older person than the reduction of muscle volume.

Interestingly, several consensus documents were released by different scientific societies and task forces at the same time [12–14]. They all presented the development of the sarcopenia condition into a bidimensional construct (i.e., mass and function reduction). However, probably because of its more accurate and detailed presentation, the EWGSOP definition became presumably the most widely adopted and largely contributed to increasing the recognition of sarcopenia. The cut-points proposed by the EWGSOP to define sarcopenia and the definition algorithm are presented in Table 2.1.

In 2013, members of the EWGSOP, together with the International Working Group on Sarcopenia (IWGS) [13] and several experts from Asia, met to discuss specific issues present with the construct of sarcopenia and to constitute the International Sarcopenia Initiative (ISI) [15]. The ISI agreed that the definitions of sarcopenia should include both muscle mass and function rather than muscle mass alone. Furthermore, it was recommended the use of standardized models and cut-points for each domain considered in the definition of sarcopenia.

In recognition of the impact that different ethnic backgrounds may have on body composition, the Asian Working Group on Sarcopenia (AWGS) [16] released a consensus in 2014 proposing specific cut-points for defining muscle mass and strength abnormalities in the Asian population (Table 2.1). The AWGS definition followed the same diagnostic approach of the EWGSOP (except for the recommendation of measuring muscle strength and gait speed as screening test). It can indeed be considered an adaptation of the EWGSOP to a different (i.e., non-European) population.

In parallel, using a completely different approach (i.e., data-driven instead of consensus statement), the Foundation for the National Institutes of Health-Sarcopenia Project (FNIH) [17] developed a new set of criteria to identify individuals with low appendicular lean mass and muscle weaknesses. The FNIH group conducted in-depth analyses taking advantage of several large cohort studies to determine the strongest predictors of mobility disability and the critical thresholds of risk. The analyses identified the low appendicular lean mass (both adjusted for body mass index and not adjusted) and poor grip strength as the most relevant criteria for capturing the two sarcopenia dimensions (Table 2.1).

More recently, the Sarcopenia Definition and Outcomes Consortium (SDOC) [18] published a position statement. Overall, the SDOC strongly agreed on the inclusion of low grip strength and slow gait speed in the definition of sarcopenia, while questioned on the use of the dual-energy X-ray absorptiometry (DXA) to assess muscle mass.

It is important to note that each definition impacts both case finding and prevalence of sarcopenia. The different diagnostic approaches, the various cut-points used to define sarcopenia, and the ethnic differences determine critical variations in

Table 2.1 Summary of different operational definitions of sarcopenia

Expert group	Cut-points for muscle mass	Cut-points for muscle strength	Cut-points for physical performance
EWGSOP1	ALM/height (m^2) using DXA: Men: <7.23 kg/m^2 Women: <5.67 kg/m^2 SMM/height (m^2) using BIA: Men: <8.87 kg/m^2 Women: <6.42 kg/m^2	Men: <30 kg Women: <20 kg	Gait speed ≤0.8 m/s
EWGSOP2	ALM Men: <20 kg Women: <15 kg ALM/height (m^2) Men: <7 kg/m^2 Women: <5.50 kg/m^2	Men: <27 kg Women: <16 kg	Gait speed ≤0.8 m/s, or Short Physical Performance Battery score ≤9, or Timed up and go ≥20 s, or 400 m walk test ≥6 min or non-completion
AWGS	ALM/height (m^2) using DXA Men: <7.0 kg/m^2 Women: <5.4 kg/m^2 SMM/height (m^2) using BIA Men: <7.0 kg/m^2 Women: <5.7 kg/m^2	Men: <26 kg Women: <18 kg	Gait speed ≤0.8 m/s
AWGS2019	ALM/height (m^2) using DXA Men: <7.0 kg/m^2 Women: <5.4 kg/m^2 SMM/height (m^2) using BIA Men: <7.0 kg/m^2 Women: <5.7 kg/m^2	Men: <28 kg Women: <18 kg	6-m walk <1.0 m/s, or Short Physical Performance Battery score ≤ 9, or 5-time chair stand test ≥12 s
IWGS	ALM/height (m^2) using DXA: Men: <7.23 kg/m^2 Women: <5.67 kg/m^2	–	Gait speed <1 m/s
FNIH	ALM/BMI (kg/m^2) using DXA Men: <0.789 Women: <0.512	Men: <26 kg Women: <16 kg	Gait speed ≤0.8 m/s
SCWD	ALM/height (m^2) using DXA <2 SD lower than apparently healthy young adults of the same ethnic group	–	Gait speed <1.0 m/s, or < 400 m in the 6-minute walking test

EWGSOP1 European Working Group on Sarcopenia in Older People, *EWGSOP2* revised version of the European Working Group on Sarcopenia in Older People, *AWGS* Asian Working Group on Sarcopenia, *AWGS2019* revised version of the Asian Working Group on Sarcopenia, *IWGS* International Working Group on Sarcopenia, *FNIH* Foundation of the National Institute of Health-Sarcopenia Project, *SCWD* Society of Sarcopenia, Cachexia and Wasting Disorders, *ALM* appendicular lean mass, *DXA* dual X-ray absorptiometry, *BIA* bioimpedence analysis, *SMM* skeletal muscle mass, *BMI* body mass index

the epidemiology of sarcopenia. Whenever a different definition is applied, with consequently varying diagnostic tools and cut-points, inevitably, the results will change, increasing the diagnostic standardization.

2.3   EWGSOP1 vs. EWGSOP2: What Is Changed?

As mentioned above, in 2010, the EWGSOP released its first consensus defining sarcopenia as a bidimensional condition characterized by low muscle mass and poor muscle function (i.e., strength or physical performance). Furthermore, three different levels of sarcopenia severity were determined:

1. Presarcopenia (i.e., presence of low muscle mass alone).
2. Sarcopenia (i.e., presence of low muscle mass combined with reduced muscle strength or physical performance).
3. Severe sarcopenia (i.e., the simultaneous presence of low muscle mass, muscle weakness, and physical impairment).

In its original consensus document, the EWGSOP also distinguished between primary and secondary sarcopenia. Primary sarcopenia was defined as the age-related muscle decline in which no other causes than aging itself can be indicated. Secondary sarcopenia was defined as that condition due to other detectable causes (e.g., pathological conditions, physical inactivity, undernutrition). The cut-points for muscle mass, strength, and physical performance suggested in the recommendations were retrieved from the existing literature. However, at that time, most of the cut-points were still primarily defined from studies that had not been designed for proposing universally applicable thresholds of risk but instead identified on specific populations. In other words, they could be argued as not sufficiently data-driven [19].

The update EWGSOP2 document was justified by the need of implementing the emerging evidence in the field and to facilitate the implementation of the research findings into the clinical practice. In this context, it cannot be ignored the recognition of sarcopenia as a formal disease with its inclusion in the ICD-10 diagnosis codebook. In the EWGSOP2 consensus, the operational definition of sarcopenia was slightly modified. In fact, sarcopenia was here presented as "a progressive and generalized skeletal muscle disorder that is associated with an increased likelihood of adverse outcomes including falls, fractures, physical disability and mortality." In other words, sarcopenia was tending to become a "disorder" (sometimes in the text "disease"), whereas it had before a rather syndromic profile [4]. The EWGSOP2 expert group also revised the cut-points for defining the abnormalities of muscle mass and strength (Table 2.1) and proposed a new algorithm for case finding. Interestingly, the proposed algorithm, identified by the acronym FACS (i.e., Find-Assess-Confirm-Severity), is structured around four steps:

1. Find. The use of the SARC-F questionnaire [20] or a clinical suspicion [21] is here recommended for detecting probable cases of sarcopenia. The SARC-F is a

screening questionnaire for sarcopenia consisting of five self-reported items (i.e., limitations in strength, walking ability, rising from a chair, climbing stairs, and history of falls). The SARC-F has been translated into many languages and has shown to be predictive of impaired physical function [22] as well as provided by excellent specificity at identifying people with sarcopenia (defined with the EWGSOP or AWGS criteria) [23].

2. Assess. The second part of the FACS is devoted to assessing muscle strength through the grip strength or chair stand tests in those previously screened as positive. At this step, the muscle weakness determines the condition of probable sarcopenia, which should pave the way towards the investigation of the underlying causes, and the design of an ad hoc intervention. Interestingly, the choice of prioritizing the assessment of muscle strength over the muscle mass quantification was motivated by the need of promoting the concept of sarcopenia in clinical practice. In fact, during the clinical routine, the evidence of muscle weakness is perceived as both more evident and relevant than the shrinking of the muscle.

3. Confirm. The next step is to confirm the diagnosis of sarcopenia through the formal assessment of the muscle quantity via DXA or bioelectrical impedance analysis (BIA, as lower level alternative) in clinical practice. The use of BIA is highly affected by the type and model of device, which requires population-specific cut off [24]. For research purposes and specialty care, the EWGSOP2 recommends the DXA, magnetic resonance imaging (MRI), and the computed tomography (CT) as standards.

4. Severity. For this final step, the EWGSOP2 explains that the assessment of physical performance (key defining criterion in the previous version of the recommendations) should determine the severity of the sarcopenia condition. For this purpose, the Short Physical Performance Battery was suggested.

In this new algorithm, it is evident how the process is redesigned, privileging the clinical implementation (as previously mentioned) and its cost-effectiveness (delaying to selected cases and specific settings the quantification of the muscle mass).

2.4   The Impact of Different Operational Definitions

The application of different operational definitions and cut-points to define sarcopenia over time has been inevitably resulting in a marked heterogeneity of the diagnostic process. Several authors reported considerable differences in both prevalence and risk factors associated with sarcopenia when different criteria are applied [23, 25–28]. In 2014, Dam et al. [25] reported that the sarcopenic condition defined according to the FNIH criteria was less prevalent (i.e., 1.3% in men and 2.3% in women) compared to the EWGSOP (i.e., 5.3% in men and 13.3% in women), and the IWGS (i.e., 5.1% in men and 11.8% in women). The authors also found a relatively low agreement among the different operational definitions. Lee et al. [28] similarly reported a higher prevalence of sarcopenia in community-dwelling older people when the condition was assessed using the EWGSOP rather than the IWGS criteria. Several studies have described that applying different criteria determines discrepancies in both prevalence and outcomes, especially when the defining models developed in Western countries are used to other regions [28, 29]. As mentioned above, because of anthropometric, ethnic, genetic, and cultural backgrounds, the traditional cut-points working for Caucasian populations seem hardly applicable to Asian populations [8, 28]. For example, Asians may have substantially higher adiposity (also in terms of abdominal and visceral fat deposition) than Western counterparts for the same body mass index [30]. Indeed, given the differences in body composition across populations, it has been argued that the defining cut-points for sarcopenia might be adjusted to the local needs and characteristics [16].

In 2016, Bahat et al. [31] defined the alternative cut-points for determining low muscle mass (i.e., 9.2 kg/m^2 in men and 7.4 kg/m^2 in women), low muscle strength (i.e., 32 kg for men and 22 kg for women), and low calf circumference (i.e., 33 cm for both men and women) in the Turkish adaptation of the EWGSOP recommendations. The Australian and New Zealand Society for Sarcopenia and Frailty Research (ANZSSFR) [32] recently published a consensus about adopting the EWGSOP criteria and the future definition of modified cut-points specific for Australian and New Zealand populations. In 2019, the AWGS updated its consensus (i.e., AWGS 2019) [33] in which the diagnostic algorithm, the protocols, and some cut-points were revised. In particular, the cut-points for muscle strength were set out at 28 kg for men and 18 kg for women. At the same time, poor physical performance was defined by a 6-m walking speed lower than 1.0 m/s, a Short Physical Performance Battery score lower than 9, or a 5-time chair stand test equal to or higher than 12 s (Table 2.1). The AWGS in this revised consensus also revised the diagnostic algorithm, distinguishing a section for community care and another for the hospital setting. Both of these two sections propose the case finding via the measurement of the calf circumference (setting sex-specific thresholds at <34 cm for men and <33 cm for women), the SARC-F score (with the critical cut-point set at ≥4), or the SARC-CalF (abnormal results defined as ≥11). As done in the EWGSOP2, the AWGS 2019 also introduced the concept of possible sarcopenia defined by low muscle strength, independently from physical performance assessment.

Just recently, Yang et al. [34] compared the EWGSOP2 criteria with those of the EWGSOP, AWGS, IWGS, and FNIH in a sample of Chinese community-dwelling older persons in order to examine the prevalence and associated risk factors of sarcopenia. They found that the prevalence of sarcopenia defined by the EWGSOP2 criteria was lower than that measured using the EWGSOP and AWGS definitions. It was also reported that the FNIH criteria were more conservative than those of the EWGSOP, EWGSOP2, AWGS, and IWGS. In fact, the FNIH criteria consider the ASM adjusted for BMI for assessing the muscle mass, which results being more selective compared to ASM adjusted for height (m^2). Hand-grip strength adjusted to body weight is also recommended to be superior to hand-grip strength in representing metabolic aspects of sarcopenia [35].

2.5 Conclusion

Over the last decade, several operational definitions for sarcopenia have been proposed across the world. The application of the different sarcopenia definitions has resulted in a marked heterogeneity in the literature, especially in studies reporting the prevalence and risk factors of sarcopenia. Given that ethnic differences determine a significant variability in body composition and lifestyle habits, it has been pointed out that unique cut-points for muscle parameters may not be readily applicable to everyone worldwide. If, on the one hand, the utility of having universal standards/targets cannot be overlooked, the need for a less stringent approach is reasonable for developing a person-centered approach, especially when dealing with the complexity of aging individuals.

References

1. Hughes VA, Frontera WR, Roubenoff R, Evans WJ, Singh MAF. Longitudinal changes in body composition in older men and women: role of body weight change and physical activity. Am J Clin Nutr. 2002;76(2):473–81.
2. Rosenberg IH. Sarcopenia: origins and clinical relevance. J Nutr. 1997;127(5 Suppl):990S–1S.
3. Delmonico MJ, Harris TB, Visser M, Park SW, Conroy MB, Velasquez-Mieyer P, et al. Longitudinal study of muscle strength, quality, and adipose tissue infiltration. Am J Clin Nutr. 2009;90(6):1579–85.
4. Cruz-Jentoft AJ, Landi F, Topinková E, Michel J-P. Understanding sarcopenia as a geriatric syndrome. Curr Opin Clin Nutr Metab Care. 2010;13(1):1–7.
5. Anker SD, Morley JE, von Haehling S. Welcome to the ICD-10 code for sarcopenia. J Cachexia Sarcopenia Muscle. 2016;7(5):512–4.
6. Molfino A, Amabile MI, Rossi Fanelli F, Muscaritoli M. Novel therapeutic options for cachexia and sarcopenia. Expert Opin Biol Ther. 2016;16(10):1239–44.
7. Vellas B, Fielding RA, Bens C, Bernabei R, Cawthon PM, Cederholm T, et al. Implications of ICD-10 for sarcopenia clinical practice and clinical trials: report by the international conference on frailty and sarcopenia research task force. J Frailty Aging. 2018;7(1):2–9.
8. Chen L-K, Lee W-J, Peng L-N, Liu L-K, Arai H, Akishita M, et al. Recent advances in sarcopenia research in Asia: 2016 update from the Asian Working Group for Sarcopenia. J Am Med Dir Assoc. 2016;17(8):767.e1–7.
9. Baumgartner RN, Koehler KM, Gallagher D, Romero L, Heymsfield SB, Ross RR, et al. Epidemiology of sarcopenia among the elderly in New Mexico. Am J Epidemiol. 1998;147(8):755–63.
10. Cruz-Jentoft AJ, Baeyens JP, Bauer JM, Boirie Y, Cederholm T, Landi F, et al. Sarcopenia: European consensus on definition and diagnosis: Report of the European Working Group on sarcopenia in older people. Age Ageing. 2010;39(4):412–23.
11. Cruz-Jentoft AJ, Bahat G, Bauer J, Boirie Y, Bruyère O, Cederholm T, et al. Sarcopenia: revised European consensus on definition and diagnosis. Age Ageing. 2019;48(1):16–31.
12. Muscaritoli M, Anker SD, Argilés J, Aversa Z, Bauer JM, Biolo G, et al. Consensus definition of sarcopenia, cachexia and pre-cachexia: joint document elaborated by Special Interest Groups (SIG) 'cachexia-anorexia in chronic wasting diseases' and 'nutrition in geriatrics'. Clin Nutr. 2010;29(2):154–9.
13. Fielding RA, Vellas B, Evans WJ, Bhasin S, Morley JE, Newman AB, et al. Sarcopenia: an undiagnosed condition in older adults. Current consensus definition: prevalence,

etiology, and consequences. International Working Group on Sarcopenia. J Am Med Dir Assoc. 2011;12(4):249–56.
14. Morley JE, Abbatecola AM, Argiles JM, Baracos V, Bauer J, Bhasin S, et al. Sarcopenia with limited mobility: an international consensus. J Am Med Dir Assoc. 2011;12(6):403–9.
15. Cruz-Jentoft AJ, Landi F, Schneider SM, Zúñiga C, Arai H, Boirie Y, et al. Prevalence of and interventions for sarcopenia in ageing adults: a systematic review. Report of the International Sarcopenia Initiative (EWGSOP and IWGS). Age Ageing. 2014;43(6):748–59.
16. Chen L-K, Liu L-K, Woo J, Assantachai P, Auyeung T-W, Bahyah KS, et al. Sarcopenia in Asia: consensus report of the Asian Working Group for Sarcopenia. J Am Med Dir Assoc. 2014;15(2):95–101.
17. Studenski SA, Peters KW, Alley DE, Cawthon PM, McLean RR, Harris TB, et al. The FNIH sarcopenia project: rationale, study description, conference recommendations, and final estimates. J Gerontol A Biol Sci Med Sci. 2014;69(5):547–58.
18. Bhasin S, Travison TG, Manini TM, Patel S, Pencina KM, Fielding RA, et al. Sarcopenia definition: the position statements of the sarcopenia definition and outcomes consortium. J Am Geriatr Soc. 2020;68(7):1410–8.
19. Marzetti E, Calvani R, Tosato M, Cesari M, Di Bari M, Cherubini A, et al. Sarcopenia: an overview. Aging Clin Exp Res. 2017;29(1):11–7.
20. Malmstrom TK, Morley JE. SARC-F: a simple questionnaire to rapidly diagnose sarcopenia. J Am Med Dir Assoc. 2013;14(8):531–2.
21. Beaudart C, Rolland Y, Cruz-Jentoft AJ, Bauer JM, Sieber C, Cooper C, et al. Assessment of muscle function and physical performance in daily clinical practice: a position paper endorsed by the European Society for Clinical and Economic Aspects of Osteoporosis, Osteoarthritis and Musculoskeletal Diseases (ESCEO). Calcif Tissue Int. 2019;105(1):1–14.
22. Cao L, Chen S, Zou C, Ding X, Gao L, Liao Z, et al. A pilot study of the SARC-F scale on screening sarcopenia and physical disability in the Chinese older people. J Nutr Health Aging. 2014;18(3):277–83.
23. Woo J, Leung J, Morley JE. Defining sarcopenia in terms of incident adverse outcomes. J Am Med Dir Assoc. 2015;16(3):247–52.
24. Alkahtani SA. A cross-sectional study on sarcopenia using different methods: reference values for healthy Saudi young men. BMC Musculoskelet Disord. 2017;18(1):119.
25. Dam T-T, Peters KW, Fragala M, Cawthon PM, Harris TB, McLean R, et al. An evidence-based comparison of operational criteria for the presence of sarcopenia. J Gerontol A Biol Sci Med Sci. 2014;69(5):584–90.
26. Kim H, Hirano H, Edahiro A, Ohara Y, Watanabe Y, Kojima N, et al. Sarcopenia: prevalence and associated factors based on different suggested definitions in community-dwelling older adults. Geriatr Gerontol Int. 2016;16(Suppl 1):110–22.
27. Han D-S, Chang K-V, Li C-M, Lin Y-H, Kao T-W, Tsai K-S, et al. Skeletal muscle mass adjusted by height correlated better with muscular functions than that adjusted by body weight in defining sarcopenia. Sci Rep. 2016;6:19457.
28. Lee W-J, Liu L-K, Peng L-N, Lin M-H, Chen L-K, ILAS Research Group. Comparisons of sarcopenia defined by IWGS and EWGSOP criteria among older people: results from the I-Lan longitudinal aging study. J Am Med Dir Assoc. 2013;14(7):528.e1–7.
29. Zeng Y, Hu X, Xie L, Han Z, Zuo Y, Yang M. The prevalence of sarcopenia in Chinese elderly nursing home residents: a comparison of 4 diagnostic criteria. J Am Med Dir Assoc. 2018;19(8):690–5.
30. Wang J, Thornton JC, Russell M, Burastero S, Heymsfield S, Pierson RN. Asians have lower body mass index (BMI) but higher percent body fat than do whites: comparisons of anthropometric measurements. Am J Clin Nutr. 1994;60(1):23–8.
31. Bahat G, Tufan A, Tufan F, Kilic C, Akpinar TS, Kose M, et al. Cut-off points to identify sarcopenia according to European Working Group on Sarcopenia in Older People (EWGSOP) definition. Clin Nutr. 2016;35(6):1557–63.

32. Zanker J, Scott D, Reijnierse EM, Brennan-Olsen SL, Daly RM, Girgis CM, et al. Establishing an operational definition of sarcopenia in Australia and New Zealand: delphi method based consensus statement. J Nutr Health Aging. 2019;23(1):105–10.

33. Chen L-K, Woo J, Assantachai P, Auyeung T-W, Chou M-Y, Iijima K, et al. Asian Working Group for Sarcopenia: 2019 consensus update on sarcopenia diagnosis and treatment. J Am Med Dir Assoc. 2020;21(3):300–307.e2.

34. Yang L, Yao X, Shen J, Sun G, Sun Q, Tian X, et al. Comparison of revised EWGSOP criteria and four other diagnostic criteria of sarcopenia in Chinese community-dwelling elderly residents. Exp Gerontol. 2020;130:110798.

35. Chun S-W, Kim W, Choi KH. Comparison between grip strength and grip strength divided by body weight in their relationship with metabolic syndrome and quality of life in the elderly. PLoS One. 2019;14(9):e0222040.

Consequences of Sarcopenia in Older People: The Epidemiological Evidence

3

Nicola Veronese and Mario Barbagallo

3.1 Introduction

Sarcopenia is traditionally defined as "*age-related muscle loss, affecting a combination of appendicular muscle mass, muscle strength, and/or physical performance measures*" [1]. An increasing body of literature suggests that sarcopenia may increase the risk of several negative outcomes, including falls [2], fractures [3], disability [4], mortality [5–7], being consequently associated also with poor quality of life [8]. At the same time, the interest in sarcopenia is also increasing beyond the perimeter of geriatric medicine [9], such as in oncology [10], cardiology [11], and respiratory medicine [12]. Emerging literature has suggested that sarcopenia can be considered as risk factor for dysphagia [13] or for gastric cancer [14].

Given this background, in this chapter, we will discuss the importance of sarcopenia as potential risk factor for negative health outcomes in older people.

3.2 Sarcopenia as Risk Factor for Falls and Fractures

It is widely known that approximately one-third of older adults fall at least once a year and a median of 4.1% of falls results in fractures [15]. Falls are associated with several negative health outcomes in older people including disability, institutionalization, and finally increased morbidity and mortality [16]. A number of risk factors have been found to predispose older adults to falls [17], and among them, poor physical performance and muscle strength, typical of sarcopenia, seem to be important [18]. Therefore, it is hardly surprising that sarcopenia could be associated with a higher risk of falls in older people [19, 20]. These epidemiological findings

N. Veronese (✉) · M. Barbagallo
Geriatric Unit, Department of Internal Medicine and Geriatrics, University of Palermo, Palermo, Italy
e-mail: mario.barbagallo@unipa.it

© Springer Nature Switzerland AG 2021
N. Veronese et al. (eds.), *Sarcopenia*, Practical Issues in Geriatrics,
https://doi.org/10.1007/978-3-030-80038-3_3

indicate the urgency for timely diagnosis and treatment of sarcopenia, since we can consider sarcopenia as a modifiable risk factor for falls and finally fractures [19, 20]. In this sense, increasing literature suggests an association between sarcopenia and fractures [21], also independent from the increased risk of falls associated with sarcopenia. Therefore, a new entity in geriatric medicine is emerging, i.e., osteosarcopenia [22]. Bone and muscle, in fact, are closely interconnected not only for their anatomical characteristics but also chemically and metabolically [22]. Moreover, some pathophysiological processes (e.g., fat infiltration and alterations in stem cell differentiation) are common to both sarcopenia and osteoporosis, therefore suggesting that sarcopenia and osteoporosis are closely linked also from a molecular point of view [23].

3.3 Sarcopenia as Risk Factor for Disability

Disability (usually defined as any restriction or lack of ability to perform an activity in the manner or within the range considered normal for a human being) is, unfortunately, a dramatic condition in older people [24]. For example, trends in the United States showed an increase in disability rate from the 1970s and into the early 1980s for most noninstitutionalized age groups [25]. Disability is associated with enormous health care costs. In the United States, for example, it is estimated that disability-associated health care expenditures accounted for 26.7% of all health care expenditures equal to $397.8 billion [26].

In epidemiological research, it was reported that sarcopenic patients have an increased risk of about three times than non-sarcopenic subjects [27], and this evidence seems to be supported by an evidence with poor risk of bias [20], meaning that sarcopenia is an important and epidemiologically strong risk factor for disability. In a seminal paper regarding this issue, it was reported that 6/7 studies included reported that sarcopenia was significantly associated with functional decline and consequently to disability [27]. Sarcopenia, in fact, is the first step of the transition from healthy aging to disability that usually passes through frailty presence [28]. This aspect opens the topic of early identification of sarcopenia, in order to avoid the progression to disability.

3.4 Sarcopenia, Hospitalization, and Mortality

The association between sarcopenia and mortality is the most explored in geriatric medicine. Again, sarcopenia was significantly and strongly associated with mortality in older people. Until 2017, 10 over 12 studies exploring this association found that sarcopenia is a risk factor for mortality and sarcopenic patients have a 4 times higher risk of death than non-sarcopenic subjects [27]. The association between sarcopenia and mortality seems not to be affected by the settings of the participants (community-dwelling versus hospitalized subjects versus nursing home residents) or to by the length of follow-up [27], and only age seems to have an impact on the results, since there was a stronger association of mortality with sarcopenia among subjects aged 79 years or older [27].

In the last years, literature supports this association without any doubt and in other contexts [29–31].

A similar association is present for sarcopenia and hospitalization [32]. Sarcopenia in old adults, in fact, has significantly higher risk of hospitalization, particularly in already hospitalized patients. Moreover, sarcopenia is associated with a longer length of stay in hospital [32], further justifying its inclusion in the ICD-10 code [33].

3.5 Sarcopenia as Risk Factor for Negative Outcomes in Surgery

A relatively novel topic that in our opinion merits a discussion is the potential association between sarcopenia and negative health outcomes in surgery [34]. We have, in fact, an important literature supporting the association between sarcopenia with postoperative complications of gastric cancer, such as postoperative ileus, and postoperative pneumonia [20, 34]. These findings were substantially confirmed in other areas of surgery including vascular surgery [35], cardiac surgery [36], and otolaryngology [37].

3.6 Conclusions

From an epidemiological perspective, sarcopenia is associated with several negative outcomes in older people. However, as shown in our chapter, we have a strong association between the presence of sarcopenia with some important negative outcomes, such as mortality and disability. At the same time, increasing literature is showing that sarcopenia is an important (and potentially modifiable) risk factor for other conditions such as for fractures and falls and in specific settings, such as in surgery, that merit further research.

References

1. Woo J. Sarcopenia. Clin Geriatr Med. 2017;33(3):305–14.
2. Landi F, Liperoti R, Russo A, Giovannini S, Tosato M, Capoluongo E, et al. Sarcopenia as a risk factor for falls in elderly individuals: results from the ilSIRENTE study. Clin Nutr. 2012;31(5):652–8. https://doi.org/10.1016/j.clnu.2012.02.007.
3. Cederholm T, Cruz-Jentoft AJ, Maggi S. Sarcopenia and fragility fractures. Eur J Phys Rehabil Med. 2013;49(1):111–7.
4. Lang T, Streeper T, Cawthon P, Baldwin K, Taaffe DR, Harris TB. Sarcopenia: etiology, clinical consequences, intervention, and assessment. Osteopor Int. 2010;21(4):543–59. https://doi.org/10.1007/s00198-009-1059-y.

5. Cesari M, Pahor M, Lauretani F, Zamboni V, Bandinelli S, Bernabei R, et al. Skeletal muscle and mortality results from the InCHIANTI study. J Gerontol A Biol Sci Med Sci. 2009;64(3):377–84. https://doi.org/10.1093/gerona/gln031.
6. Gariballa S, Alessa A. Sarcopenia: prevalence and prognostic significance in hospitalized patients. Clin Nutr. 2013;32(5):772–6. https://doi.org/10.1016/j.clnu.2013.01.010.
7. Perkisas S, De Cock A-M, Vandewoude M, Verhoeven V. Prevalence of sarcopenia and 9-year mortality in nursing home residents. Aging Clin Exp Res. 2019;31(7):951–9.
8. Rizzoli R, Reginster JY, Arnal JF, Bautmans I, Beaudart C, Bischoff-Ferrari H, et al. Quality of life in sarcopenia and frailty. Calcif Tissue Int. 2013;93(2):101–20. https://doi.org/10.1007/s00223-013-9758-y.
9. Dent E, Morley J, Cruz-Jentoft A, Arai H, Kritchevsky S, Guralnik J, et al. International clinical practice guidelines for sarcopenia (ICFSR): screening, diagnosis and management. J Nutr Health Aging. 2018;22(10):1148–61.
10. Chindapasirt J. Sarcopenia in cancer patients. Asian Pac J Cancer Prev. 2015;16(18):8075–7.
11. von Haehling S. Muscle wasting and sarcopenia in heart failure: a brief overview of the current literature. ESC Heart Fail. 2018;5(6):1074–82. https://doi.org/10.1002/ehf2.12388.
12. Jones SE, Maddocks M, Kon SS, Canavan JL, Nolan CM, Clark AL, et al. Sarcopenia in COPD: prevalence, clinical correlates and response to pulmonary rehabilitation. Thorax. 2015;70(3):213–8. https://doi.org/10.1136/thoraxjnl-2014-206440.
13. Cha S, Kim W-S, Kim KW, Han JW, Jang HC, Lim S, et al. Sarcopenia is an independent risk factor for dysphagia in community-dwelling older adults. Dysphagia. 2019;34(5):692–7.
14. Kim YM, Kim J-H, Baik SJ, Chun J, Youn YH, Park H. Sarcopenia and sarcopenic obesity as novel risk factors for gastric carcinogenesis: a health checkup cohort study. Front Oncol. 2019;9:1249.
15. Bergen G, Stevens MR, Burns ER. Falls and fall injuries among adults aged≥ 65 years—United States, 2014. Morb Mortal Wkly Rep. 2016;65(37):993–8.
16. Terroso M, Rosa N, Marques AT, Simoes R. Physical consequences of falls in the elderly: a literature review from 1995 to 2010. Eur Rev Aging Phys Act. 2014;11(1):51–9.
17. Stubbs B, Brefka S, Denkinger MD. What works to prevent falls in community-dwelling older adults? Umbrella review of meta-analyses of randomized controlled trials. Phys Ther. 2015;95(8):1095–110.
18. Ikegami S, Takahashi J, Uehara M, Tokida R, Nishimura H, Sakai A, et al. Physical performance reflects cognitive function, fall risk, and quality of life in community-dwelling older people. Sci Rep. 2019;9(1):1–7.
19. Yeung SS, Reijnierse EM, Pham VK, Trappenburg MC, Lim WK, Meskers CG, et al. Sarcopenia and its association with falls and fractures in older adults: a systematic review and meta-analysis. J Cachexia Sarcopenia Muscle. 2019;10(3):485–500.
20. Veronese N, Demurtas J, Soysal P, Smith L, Torbahn G, Schoene D, et al. Sarcopenia and health-related outcomes: an umbrella review of observational studies. Eur Geriatr Med. 2019;10:853–62.
21. Huang P, Luo K, Xu J, Huang W, Yin W, Xiao M, et al. Sarcopenia as a risk factor for future HIP fracture: a meta-analysis of prospective cohort studies. J Nutr Health Aging. 2021;25(2):183–8.
22. Hirschfeld H, Kinsella R, Duque G. Osteosarcopenia: where bone, muscle, and fat collide. Osteoporos Int. 2017;28(10):2781–90.
23. Levinger I, Phu S, Duque G. Sarcopenia and osteoporotic fractures. Clin Rev Bone Miner Metab. 2016;14(1):38–44.
24. Ostir GV, Carlson JE, Black SA, Rudkin L, Goodwin JS, Markides KS. Disability in older adults: prevalence, causes, and consequences. Behav Med. 1999;24(4):147–56.
25. Manton KG, Corder L, Stallard E. Chronic disability trends in elderly United States populations: 1982–1994. Proc Natl Acad Sci. 1997;94(6):2593–8.
26. Centers for Disease Control and Prevention (CDC). Prevalence of disabilities and associated health conditions among adults—United States, 1999. MMWR Morb Mortal Wkly Rep. 2001;50(7):120.

27. Beaudart C, Zaaria M, Pasleau F, Reginster JY, Bruyere O. Health outcomes of sarcopenia: a systematic review and meta-analysis. PLoS One. 2017;12(1):e0169548. https://doi.org/10.1371/journal.pone.0169548.
28. Topinková E. Aging, disability and frailty. Ann Nutr Metab. 2008;52(Suppl 1):6–11. https://doi.org/10.1159/000115340.
29. Bayraktar E, Tasar PT. Relationship between sarcopenia and mortality in elderly inpatients. Eurasian J Med. 2020;52(1):29–33. https://doi.org/10.5152/eurasianjmed.2020.19214.
30. Lin Y-L, Liou H-H, Wang C-H, Lai Y-H, Kuo C-H, Chen S-Y, et al. Impact of sarcopenia and its diagnostic criteria on hospitalization and mortality in chronic hemodialysis patients: a 3-year longitudinal study. J Formos Med Assoc. 2020;119(7):1219–29.
31. Rippberger PL, Emeny RT, Mackenzie TA, Bartels SJ, Batsis JA. The association of sarcopenia, telomere length, and mortality: data from the NHANES 1999–2002. Eur J Clin Nutr. 2018;72(2):255–63. https://doi.org/10.1038/s41430-017-0011-z.
32. Zhao Y, Zhang Y, Hao Q, Ge M, Dong B. Sarcopenia and hospital-related outcomes in the old people: a systematic review and meta-analysis. Aging Clin Exp Res. 2019;31(1):5–14. https://doi.org/10.1007/s40520-018-0931-z.
33. Anker SD, Morley JE, von Haehling S. Welcome to the ICD-10 code for sarcopenia. J Cachexia Sarcopenia Muscle. 2016;7(5):512–4.
34. Yang Z, Zhou X, Ma B, Xing Y, Jiang X, Wang Z. Predictive value of preoperative sarcopenia in patients with gastric cancer: a meta-analysis and systematic review. J Gastrointest Surg. 2018;22(11):1890–902. https://doi.org/10.1007/s11605-018-3856-0.
35. Waduud M, Wood B, Keleabetswe P, Manning J, Linton E, Drozd M, et al. Influence of psoas muscle area on mortality following elective abdominal aortic aneurysm repair. Br J Surg. 2019;106(4):367–74.
36. Visser M, van Venrooij LM, Vulperhorst L, de Vos R, Wisselink W, van Leeuwen PA, et al. Sarcopenic obesity is associated with adverse clinical outcome after cardiac surgery. Nutr Metab Cardiovasc Dis. 2013;23(6):511–8.
37. Stone L, Olson B, Mowery A, Krasnow S, Jiang A, Li R, et al. Association between sarcopenia and mortality in patients undergoing surgical excision of head and neck cancer. JAMA Otolaryngol Head Neck Surg. 2019;145(7):647–54.

Emerging Markers for Sarcopenia

4

Shaun Sabico and Abdullah M. Alguwaihes

4.1 Introduction

In the past decade, there has been an obvious exponential progress in both interest and literature on sarcopenia, largely driven after a consensus operational definition has been published in 2010 [1]. The clear growth in sarcopenia research has eventually led to its recognition as an independent disease replete with its own code in ICD-10-CM (M62.84) [2, 3]. This milestone has opened wider doors for more clinical investigations and increased enthusiasm from major clinical institutions and pharmaceutical companies. As is true with any disease entity, it is imperative to understand the pathophysiology of sarcopenia, its relationship between measurable biological processes and its associations with clinical outcomes. To achieve this, there needs to be an in-depth study of genetic and serological biomarkers specific to sarcopenia. This will not only deepen our still developing knowledge on sarcopenia but more so lead to the unfolding of new treatments.

Biomarker is a generic term referring to a wide subgroup of clinical signs or objective indications of a clinical state detected from patients which can be measured accurately and reproducibly [4]. The term biomarker is defined as "*a characteristic that is objectively measured and evaluated as an indicator of normal biological processes, pathogenic processes, or pharmacologic responses to a therapeutic intervention*" by the National Institutes of Health Biomarkers Definitions Working Group in 1998 [5]. Fortunately, sarcopenia's intricate link with aging has

S. Sabico (✉)
Chair for Biomarkers of Chronic Diseases, Biochemistry Department, College of Science, King Saud University, Riyadh, Saudi Arabia
e-mail: ssabico@ksu.edu.sa

A. M. Alguwaihes
Division of Endocrinology, Department of Internal Medicine, College of Medicine, King Saud University, Riyadh, Saudi Arabia
e-mail: aalguwaihes@ksu.edu.sa

© Springer Nature Switzerland AG 2021
N. Veronese et al. (eds.), *Sarcopenia*, Practical Issues in Geriatrics,
https://doi.org/10.1007/978-3-030-80038-3_4

provided a foundational platform upon which emerging and overlapping biomarkers for frailty and sarcopenia can be extracted, since the age-related decrease in skeletal muscle mass and strength that are indicative of sarcopenia are common and significant risk factors for disability and mortality in aging. The biomarkers for aging, as defined by the American Federation for Aging Research (AFAR), must (a) predict an individual's physiological, cognitive, and physical function in an age-related way, future onset of age-related conditions and diseases, and do so independently of chronological age; (b) be testable and not harmful to test subjects, technically simple but accurate and reproducible, and (c) work in laboratory animals as well as humans [6]. It is important to emphasize that despite the advances in geriatric research, there is still no gold standard or benchmark tool for measuring healthy aging, and no single biomarker has yet qualified as a sensitive and specific parameter for both aging and sarcopenia [7]. Case in point is telomere length, the gene sequence at chromosomal ends that preserves genomic integrity, is widely known to be a biomarker of aging [8]. However, alterations such as lengthening of telomere lengths failed to offer advantages in age-related outcomes [8] and had none to inconsistent effects on mortality among elderly patients with sarcopenia [9], suggesting that a single biomarker cannot be considered a meaningful biological indicator for complex, multifactorial age-related complications, including sarcopenia and frailty [10]. In this chapter, an overview of established biomarkers of sarcopenia is discussed, as well as emerging biomarkers that can be used for future clinical investigations.

4.2 Traditional Biomarkers of Sarcopenia

The first biomarkers for sarcopenia, as expected, were heavily concentrated on its operational definition which included imaging techniques that can accurately assess muscle mass and strength decline. The International Working Group on Sarcopenia enumerated the first major diagnostic markers for sarcopenia for use in clinical trials as listed in Table 4.1 which also included nonspecific muscle markers [11]. The list does not include questionnaire-based screening tools such as the SARC-F, which, on its own, is an excellent and easiest available tool requiring no special equipment and endorsed by major global geriatric associations [12, 13].

The joint assessment of muscle mass and strength, while fundamental to the diagnosis of sarcopenia, is still limited by the lack of consensus on thresholds that will clearly distinguish normal from aberrant muscle aging [14, 15]. Furthermore, the wide range of techniques that can be used to measure muscle mass also complicate diagnosis as values differ, although this has been addressed with the endorsement of dual-energy X-ray absorptiometry as a reference standard (not as a gold standard) [16]. To compensate for this, additional measurements, such as serologic or biofluid markers, are necessary and potentially critical, in facilitating management and prediction of prognosis for individuals with sarcopenia. In the journey to discover these biomarkers, experts in the field of geriatrics acknowledge that key processes overlap between aging and age-related diseases, including sarcopenia.

Table 4.1 Markers for sarcopenia for use in prospective investigations (arranged according to significance)

Characteristic	Screening	Baseline	Assessment End point
Muscle specific			
Function (physical performance, muscle strength, disability)	***	***	***
Mass			
• Bioelectrical impedance analysis (BIA)	***	***	***
• Dual-energy X-ray absorptiometry (DXA)	***	**	**
• Computerized tomography (CT)	**	***	***
• Magnetic resonance imaging (MRI)	**	***	***
• Echography	**	**	**
• Electrical impedance myography	*	**	**
• Anthropometry	*		
Non-muscle specific			
Pathogenesis			
• Inflammation	**	**	**
• Oxidative damage	**	**	**
• Antioxidants	**	**	**
• Apoptosis	*	**	**
Nutrition (albumin, hemoglobin, urinary creatinine, etc.)	***	**	**
Hormones (dehydroepiandrosterone, testosterone, insulin-like growth factor 1, etc.)	**	**	**

Note: * maybe useful but severely limited; ** suitable for use; *** recommended. Recreated, as adopted from Cesari and colleagues [11]

Central to this is inflammation, or *inflamm-aging*, which is the by-product a chronic, sterile, low-grade inflammation that cumulatively damages the innate immune system and metabolism over time [17]. The following subsections below highlight the biomarkers used for sarcopenia research, most of which are yet to be translated into real-time clinical practice. A summary of the biomarkers mentioned is provided in Fig. 4.1.

4.3 Inflammatory Biomarkers

Pro-inflammatory markers are one of the most studied groups of biomarkers in relation to both aging and sarcopenia, particularly the acute phase reactants. In a recent systematic review and meta-analysis gathered from inception until June 2020 involving 168 articles (149 cross-sectional and 19 prospective studies) and having a total of 89,194 participants, elevated levels of C reactive protein (CRP), interleukin-6 (IL-6), and tumor necrosis factor-alpha (TNF-α) were found to be inversely associated with lower handgrip and knee extension strength independent of sarcopenia status. Furthermore, while these associations were also significantly associated with progressive decline in muscle strength and mass, the strength of associations vary widely depending on the population of sex of participants [18]. In elderly patients with recent hip fracture stratified according to presence of sarcopenia, these

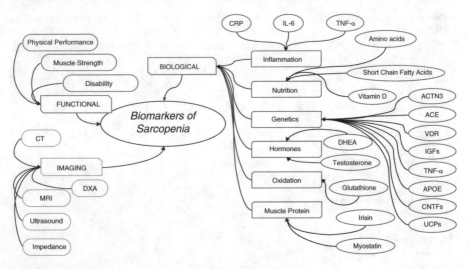

Fig. 4.1 Functional, imaging, and biological markers of sarcopenia

significant inverse associations appear to be lost, with the exception of TNF-α being significantly lower among those with sarcopenia than those without, suggesting impaired immune response in the elderly as demonstrated by fracture-related early inflammation being hampered by sarcopenia [19].

4.4   Nutritional Biomarkers

Adequate nutrition plays an important role in the maintenance of muscle health. Guidelines have been developed taking into consideration specific intakes of protein such as leucine and creatine which may not only slow muscle mass loss but also enhance muscle strength among individuals with sarcopenia [20], and major food groups such as vegetables and fruit consumption do not seem to be associated with the disease, at least among individuals coming from low- to middle-income nations [21]. Despite recommendations, investigations on dietary intake and muscle function appear limited and under focused as opposed to physical activity in the prevention of sarcopenia [22, 23].

The "BIOmarkers associated with Sarcopenia and PHysical frailty in EldeRly pErsons" (BIOSPHERE) study is a large-scale study conceived to search for novel biomarkers that can be used to detect, monitor, and obtain information that can aid in the identification of meaningful targets for the prevention and/or therapeutic interventions of sarcopenia and physical frailty [24, 25]. In their study which used metabolomics, patients with physical frailty and sarcopenia were observed to have higher circulating levels of asparagine, aspartic acid, citrulline, ethanolamine, glutamic acid, sarcosine, and taurine. In parallel, higher concentrations of alpha amino butyric acid and methionine were seen in controls [24]. Furthermore, a link between a poor-quality protein diet and impaired mitochondrial quality control mechanism was observed [24]. These results were echoed by the Maastricht Sarcopenia study (MaSS) in which several branched-chain amino acids including vitamin D were observed to be decreased in direct association with lower muscle mass and strength in older adults [26].

Micronutrient deficiencies, vitamin D in particular, have been found to be related to a number of diseases commonly observed among the elderly people, including sarcopenia [27]. The discovery of vitamin D receptors (VDRs) in several tissues including the muscles has gained considerable interest, and VDR levels were in fact observed to decline in muscles with age, as well as circulating vitamin D being associated with functional decline and muscle atrophy [28]. Despite several guidelines however advocating vitamin D supplementation in the elderly [26, 29], concrete beneficial effects as a standalone supplement such as suppression of muscle atrophy and increased muscle strength are questionable [29], and may be more beneficial in combination with protein [30].

4.5 Genetic Biomarkers

The identification of candidate gene biomarkers for sarcopenia was based on the rationale that skeletal muscle traits are highly heritable by as much as 80% [31]. To date, there has been a clear lack of genome-wide association studies in sarcopenia. Nevertheless, a recent systematic review, which is the first to explore genetic associations with muscle phenotypes in the elderly, was able to demonstrate (based on available evidence from January 2004 to March 2019) several compelling evidence of associations from select genotypes taken from a total of 38,112 participants above 50 years old across 54 studies [32]. A summary of these genes is enumerated in Table 4.2.

Table 4.2 Summary of gene markers associated with muscle phenotypes in the elderly

Gene	
ACTN3 (Sprint Gene)	Encodes ACTN3 protein which is crucial for muscle strength
ACE	Expressed in skeletal muscle endothelial cells; expression is highly determined by ethnicity
VDR	Known to stimulate muscle protein synthesis through messenger RNA transcription
IGF1 and IGFBP3	Low levels of IGF1 seen in elderly and IGFBP3 is the most effective stimulator of IGF1
TNF-α	Integral mediator of the inflammatory response to muscle damage
APOE	E4 allele associated with unfavorable muscle traits
CNTF and CNTFR	Located in glial cells, limits muscle atrophy by denervation
UCP2 and UCP3	Mitochondrial transporters, active in later stages in life

Note: Summarized information based on the review of Pratt and colleagues [32]. *ACTN3* actinin alpha 3, *ACE* angiotensin converting enzyme, *VDR* vitamin D receptor, *IGF1* insulin growth factor 1, *IGFBP3* insulin growth factor binding protein 3, *TNF-α* tumor necrosis factor alpha, *APOE* apolipoprotein E, *CNTF* ciliary neutrophic factor, *CNTFR* ciliary neutrophic factor receptor, *UCP* uncoupling protein

4.6   Hormones

A considerable decline in several hormones, notably the sex hormones, testosterone, and dehydroepiandrosterone (DHEA), as well as growth hormones and insulin-like growth factors, characterizes the altered metabolic profile of individuals with sarcopenia [33]. Treatment with testosterone was observed to increase types I and II muscle fibers, and while this remains promising, the side effects such as increased risk for cardiovascular disease are a cause for concern [34]. Several proteins which are also now being considered as hormones, such as adipocytokines and myokines, shed light on the cross talks between adipose and muscle physiology [35]. These cluster of hormones may soon be the next generation of biomarkers for sarcopenia and will not be dealt in detail in this chapter given the limited information available. However, "hormones" derived from muscle tissues such as myostatin and irisin deserve special mention, as preliminary evidence has shown significant associations that support the adipose-bone-muscle cross talk [36]. Irisin is directly correlated with muscle mass and strength and has been observed to be highly heritable [37]. In contrast, myostatin is mainly expressed in skeletal muscle tissues and is a negative regulator of muscle mass [38]. Both muscle hormones are affected by physical activity and possess anti-inflammatory effects, making them promising targets in the development of aging and/or sarcopenia drugs [39].

4.7   Biomarkers of Oxidation

The free-radical theory of aging states that oxidative stress is a major factor initiating the onset of age-related conditions by stimulating several alterations in key cellular components. While innate defenses exist for lowering the risk of detrimental effects, their ability to thwart the persistent production of reactive oxygen species becomes increasingly incompetent with aging [40]. In a recent review ascertaining the association of longevity with oxidative stress, centenarians (individuals above 100 years old) presented significantly lower superoxide dismutase and elevated glutathione reductase activities with lower susceptibility to lipid peroxidation than elderly controls [41]. Glutathione deficiency in the elderly was also observed to initiate a unique cycle connecting mitochondrial oxidation to protein catabolism, contributing to sarcopenia [42].

4.8   Conclusion

In summary, research on the different biomarkers for sarcopenia is still a work in progress. From discovery, validation, and standardization, it will take a while before several biomarkers for sarcopenia can actually make it to clinical settings. Given the multidimensional processes involved in sarcopenia, it is essential to conduct well-designed studies with results that are reproducible, as most findings from new and emerging biomarkers are promising, but remain suggestive. The biomarkers presented in this chapter are far from exhaustive as new markers are added in the literature over time. The chapter nevertheless gives a snapshot of some of the well-established biomarkers, and the emerging ones that are more likely to be used in the years to come. Future investigations are recommended to involve clustering of these biomarkers using the "omics" approach as this may yield more accurate predictions and mechanistic insights.

References

1. Cruz-Jentoft AJ, Baeyens JP, Bauer JM, Boirie Y, Cederholm T, Landi F, Martin FC, Michel JP, Rolland Y, Schneider SM, Topinková E, Vandewoude M, Zamboni M, European Working Group on Sarcopenia in Older People. Sarcopenia: European consensus on definition and diagnosis: report of the European Working Group on Sarcopenia in Older People. Age Ageing. 2010;39(4):412–23.
2. Cao L, Morley JE. Sarcopenia is recognized as an independent condition by an international classification of disease, tenth revision, clinical modification (ICD-10-CM) code. J Am Med Dir Assoc. 2016;17(8):675–7.
3. Anker SD, Morley JE, von Haehling S. Welcome to the ICD-10 code for sarcopenia. J Cachexia Sarcopenia Muscle. 2016;7(5):512–4.
4. Strimbu K, Tavel JA. What are biomarkers? Curr Opin HIV AIDS. 2010;5(6):463–6.
5. Biomarkers Definitions Working Group. Biomarkers and surrogate endpoints: preferred definitions and conceptual framework. Clin Pharmacol Ther. 2001;69(3):89–95.
6. Johnson TE. Recent results: biomarkers of aging. Exp Gerontol. 2006;41(12):1243–6.
7. Wagner KH, Cameron-Smith D, Wessner B, Franzke B. Biomarkers of aging: from function to molecular biology. Nutrients. 2016;8(6):338.
8. Epel ES, Blackburn EH, Lin J, Dhabhar FS, Adler NE, Morrow JD, Cawthon RM. Accelerated telomere shortening in response to life stress. Proc Natl Acad Sci U S A. 2004;101(49):17312–5.
9. Kuo CL, Pilling LC, Kuchel GA, Ferrucci L, Melzer D. Telomere length and aging-related outcomes in humans: a Mendelian randomization study in 261,000 older participants. Aging Cell. 2019;18(6):e13017.
10. Rippberger PL, Emeny RT, Mackenzie TA, Bartels SJ, Batsis JA. The association of sarcopenia, telomere length, and mortality: data from the NHANES 1999-2002. Eur J Clin Nutr. 2018;72(2):255–63.
11. Cesari M, Fielding RA, Pahor M, Goodpaster B, Hellerstein M, van Kan GA, Anker SD, Rutkove S, Vrijbloed JW, Isaac M, Rolland Y, M'rini C, Aubertin-Leheudre M, Cedarbaum JM, Zamboni M, Sieber CC, Laurent D, Evans WJ, Roubenoff R, Morley JE, Vellas B, International Working Group on Sarcopenia. Biomarkers of sarcopenia in clinical trials-recommendations from the International Working Group on Sarcopenia. J Cachexia Sarcopenia Muscle. 2012;3(3):181–90.
12. Malmstrom TK, Morley JE. SARC-F: a simple questionnaire to rapidly diagnose sarcopenia. J Am Med Dir Assoc. 2013;14(8):531–2.
13. Morley JE, Sanford AM. Editorial: screening for sarcopenia. J Nutr Health Aging. 2019;23(9):768–70.
14. Marzetti E. Editorial: imaging, functional and biological markers for sarcopenia: the pursuit of the golden ratio. J Frailty Aging. 2012;1(3):97–8.
15. Calvani R, Marini F, Cesari M, Tosato M, Anker SD, von Haehling S, Miller RR, Bernabei R, Landi F, Marzetti E, SPRINTT consortium. Biomarkers for physical frailty and sarcopenia: state of the science and future developments. J Cachexia Sarcopenia Muscle. 2015;6(4):278–86.
16. Buckinx F, Landi F, Cesari M, Fielding RA, Visser M, Engelke K, Maggi S, Dennison E, Al-Daghri NM, Allepaerts S, Bauer J, Bautmans I, Brandi ML, Bruyère O, Cederholm T, Cerreta F, Cherubini A, Cooper C, Cruz-Jentoft A, McCloskey E, Dawson-Hughes B, Kaufman

JM, Laslop A, Petermans J, Reginster JY, Rizzoli R, Robinson S, Rolland Y, Rueda R, Vellas B, Kanis JA. Pitfalls in the measurement of muscle mass: a need for a reference standard. J Cachexia Sarcopenia Muscle. 2018;9(2):269–78.

17. Franceschi C, Garagnani P, Parini P, Giuliani C, Santoro A. Inflammaging: a new immune-metabolic viewpoint for age-related diseases. Nat Rev Endocrinol. 2018;14(10):576–90.

18. Tuttle CSL, Thang LAN, Maier AB. Markers of inflammation and their association with muscle strength and mass: a systematic review and meta-analysis. Ageing Res Rev. 2020;64:101185.

19. Sánchez-Castellano C, Martín-Aragón S, Bermejo-Bescós P, Vaquero-Pinto N, Miret-Corchado C, Merello de Miguel A, Cruz-Jentoft AJ. Biomarkers of sarcopenia in very old patients with hip fracture. J Cachexia Sarcopenia Muscle. 2020;11(2):478–86.

20. Morley JE, Argiles JM, Evans WJ, Bhasin S, Cella D, Deutz NE, Doehner W, Fearon KC, Ferrucci L, Hellerstein MK, Kalantar-Zadeh K, Lochs H, MacDonald N, Mulligan K, Muscaritoli M, Ponikowski P, Posthauer ME, Rossi Fanelli F, Schambelan M, Schols AM, Schuster MW, Anker SD, Society for Sarcopenia, Cachexia, and Wasting Disease. Nutritional recommendations for the management of sarcopenia. J Am Med Dir Assoc. 2010;11(6):391–6.

21. Koyanagi A, Veronese N, Solmi M, Oh H, Shin JI, Jacob L, Yang L, Haro JM, Smith L. Fruit and vegetable consumption and sarcopenia among older adults in low- and middle-income countries. Nutrients. 2020;12(3):706.

22. Beaudart C, Dawson A, Shaw SC, Harvey NC, Kanis JA, Binkley N, Reginster JY, Chapurlat R, Chan DC, Bruyère O, Rizzoli R, Cooper C, Dennison EM, IOF-ESCEO Sarcopenia Working Group. Nutrition and physical activity in the prevention and treatment of sarcopenia: systematic review. Osteoporos Int. 2017;28(6):1817–33.

23. Cereda E, Veronese N, Caccialanza R. The final word on nutritional screening and assessment in older persons. Curr Opin Clin Nutr Metab Care. 2018;21(1):24–9.

24. Calvani R, Picca A, Marini F, Biancolillo A, Cesari M, Pesce V, Lezza AMS, Bossola M, Leeuwenburgh C, Bernabei R, Landi F, Marzetti E. The "BIOmarkers associated with sarcopenia and PHysical frailty in EldeRly pErsons" (BIOSPHERE) study: rationale, design and methods. Eur J Intern Med. 2018;56:19–25.

25. Calvani R, Marini F, Cesari M, Tosato M, Picca A, Anker SD, von Haehling S, Miller RR, Bernabei R, Landi F, Marzetti E, SPRINTT Consortium. Biomarkers for physical frailty and sarcopenia. Aging Clin Exp Res. 2017;29(1):29–34.

26. Ter Borg S, Luiking YC, van Helvoort A, Boirie Y, Schols JMGA, de Groot CPGM. Low levels of branched chain amino acids, eicosapentaenoic acid and micronutrients are associated with low muscle mass, strength and function in community-dwelling older adults. J Nutr Health Aging. 2019;23(1):27–34.

27. Skaaby T, Thuesen BH, Linneberg A. Vitamin D, sarcopenia and aging. In: Giustina A, Bliezikian JP, editors. Vitamin D in clinical medicine, vol. 50. Basel: Karger; 2018. p. 177–88. Front Horm Res.

28. Abiri B, Vafa M. Vitamin D and muscle sarcopenia in aging. Methods Mol Biol. 2020;2138:29–47.

29. Uchitomi R, Oyabu M, Kamei Y. Vitamin D and sarcopenia: potential of vitamin D supplementation in sarcopenia prevention and treatment. Nutrients. 2020;12(10):3189.

30. Gkekas NK, Anagnostis P, Paraschou V, Stamiris D, Dellis S, Kenanidis E, Potoupnis M, Tsiridis E, Goulis DG. The effect of vitamin D plus protein supplementation on sarcopenia: a systematic review and meta-analysis of randomized controlled trials. Maturitas. 2021;145:56–63.

31. Roth SM. Genetic aspects of skeletal muscle strength and mass with relevance to sarcopenia. Bonekey Rep. 2012;1:58.

32. Pratt J, Boreham C, Ennis S, Ryan AW, De Vito G. Genetic associations with aging muscle: a systematic review. Cell. 2019;9(1):12.

33. Curcio F, Ferro G, Basile C, Liguori I, Parrella P, Pirozzi F, Della-Morte D, Gargiulo G, Testa G, Tocchetti CG, Bonaduce D, Abete P. Biomarkers in sarcopenia: a multifactorial approach. Exp Gerontol. 2016;85:1–8.

34. Shin MJ, Jeon YK, Kim IJ. Testosterone and sarcopenia. World J Mens Health. 2018;36(3):192–8.
35. Wilhelmsen A, Tsintzas K, Jones SW. Recent advances and future avenues in understanding the role of adipose tissue cross talk in mediating skeletal muscle mass and function with ageing. Geroscience. 2021;43(1):85–110. https://doi.org/10.1007/s11357-021-00322-4.
36. Vicenti G, Bortone I, Bizzoca D, Sardone R, Belluati A, Solarino G, Moretti B. Bridging the gap between serum biomarkers and biomechanical tests in musculoskeletal ageing. J Biol Regul Homeost Agents. 2020;34(4 Suppl 3):263–74.
37. Al-Daghri NM, Al-Attas OS, Alokail MS, Alkharfy KM, Yousef M, Vinodson B, Amer OE, Alnaami AM, Sabico S, Tripathi G, Piya MK, McTernan PG, Chrousos GP. Maternal inheritance of circulating irisin in humans. Clin Sci (Lond). 2014;126(12):837–44.
38. Paris MT, Bell KE, Mourtzakis M. Myokines and adipokines in sarcopenia: understanding cross-talk between skeletal muscle and adipose tissue and the role of exercise. Curr Opin Pharmacol. 2020;52:61–6.
39. Gomarasca M, Banfi G, Lombardi G. Myokines: the endocrine coupling of skeletal muscle and bone. Adv Clin Chem. 2020;94:155–218.
40. Fougere B, van Kan GA, Vellas B, Cesari M. Redox systems, antioxidants and sarcopenia. Curr Protein Pept Sci. 2018;19(7):643–8.
41. Belenguer-Varea Á, Tarazona-Santabalbina FJ, Avellana-Zaragoza JA, Martínez-Reig M, Mas-Bargues C, Inglés M. Oxidative stress and exceptional human longevity: systematic review. Free Radic Biol Med. 2020;149:51–63.
42. Sekhar RV, Hsu J, Jahorr F, Chacko S, Kumar P, Liu C. Glutathione, mitochondrial defects, and a unique metabolic cycle in older humans: implications for sarcopenia. Innov Aging. 2019;3(1):S256.

Screening for Sarcopenia

5

M. Locquet and Charlotte Beaudart

5.1   Introduction

It is now recognized that sarcopenia represents an important health concern. Indeed, accumulating evidence have suggested that the prevalence of sarcopenia is currently high; approximately 10% of older individuals around the world are suffering from sarcopenia [1]. This prevalence could significantly increase over the next few decades from 10.9 in 2016 to 18.7 million in 2045 [2]. The importance of sarcopenia in terms of public health is also highlighted by researchers who have suggested that untreated sarcopenia engenders objective and measurable detrimental health consequences such as falls, fractures, disabilities, hospitalizations, and, ultimately, death [3]. Finally, the financial burden linked to sarcopenia is not negligible. A recent systematic review showed that individuals with sarcopenia tend to have higher health care expenditures than non-sarcopenic subjects [4].

The impact of sarcopenia on public health is therefore significant. However, at present, this disease is often only highlighted when an adverse health event arises or worsens, such as functional repercussions linked to the disease (e.g., falls, fractures,

M. Locquet
WHO Collaborating Center for Public Health Aspects of Musculo-Skeletal Health and Ageing, Division of Public Health, Epidemiology and Health Economics, University of Liège, Liège, Belgium

C. Beaudart (✉)
WHO Collaborating Center for Public Health Aspects of Musculo-Skeletal Health and Ageing, Division of Public Health, Epidemiology and Health Economics, University of Liège, Liège, Belgium

Department of Health Services Research, University of Maastricht, Maastricht, Netherlands
e-mail: c.beaudart@uliege.be

© Springer Nature Switzerland AG 2021
N. Veronese et al. (eds.), *Sarcopenia*, Practical Issues in Geriatrics,
https://doi.org/10.1007/978-3-030-80038-3_5

loss of autonomy, physical disabilities). This is where the advantage of a screening comes in; it offers the possibility to act at an early stage, or a latent phase, of the disease. If clinicians can detect individuals at risk of sarcopenia in a susceptible group (i.e., older adults), before they become sarcopenic, then they can act proactively by preventing downstream adverse health consequences. Two avenues are currently being considered to prevent sarcopenia, based on early screening. First, as shown in a recent umbrella review [5], exercise interventions (i.e., resistance training, multimodal exercise, blood flow restriction) are beneficial in improving muscle strength and limiting sedentary lifestyle. Second, nutritional supplementation seems to have an impact on muscle mass and function and could be interesting in preventing sarcopenia [6].

Screening in the area of sarcopenia could also, in select population, avoid cumbersome diagnostic procedures that are long and costly for the patient and the society. Indeed, the screening test, not only being safe and inexpensive, is also intended to be simpler and faster than diagnostic processes. It allows to differentiate, with a certain error rate, healthy versus sick subjects. It will therefore facilitate identification of patients who will benefit the most from early diagnostic procedures. To meet the different screening objectives, different sarcopenia screening tools have been validated in the scientific literature.

5.2   Part 1. Existing Screening Tools for Sarcopenia

5.2.1   Introduction

As mentioned above, because current methods for diagnosing sarcopenia are complex to implement in daily practice, simplified methods have been developed by different authors, not to replace a complete clinical diagnosis of sarcopenia but to offer an easy way for a first screening of patients at risk of sarcopenia. If the screening test revealed to be positive, more sophisticated assessment of sarcopenia can be performed. Consideration of possible sarcopenia in daily practice has been proposed for older individuals (e.g., >65 years) with signs or symptoms suggestive of the condition both in primary care and in specialized clinical settings [7]. Indeed, there are no obvious symptoms of early sarcopenia, and patients with sarcopenia are often unaware of their disease until the decline in strength and physical performance becomes severe, resulting in physical and functional dependence [8]. Screening to detect sarcopenia before the occurrence of physical disability is thus of great importance to prevent this dependence.

Several methods are proposed to perform a simple, rapid, and inexpensive identification of patients at risk. These methods are listed below, and the evidence-based literature data available on their respective screening performance are presented in the next chapter.

5.2.2   Summary of Existing Screening Tools

5.2.2.1 SARC-F Questionnaire

The SARC-F [9] is a 5-item questionnaire used to determine the level of difficulty experienced by an individual. It ranks five components: strength, assistance in walking, rise from a chair, climb stairs, and falls, with a three-level score range of 0–2 points for each item. The total score ranges from 0 to 10, with ≥4 points indicating a risk of sarcopenia. Many different studies tested SARC-F as a screening tool for sarcopenia and, despite some small variances, consensually reported a high specificity but a low sensitivity. In 2019, Ida et al. published a meta-analysis on SARC-F accuracy which involved seven studies and 12,800 individuals [10]. The pooled sensitivity was 21% and the pooled specificity was 90%, confirming that this questionnaire has a very good performance for identifying patients not at risk of sarcopenia and therefore, those who should not undergo further testing for confirming a diagnosis of sarcopenia.

5.2.2.2 Calf Circumference

Calf circumference is an anthropometric measurement that should be performed with the patient sitting on a chair and holding his bare foot down, holding the leg folded to 90°. The calf circumference has to be measured at its widest point, without tightening (Fig. 5.1).

Many works have suggested that calf circumference could be used as a proxy of appendicular muscle mass. Given this observation, several authors considered calf circumference in their analyses as a measure of sarcopenia. In 2003, Rolland et al. [11] demonstrated that a calf circumference under 31 cm was the best clinical indicator for sarcopenia, with a sensitivity of 44.3% and a specificity of 91.4% in a population of women aged 70 years and older. In a cohort of Korean adults aged 70 years and older, Kim et al. suggested in 2018 a cut-off of 32 cm as the best compromise between sensitivity and specificity in regard of a diagnosis of sarcopenia (men: sensitivity 75%, specificity 83%; women: sensitivity 85%, specificity 57%).

5.2.2.3 SARC-CalF

Because of the low sensitivity of the SARC-F questionnaire, different groups of researchers suggested to combine the SARC-F questionnaire with the measurement of the calf circumference and that this combination may significantly improve the diagnostic accuracy of the SARC-F and especially the sensitivity. In 2016, Barbosa-Silva et al. [12] first tested this procedure and demonstrated a sensitivity for the diagnosis of sarcopenia that increased from 33.3% using the SARC-F alone to 66.7% using the combined SARC-F and calf circumference, also called SARC-CalF. Later, Yang et al. [13] also tested this method in a sample of 384 Chinese participants aged 60 years and older. The sensitivity of the SARC-F alone was 29.5% and increased to 60.7% for the SARC-CalF. Specificity remained very high

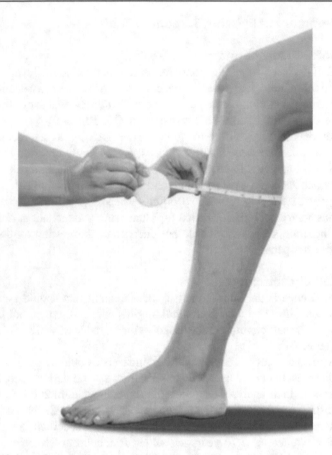

Fig. 5.1 Calf circumference measurement

in both studies. Very recently, a meta-analysis, including five studies and 1127 participants (Barbosa-Silva and Yang included), indicated a sensitivity of 58% and a specificity of 87% for the SARC-CalF as compared with the European Working Group on Sarcopenia in Older People (EWGSOP) diagnosis criteria confirming the idea of combining both screening tools for a better accuracy [14].

5.2.2.4 MSRA: Mini Sarcopenia Risk Assessment
The Mini Sarcopenia Risk Assessment (MSRA) questionnaire is composed of seven questions and investigates anamnestic and nutritional characteristics related to the risk of sarcopenia onset (age, protein and dairy products consumption, number of meals per day, physical activity level, number of hospitalizations, and weight loss in the last year). A smaller version composed of only five questions also exists. Rossi et al. [15] developed and tested this questionnaire as a screening tool for sarcopenia against EWGSOP diagnosis criteria among 274 community-dwelling people aged 65 years and older. Their results suggested that with the 7-item version of the

MSRA, patients with a score of 30 or less had five times greater risk of being sarcopenic, with a sensitivity of 80.4% and a specificity of 50.1%. Because two items showed nonsignificant diagnostic power, they also tested the 5-item version and demonstrated an equivalent sensitivity but a higher specificity (60.4%).

5.2.2.5 Ishii Score

A multivariate model has been developed in 2014 by Ishii et al. [16] to screen for the risk of sarcopenia. It uses three variables: age, grip strength, and calf circumference. A score is assigned to each parameter, and the summary score indicates the likelihood of having sarcopenia. A score >105 and >120 in men and women, respectively, identifies people with a high probability of having sarcopenia. Authors highlighted a sensitivity of 75.5% for women and 84.9% for men and a specificity of 92% for women and 88.2% for men based on the EWGSOP diagnosis criteria.

5.2.2.6 Equation of Yu

In 2015, Yu et al. also proposed a prediction equation based on four parameters to estimate low muscle mass. The prediction equation included weight, body mass index, age, and sex. Combined with a grip strength <30 kg, the sensitivity of the proposed equation in predicting sarcopenia was 57.5% and 57.1% in men and women, respectively, and the specificity was 99.5% in men and 94.7% in women.

5.2.2.7 Screening Grid of Goodman

The screening grid of Goodman et al. [17] is a practical tool built on three parameters: age, body mass index (BMI), and sex. Sex-specific grids provide the probability of having low muscle mass depending on the age and the BMI of the individual. The authors consider that, in women, a probability greater than 80% is indicative of low muscle mass (and therefore at risk of sarcopenia). In men, as soon as the probability exceeds 70%, a low muscle mass is considered present. The authors validated their tool in a sample of 200 subjects from the National Health and Nutrition Examination Surveys (NHANES) cohort. In their validation sample, the sensitivity of the instrument was 81.6% for men and 90.6% for women. As for specificity, it reached 66.2% in both sexes.

5.2.2.8 Chair Stand Test

The chair stand test consists of instructing patients to cross their arms over their chest and to stand up and sit down, five times, from a chair as fast as possible. The time is measured in seconds. In 2016, Pinheiro et al. [18] described a positive association between the results of this test and the diagnosis of sarcopenia, considering it as a performant screening test for sarcopenia. For each 1 s increment in the test performance, they highlighted that the sarcopenia's probability was increased by 8% in women aged 60 years and older. They also found that the best results for this test to maximize sensitivity and specificity in regards to the clinical diagnosis was 13 s. This means that patients that performed the chair stand test in >13 s could be identified as at high risk of sarcopenia with a sensitivity of 85.7% and a specificity of 53.2%.

5.2.2.9 Yubi-Wakka (Finger-Ring) Test

The "Yubi-wakka" test is a sarcopenia screening procedure proposed by Tanaka et al. [19] in 2018 that checks whether the maximum nondominant calf circumference is bigger than the individual's own finger-ring circumference, which is formed by the thumb and forefinger of both hands. Individuals' calf circumference could then be "bigger," "just fits," or "smaller" based on a comparison with the finger-ring circumference. Authors did not provide sensitivity and specificity values in their paper but highlighted that individuals in the "smaller" group had a 6.6-fold higher prevalence of sarcopenia and individuals in the "just fit" group had a 2.4-fold higher prevalence of sarcopenia than the "bigger" group. Later, Beaudart et al. assessed this screening test in the SarcoPhAge study [20] and revealed a sensitivity of 46.9% and a specificity of 78.3% for the "smaller" group as compared with the EWGSOP2 criteria [21] (data not published).

5.2.2.10 GripBMI

The GripBMI screening tool, proposed in 2020 by Churilov et al. [22], uses the combined EWGSOP2 [21] recommended low grip strength cut offs and body mass index of less than 25. Authors found a sensitivity of 83% and a specificity of 96% using this technique among 277 post-acute rehabilitation inpatients.

5.2.2.11 TRSS: Taiwan Risk Score for Sarcopenia

Very recently, Tseng et al. [23] developed a prediction model called Taiwan Risk Score for Sarcopenia (TRSS). On a sample of 1025 subjects, they found that based on seven items, for instance, age, female sex, receiving social assistance pension, absence of exercise, being underweight, abnormal fasting glucose levels, and abnormal creatinine levels, the TRSS could be used as a screening tool for sarcopenia with a sensitivity of 71.8% and a specificity of 71.1%. This model, which requires serum biomarkers, is suggested to be a cost-effective screening tool for sarcopenia.

5.2.2.12 Red Flag Method

Although not strictly a screening tool, the "Red Flag" method developed by Beaudart et al. in 2016 [24] is proving to be an interesting method for the physician, easily integrated into clinical practice. Indeed, the method consists in identifying, during a usual consultation, the manifestations of sarcopenia. The authors suggest three distinct evaluations made up of several elements each considered as a "Red Flag":

– Clinical observation: General weakness of the individual, visual identification of loss of muscle mass, low walking speed;
– Individuals' presenting features: Loss of weight, loss of muscle strength, general weakness, fatigue, falls, mobility impairment, loss of energy, difficulties in physical activity, or activity of daily living;
– Clinical assessment: Nutrition, body weight, physical activity.

The clinical assessment of nutrition and physical activity can be done in a simple way (e.g., question on protein intake, question on the level of inactivity) and also by using more demanding tools such as the Mini-Nutritional Assessment [25] (for nutrition) or the Minnesota [26] (for physical activity).

If this strategy identifies a "Red Flag," then one can suggest the potential presence of sarcopenia. From this observation, further diagnostic procedures can be implemented.

5.3 Part 2. Performance Comparison of the Screening Tools for Sarcopenia

5.3.1 Introduction

There are many tools to screen for sarcopenia. Therefore, an important step must be undertaken to help the clinician in the choice of which one is most appropriate. Indeed, it is important to compare mathematically the performance of the different screening tools, through evidence-based screening studies. In general, this type of study will compare the performance of the different tools via several indicators:

– Sensitivity: or the proportion of subjects who actually present sarcopenia (based on the reference diagnosis) that have been correctly identified as sarcopenic using the screening tool (i.e., positive screening test).
– Specificity: or the proportion of subjects who are not actually affected by sarcopenia (based on the reference diagnosis) that have been correctly identified as non-sarcopenic using the screening tool (i.e., negative screening test).
– Positive predictive value (PPV): or the probability of presenting sarcopenia in case of a positive screening test.
– Negative predictive value (NPV): or the probability of not suffering from sarcopenia in case of a negative screening test.
– Area under the curve (AUC) via receiver operating characteristics (ROC) analysis: or the capacity of the screening test to distinguish those at risk of sarcopenia from those not at risk. The AUCs of each screening methods can be statistically compared using a statistical test to verify that the AUCs of the different screening tools differ significantly between them.

Several researchers have studied the question of the comparative performance of screening tools. We will summarize it in this chapter. Four main studies compared the performance of a large number of sarcopenia screening tools. That will be the subject of our first paragraph. The other studies presented a comparison of the primary tool used in screening for sarcopenia, the SARC-F [9], with one and only one other method. This will be the subject of our second paragraph.

5.3.2   Head-to-Head Comparisons of the Performance of Multiple Sarcopenia Screening Tools

The study comparing the most screening tools at a time is the study performed by Locquet et al. [27], conducted in 2018, involving 306 community-dwelling older subjects, mean age 74.8 ± 5.9 years. Five screening methods were studied: the two-stage algorithm of the EWGSOP [28], the SARC-F [9], the screening grid of Goodman [29], the score chart of Ishii [16], and the equation of Yu [30]. The authors carried out a sensitivity analysis indicating as a reference diagnosis five operational definitions of sarcopenia: that of the European Working Group on Sarcopenia in Older people (EWSOP) [28], that of the International Working Group on Sarcopenia (IWGS) [31], that of the Society on Sarcopenia, Cachexia and Wasting disorders (SSCWD) [32], that of the Asian Working Group and Sarcopenia (AWGS) [33], and that of the Foundation of the National Institute of Health (FNIH) [34]. While the sensitivity and PPV of the screening tests were low in most cases, the specificity and the NPV were very high for all screening tests, regardless of the standard diagnostic definition employed (e.g., specificity ranging from 60% to 91.1% and NPV ranging from 87.2% to 100%). All the screening tools were able to distinguish between those at risk of sarcopenia and those not at risk of sarcopenia (all AUCs significantly superior to 0.5) with the best performance provided by the screening instrument of Ishii, with an AUC rising to 0.914. In conclusion, for individuals who were not affected by sarcopenia, screening tests performed well. The high specificity of the screening equalled a high true-negative rate. These kinds of screening tests with high specificity offer the advantage of avoiding unnecessary resource-consuming diagnostic investigations in the subset of individuals classified as negative. Furthermore, individuals screened negative for sarcopenia can be confident because there is a probability equal to or higher than 87.2% (i.e., value of the NPV) of not suffering from sarcopenia. However, the ideal screening test is one that would allow the distinction, without error, between the positives and the negatives. In real-world conditions, the best test is the one that optimizes its sensitivity and specificity simultaneously. In the study of Locquet et al. [35], this test was the equation of Ishii et al. [16], (i.e., equation including age, grip strength, and calf circumference information) which offered the best ratio sensitivity–specificity (i.e., an AUC rising to 0.914).

This study already provides relevant information on the comparison of screening tests for sarcopenia, but its main weakness is that it did not consider all the screening tests available in the field of sarcopenia. Another study will then allow us to complete our first observations: that of Yang et al. [36], dating from the year 2019. It should be noted here that the population of interest is different; these were 277 older people living in a nursing home, mean age 81.6 ± 3.3 years. The screening tools considered were the SARC-F [9], SARC-CalF [12], MSRA-5 [37], and MSRA-7 [37]. Four gold standards (i.e., diagnosis references) were proposed to compute sensitivity analyses: that of EWGSOP [28], that of IWGS [31], that of

AWGS [33], and that of FNIH [34]. The sensitivity of the four different screening tests was low or medium, depending on the diagnostic definition used (i.e., sensitivity ranging from 17.8% to 64.4%). The specificity was excellent in all cases, it started at 80% to reach 98.4%. The poorest performance in discriminating people at risk from those not at risk for sarcopenia was that obtained by the MSRA-7 (i.e., AUC of 0.681). The skills of the SARC-F and the MSRA-5 did not differ significantly while the best performance was obtained by the SARC-CalF, with an excellent AUC of maximum 0.867. Again, we can see that all of the screening tools studied performed well to identify subjects not at risk of sarcopenia (i.e., high specificity). All the tools also made it possible to distinguish with satisfaction the individuals at risk of sarcopenia from those not at risk. The best performance was that of the SARC-CalF tool, which, therefore, seems quite suitable for screening for sarcopenia in a nursing home.

Another study [38], conducted in 2020 on 100 older people, but living in community, confirms these latest results. Indeed, after comparing the same screening tools (SARC-F, SARC-CalF, MSRA-5, and MSRA-7) according to six different diagnostic criteria, the authors conclude that the MSRA-7 has the smallest AUC and the SARC-CalF is the most suitable screening tools for sarcopenia in older community-dwelling individuals.

Finally, a last study [39] proposed a comparison of three screening tools for sarcopenia: calf circumference, SARC-F, and SARC-CalF referred to the AWGS diagnosis reference. The study was conducted in 1050 community-dwelling individuals. The notable difference with the other studies is, that for once, a screening instrument offered a great sensitivity (81.5% for the calf circumference). The calf circumference test obtained the best AUC (0.790).

However, the SARC-F remains recommended by scientific societies in the field of sarcopenia [21, 40]. Therefore, this has been studied a lot in order to determine its screening accuracy. A recent meta-analysis demonstrates excellent specificity (pooled specificity = 0.90 (95% CI, 0.83–0.94), despite low sensitivity. The authors therefore conclude that the tool is effective in detecting individuals who should resort to a further diagnosis. Many other studies have therefore sought to compare the performance of this SARC-F, specifically, with other screening tools.

5.3.3   Performance Comparison of the SARC-F with Other Sarcopenia Screening Tools

A list of the different studies comparing the SARC-F with another tool is available in Table 5.1. On this topic, six studies have been published. All the studies showed that the two tools were effective in distinguishing individuals at risk from those not at risk of sarcopenia. In general, when the SARC-F was enhanced with calf circumference or EBM, it returned better screening accuracy. Ishii's score was also very powerful.

Table 5.1 Studies about the comparison of the performance of SARC-F versus another screening tool for sarcopenia

Screening tests compared	Population	Reference standard(s)	Performance indicators			Conclusion
			Sensitivity (%)	Specificity (%)	AUCs	
SARC-F versus SARC-CalF Yang et al. [13]	384 community-dwelling older adults aged 60 years or older	EWGSOP AWGS IWGS FNIH	SARC-F: 19.8–30.5 SARC-CalF: 42.7–60.7	SARC-F: 95.6–98.2 SARC-CalF: 90.6–95.5	SARC-F: 0.790–0.890 SARC-CalF: 0.830–0.920	SARC-CalF offered better sensitivity than SARC-F and better distinguished those at risk from those not at risk of sarcopenia (better diagnostic accuracy)
SARC-F versus SARC-CalF Bahat et al. [41]	207 community-dwelling older adults aged 65 years or older	EWGSOP FNIH IWGS SSCWD	SARC-F: 25.0–50.0 SARC-CalF: 15.7–50.0	SARC-F: 81.4–82.4 SARC-CalF: 90.0–90.6	SARC-F: 0.522–0.701 SARC-CalF: 0.682–836	SARC-CalF presented equal sensitivity than SARC-F and better specificity. Therefore, SARC-CalF offered better screening accuracy
SARC-F versus SARC-CalF Fu et al. [42]	309 patients with cancer, mean age 54.7 ± 11.3 years old	Western and eastern diagnostic criteria based on lumbar spine skeletal muscle index (cm²/m²)	SARC-F: 22.4 and 32.1 SARC-CalF: 55.1 and 66.6	SARC-F: 92.1 and 90.7 SARC-CalF: 76.4 and 70.1	SARC-F: 0.680 and 0.700 SARC-CalF: 0.700 and 0.750	In cancer patients, SARC-CalF allowed to increase sensitivity and overall screening accuracy

SARC-F versus MSRA-5 Yang et al. [43]	384 community-dwelling older adults aged 60 years or older	AWGS	SARC-F: 29.5 MSRA-5: 90.2	SARC-F: 98.1 MSRA-5: 70.6	SARC-F: 0.890[a] MSRA-5: 0.850[a]	SARC-F and MSRA-5 demonstrated similar abilities to distinguish those at risk of sarcopenia from those not at risk
SARC-F versus Ishii score Li et al. [44]	138 hospitalized patients aged 60 years and older	AWGS	Not mentioned	Not mentioned	SARC-F: 0.640 Ishii score: 0.780	SARC-F and Ishii score allowed a satisfying screening accuracy, the Ishii score performing a little bit better
SARC-F versus SARC-F + EBM[b] derivation Kurita et al. [45]	959 adult patients with musculoskeletal disease	AWGS EWGSOP2[c]	SARC-F: 41.7 SARC-F + EBM: 77.8	SARC-F: 68.5 SARC-F + EBM: 69.6	SARC-F: 0.557 SARC-F + EBM: 0.824	SARC-F + EBM performed better in screening accuracy even if SARC-F alone already showed good discriminatory abilities

[a]Not significantly different
[b]EBM *elderly and body mass information*
[c]Revised consensus definition of the EWGSOP [21]

5.3.4 Further Considerations Regarding the Performance of Screening Methods

As we have seen, some screening tools seemed to perform better than others. Two important points must, however, attract our attention. First, the studies presented here have different settings and are performed on different samples. Therefore, a large screening accuracy study, especially designed to compare the performance of sarcopenia screening tools whatever the population, should be carried out while being exhaustive in terms of the various existing screening tests but also in terms of the different diagnosis definitions of sarcopenia that could be used as gold standard. Second, and also an important consideration, is that it is essential to determine, mathematically and statistically, which screening tool is the most efficient, but this tool must also meet four other qualities other than that of statistical superiority:

1. Ease of implementation.
2. Reliability (results must be reproducible).
3. Acceptability by the population.
4. Validity (sensitivity, specificity, PPV, NPV, AUC).

For the score chart of Ishii, for example, the complicated calculations that it implies limit its use in clinical settings (quality criteria 1 not met). This screening tool is ultimately close to a diagnosis technique since muscle strength (using a hand dynamometer) and muscle mass (using anthropometry) have to be measured. Therefore, we lose the targeted advantage of screening tests, which is to limit the use of relatively resource-consuming diagnostic techniques in individuals. We can also put this argument forward for the SARC-CalF which already requires an anthropometric measurement as for the SARC-F + EBM.

Therefore, different working groups on sarcopenia (the EWGSOP and the Society on Sarcopenia, Cachexia and Wasting Disorder) decided on the question of the most appropriate screening test. The screening method of the SARC-F was chosen by these groups as the best method for two reasons. First, the SARC-F had high specificity regardless of the definition of sarcopenia that was used, as evidenced by numerous studies. Second, by its five simple questions reflecting the five symptoms usually associated with sarcopenia, the SARC-F is favored due to its rapidity and simplicity of application that does not require specific resources for clinicians. The project of translation and cross-cultural adaptation of the SARC-F in numerous languages around the world is currently ongoing [46]. However, even if not easily implemented, the equation of Ishii et al. for screening sarcopenia has been proposed by the EWGSOP as an alternative for clinicians who are seeking a more formal case-finding tool and who have the time to adopt the calculations and assessments required by this equation.

In future researches, it would be interesting to underline the importance of screening by testing the hypothesis that individuals who are identified as at risk of sarcopenia by the screening method will present more morbid events than those who are not at risk, as it has been demonstrated for the SARC-F [44]. Another step will then be to investigate whether early detection of sarcopenia will ultimately reduce the consequences of the disease. A screening strategy should indeed be effective in reducing mortality and morbidity.

References

1. Shafiee G, Keshtkar A, Soltani A, Ahadi Z, Larijani B, Heshmat R. Prevalence of sarcopenia in the world: a systematic review and meta-analysis of general population studies. J Diabetes Metab Disord. 2017;16(1):21. https://doi.org/10.1186/s40200-017-0302-x.
2. Ethgen O, Tchoconte C, Beaudart C, Buckinx F, Reginster J-Y, Bruyère O. The future prevalence of sarcopenia in Europe. Osteoporos Int. 2016;27(Suppl 1):53–4.
3. Beaudart C, Zaaria M, Pasleau F, Reginster J-Y, Bruyère O. Health outcomes of sarcopenia: a systematic review and meta-analysis. PLoS One. 2017;12(1):e0169548. https://doi.org/10.1371/journal.pone.0169548.
4. Janssen I, Shepard DS, Katzmarzyk PT, Roubenoff R. The healthcare costs of sarcopenia in the United States. J Am Geriatr Soc. 2004;52(1):80–5.
5. Beckwée D, Delaere A, Aelbrecht S, et al. Exercise interventions for the prevention and treatment of sarcopenia. A systematic umbrella review. J Nutr Health Aging. 2019;23(6):494–502. https://doi.org/10.1007/s12603-019-1196-8.
6. Beaudart C, Dawson A, Shaw SC, et al. Nutrition and physical activity in the prevention and treatment of sarcopenia: systematic review. Osteoporos Int. 2017;28(6):1817–33. https://doi.org/10.1007/s00198-017-3980-9.
7. Beaudart C, McCloskey E, Bruyère O, et al. Sarcopenia in daily practice: assessment and management. BMC Geriatr. 2016;16(1):170. https://doi.org/10.1186/s12877-016-0349-4.
8. Visvanathan R, Chapman I. Preventing sarcopaenia in older people. Maturitas. 2010;66(4):383–8. https://doi.org/10.1016/j.maturitas.2010.03.020.
9. Malmstrom TK, Morley JE, Haren MT, et al. SARC-F: a simple questionnaire to rapidly diagnose sarcopenia. J Am Med Dir Assoc. 2013;14(8):531–2. https://doi.org/10.1016/j.jamda.2013.05.018.
10. Ida S, Kaneko R, Murata K. SARC-F for screening of sarcopenia among older adults: a meta-analysis of screening test accuracy. J Am Med Dir Assoc. 2018;19(8):685–9. https://doi.org/10.1016/j.jamda.2018.04.001.
11. Rolland Y, Lauwers-Cances V, Cournot M, et al. Sarcopenia, calf circumference, and physical function of elderly women: a cross-sectional study. J Am Geriatr Soc. 2003;51(8):1120–4. https://doi.org/10.1046/j.1532-5415.2003.51362.x.
12. Barbosa-Silva TG, Menezes AMB, Bielemann RM, Malmstrom TK, Gonzalez MC. Enhancing SARC-F: improving sarcopenia screening in the clinical practice. J Am Med Dir Assoc. 2016;17(12):1136–41. https://doi.org/10.1016/j.jamda.2016.08.004.
13. Yang M, Hu X, Xie L, et al. Screening sarcopenia in community-dwelling older adults: SARC-F vs SARC-F combined with calf circumference (SARC-CalF). J Am Med Dir Assoc. 2018;19(3):277.e1–8. https://doi.org/10.1016/j.jamda.2017.12.016.
14. Mo Y, Dong X, Wang XH. Screening accuracy of SARC-F combined with calf circumference for sarcopenia in older adults: a diagnostic meta-analysis. J Am Med Dir Assoc. 2020;21(2):288–9. https://doi.org/10.1016/j.jamda.2019.09.002.
15. Rossi AP, Micciolo R, Rubele S, et al. Assessing the risk of sarcopenia in the elderly: the mini sarcopenia risk assessment (MSRA) questionnaire. J Nutr Heal Aging. 2017;21(6):743–9. https://doi.org/10.1007/s12603-017-0921-4.
16. Ishii S, Tanaka T, Shibasaki K, et al. Development of a simple screening test for sarcopenia in older adults. Geriatr Gerontol Int. 2014;14(Suppl 1):93–101. https://doi.org/10.1111/ggi.12197.

17. Goodman MJ, Ghate SR, Mavros P, et al. Development of a practical screening tool to predict low muscle mass using NHANES 1999-2004. J Cachexia Sarcopenia Muscle. 2013;4(3):187–97. https://doi.org/10.1007/s13539-013-0107-9.

18. Pinheiro PA, Carneiro JAO, Coqueiro RS, Pereira R, Fernandes MH. "Chair stand test" as simple tool for sarcopenia screening in elderly women. J Nutr Heal Aging. 2016;20(1):56–9. https://doi.org/10.1007/s12603-016-0676-3.

19. Tanaka T, Takahashi K, Akishita M, Tsuji T, Iijima K. "Yubi-wakka" (finger-ring) test: a practical self-screening method for sarcopenia, and a predictor of disability and mortality among Japanese community-dwelling older adults. Geriatr Gerontol Int. 2018;18(2):224–32. https://doi.org/10.1111/ggi.13163.

20. Beaudart C, Reginster JY, Petermans J, et al. Quality of life and physical components linked to sarcopenia: the SarcoPhAge study. Exp Gerontol. 2015;69 https://doi.org/10.1016/j.exger.2015.05.003.

21. Cruz-Jentoft AJ, Bahat G, Bauer J, et al. Sarcopenia: revised European consensus on definition and diagnosis. Age Ageing. 2018; https://doi.org/10.1093/ageing/afy169.

22. Churilov I, Churilov L, Brock K, Murphy D, MacIsaac RJ, Ekinci EI. GripBMI – a fast and simple sarcopenia screening tool in post acute inpatient rehabilitation. Clin Nutr. 2021;40:1022–7. https://doi.org/10.1016/j.clnu.2020.06.034.

23. Tzyy-Guey T, Lu CK, Yu-Han H, Shu-Chuan P, Chi-Jung T, Lee MC. Development of Taiwan risk score for sarcopenia (TRSS) for sarcopenia screening among community-dwelling older adults. Int J Environ Res Public Health. 2020;17(8):1–10. https://doi.org/10.3390/ijerph17082859.

24. Beaudart C, McCloskey E, Bruyère O, et al. Sarcopenia in daily practice: assessment and management. BMC Geriatr. 2016;16(1):1–10. https://doi.org/10.1186/s12877-016-0349-4.

25. Cereda E. Mini nutritional assessment. Curr Opin Clin Nutr Metab Care. 2012;15(1):29–41. https://doi.org/10.1097/MCO.0b013e32834d7647.

26. Elosua R, Marrugat J, Molina L, Pons S, Pujol E. Validation of the Minnesota leisure time physical activity questionnaire in Spanish men. Am J Epidemiol. 1994;139(12):1197–209. https://doi.org/10.1093/oxfordjournals.aje.a116966.

27. Locquet M, Beaudart C, Reginster J-Y, Petermans J, Bruyère O. Comparison of the performance of five screening methods for sarcopenia. Clin Epidemiol. 2018;10:71–82. https://doi.org/10.2147/CLEP.S148638.

28. Cruz-Jentoft AJ, Baeyens JP, Bauer JM, et al. Sarcopenia: European consensus on definition and diagnosis: report of the European working group on sarcopenia in older people. Age Ageing. 2010;39(4):412–23. https://doi.org/10.1093/ageing/afq034.

29. Goodman MJ, Ghate SR, Mavros P, et al. Development of a practical screening tool to predict low muscle mass using NHANES 1999-2004. J Cachexia Sarcopenia Muscle. 2013;4(3):187–97. https://doi.org/10.1007/s13539-013-0107-9.

30. Yu S, Appleton S, Chapman I, et al. An anthropometric prediction equation for appendicular skeletal muscle mass in combination with a measure of muscle function to screen for sarcopenia in primary and aged care. J Am Med Dir Assoc. 2015;16(1):25–30. https://doi.org/10.1016/j.jamda.2014.06.018.

31. Fielding RA, Vellas B, Evans WJ, et al. Sarcopenia: an undiagnosed condition in older adults. Current consensus definition: prevalence, etiology, and consequences. International Working Group on Sarcopenia. J Am Med Dir Assoc. 2011;12(4):249–56. https://doi.org/10.1016/j.jamda.2011.01.003.

32. Morley JE, Abbatecola AM, Argiles JM, et al. Sarcopenia with limited mobility: an international consensus. J Am Med Dir Assoc. 2011;12(6):403–9. https://doi.org/10.1016/j.jamda.2011.04.014.

33. Chen L-K, Liu L-K, Woo J, et al. Sarcopenia in Asia: consensus report of the Asian Working Group for Sarcopenia. J Am Med Dir Assoc. 2014;15(2):95–101. https://doi.org/10.1016/j.jamda.2013.11.025.

34. Studenski SA, Peters KW, Alley DE, et al. The FNIH sarcopenia project: rationale, study description, conference recommendations, and final estimates. Journals Gerontol Ser A Biol Sci Med Sci. 2014;69(5):547–58. https://doi.org/10.1093/gerona/glu010.
35. Locquet M, Beaudart C, Reginster J-Y, Petermans J, Bruyère O. Comparison of the performance of five screening methods for sarcopenia. Clin Epidemiol. 2018;10:71–82. https://doi.org/10.2147/CLEP.S148638.
36. Yang M, Lu J, Jiang J, Zeng Y, Tang H. Comparison of four sarcopenia screening tools in nursing home residents. Aging Clin Exp Res. 2019;31(10):1481–9. https://doi.org/10.1007/s40520-018-1083-x.
37. Rossi AP, Micciolo R, Rubele S, et al. Assessing the risk of sarcopenia in the elderly: The Mini Sarcopenia Risk Assessment (MSRA) questionnaire. J Nutr Heal Aging. 2017;21(6):743–9. https://doi.org/10.1007/s12603-017-0921-4.
38. Krzymińska-Siemaszko R, Tobis S, Lewandowicz M, Wieczorowska-Tobis K. Comparison of four sarcopenia screening questionnaires in community-dwelling older adults from Poland using six sets of international diagnostic criteria of sarcopenia. PLoS One. 2020;15(4):e0231847. https://doi.org/10.1371/journal.pone.0231847.
39. Mo YH, Zhong J, Dong X, et al. Comparison of three screening methods for sarcopenia in community-dwelling older persons. J Am Med Dir Assoc. 2021;22:746–750.e1. https://doi.org/10.1016/j.jamda.2020.05.041.
40. Bauer J, Morley JE, AMWJ S, et al. Sarcopenia: a time for action. An SCWD Position Paper. J Cachexia Sarcopenia Muscle. 2019;10:956–61. https://doi.org/10.1002/jcsm.12483.
41. Bahat G, Oren MM, Yilmaz O, Kiliç C, Aydin K, Karan MA. Comparing sarc-f with sarc-calf to screen sarcopenia in community living older adults. J Nutr Heal Aging. 2018;22(9):1034–8. https://doi.org/10.1007/s12603-018-1072-y.
42. Fu X, Tian Z, Thapa S, et al. Comparing SARC-F with SARC-CalF for screening sarcopenia in advanced cancer patients. Clin Nutr. 2020;39:3337–45. https://doi.org/10.1016/j.clnu.2020.02.020.
43. Yang M, Hu X, Xie L, et al. Comparing mini sarcopenia risk assessment with SARC-F for screening sarcopenia in community-dwelling older adults. J Am Med Dir Assoc. 2019;20(1):53–7. https://doi.org/10.1016/j.jamda.2018.04.012.
44. Li M, Kong Y, Chen H, Chu A, Song G, Cui Y. Accuracy and prognostic ability of the SARC-F questionnaire and Ishii's score in the screening of sarcopenia in geriatric inpatients. Braz J Med Biol Res. 2019;52(9):e8204. https://doi.org/10.1590/1414-431x20198204.
45. Kurita N, Wakita T, Kamitani T, Wada O, Mizuno K. SARC-F validation and SARC-F+EBM derivation in musculoskeletal disease: the SPSS-OK Study. J Nutr Heal Aging. 2019;23(8):732–8. https://doi.org/10.1007/s12603-019-1222-x.
46. Bahat G, Yilmaz O, Oren MM, et al. Cross-cultural adaptation and validation of the SARC-F to assess sarcopenia: methodological report from European Union Geriatric Medicine Society Sarcopenia Special Interest Group. Eur Geriatr Med. 2018;9(1):23–8. https://doi.org/10.1007/s41999-017-0003-5.

Radiological Evaluation of Muscle Mass

6

Luciana La Tegola and Giuseppe Guglielmi

6.1 Introduction

In recent years, the importance of muscle mass has been emphasized in numerous conditions [1–3]. The reduction of muscle mass, the decreasing of muscle strength, and the declining of physical performance fall under the definition of sarcopenia [4], a geriatric syndrome associated with increased risk of disability, poor quality of life, and hospitalization [5].

As the elderly population increases, sarcopenia is expected to be one of the major public health problems [6] and therefore, has become a topic of clinical interest.

There is still no general consensus about the definition of sarcopenia; however, according the latest consensus of the European working group on sarcopenia in older people (EWGSOP2) [4], the suspicion of probable sarcopenia is linked to a reduction in muscle strength, while the diagnostic confirmation comes from the detection of a poor muscle quality or quantity, so radiological assessment of skeletal muscle in terms of size, mass, fatty infiltration, and inflammatory states plays an important role in the diagnostic process and in the treatment response [4].

The most used imaging techniques for body composition assessment in daily clinical practice and for research purposes are dual-energy X-ray absorptiometry (DXA), computed tomography (CT), and magnetic resonance imaging (MRI). Ultrasonography (US) is limited to some epidemiological studies [7, 8]. In this chapter, we will briefly discuss these methods.

L. La Tegola
Department of Clinical and Experimental Medicine, Foggia University School of Medicine, Foggia, Italy

G. Guglielmi (✉)
Department of Clinical and Experimental Medicine, Foggia University School of Medicine, Foggia, Italy

Radiology Unit, "Dimiccoli" Hospital, Barletta, Italy
e-mail: giuseppe.guglielmi@unifg.it

© Springer Nature Switzerland AG 2021
N. Veronese et al. (eds.), *Sarcopenia*, Practical Issues in Geriatrics,
https://doi.org/10.1007/978-3-030-80038-3_6

6.2   US

Ultrasonography is a well-known technique characterized by low costs and wide accessibility. It allows a regional assessment of muscle quantity (through the measurement of muscle thickness and cross-sectional area) and muscle quality (through the evaluation of echogenicity) with high inter/intra-operator reproducibility [9]. Both size and echo intensity are associated with muscle strength, as demonstrated in several studies focusing on the association between ultrasound muscle measurements and strength. Strasser et al. demonstrated that sarcopenia can be monitored through vastus medialis muscle thickness measurement and that there is a high correlation between muscle thickness and isometric maximum voluntary contraction force [10].

Main limitations of US in the study of muscle mass are represented by the lack of site-specific cut off, lack of standardization, and requirement of technical preparation of the operator; for these reasons, its application in sarcopenia diagnostic algorithm is limited.

6.3   CT

CT is a tomographic imaging technique based on the different degree of attenuation of X-rays in the passage through the tissues of the body. It is routinely performed in many conditions, particularly for staging and follow-up of cancer, and so it can allow the assessment of BC in this occasion without performing other examinations.

The assessment of body composition (BC) with CT can be carried out both at the level of the entire body through manual or semiautomatic segmentation software and at the level of a single slice with high accuracy and strong correlation with whole-body lean mass and fat mass [11].

The main parameter on a CT scan that give information on muscle mass is the Cross-Sectional Area (CSA, cm^2) measurement of skeletal muscles, while quality muscle assessment is obtained by the estimation of fatty infiltration, or intermuscular adipose tissue (IMAT). Normally the muscle density values are between 40 and 100 Hounsfield Unit (HU). A reduction in the average density values calculated in a region of interest (ROI) up to 0–30 HU is indicative of myosteatosis (Fig. 6.1), but the lack of validated thresholds to put the diagnosis of sarcopenia represents a limit.

In addition to this, other limits of CT are the high dose of radiation exposure, high costs, and not executability in severe obesity.

An alternative to CT is the peripheral quantitative computed tomography (pQCT) which enables, through tomographic images, quantification of three-dimensional tissue structure and skeletal muscle assessment with lower exposure dose and lower cost than CT. The muscle density values are between 65 and 90 mg/cm^3 [12]; in fatty infiltration the values decrease.

The pqCT scanner is small so that the study of muscle mass can only be performed at a peripheral level; the latest scanners allow to study up to the mid-thigh

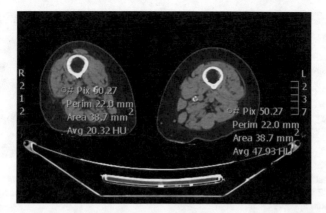

Fig. 6.1 Axial CT image of the mid-thigh of an 84 years old woman. Note the different average (Avg) of the density values in the ROIs; in the right thigh, there is greater fatty infiltration (on the right Avg 20 HU about, on the left about 48 HU)

level, and this obviously represents a limit of muscle assessment; moreover, also in this case, there is no validated protocol [13].

6.4   MRI

MR produces tomographic images by interaction between radiofrequency waves and nuclei of the cellular elements, principally hydrogen in water and fat; it allows to measure muscle mass and fat mass with high accuracy, thanks to multiparametricity and high contrast resolution. With CT, it is considered the reference standard imaging modality to assess muscle quantity and quality [14].

Lots of sequences can be useful in BC; among these Dixon, imaging plays an important role. It is a multiecho gradient-echo sequence that obtains from a single acquisition water-only and fat-only images allowing a quantitative assessment of myosteatosis [15].

Moreover, with MR it is possible to get other muscle quality information such as edema, fibrosis, elasticity, and contractility which correlate with decrease of muscle quality and so with sarcopenia [16].

MR is considered a promising technique in sarcopenia and does not require ionizing radiation, but its use today is limited to research, because of high costs, scarce availability, complex post-processing, and lack of standardization (Fig. 6.2).

6.5   DXA

DXA is the most commonly used technique in clinical routine for body composition. It is based on a three-compartment model of body composition (bone, fat, and lean mass) obtained by the attenuation that a beam of X photons at two different

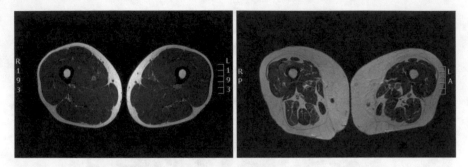

Fig. 6.2 Axial T1 weighted MRI images of the thighs of two patients of different ages. On the left a patient of 32 years, on the right a patient of 76 years. The adipose infiltration of the muscles in the older patient appears clear

energy levels undergoes through the body tissues. The reference parameter for the sarcopenia assessment is ALMI, Appendicular Lean Mass Index. It is a parameter derived from measuring the skeletal muscle mass at the limbs, where is represented the 75% of the skeletal muscle mass of the whole body, proportionate to the height squared (ALM/height^2) [17]. ALMI, as demonstrated in several studies [13, 18], is highly correlated to the skeletal muscle volume measured with the CT and the MR, considered the reference standard techniques (Fig. 6.3).

The latest recommendations issued in 2018 by the European Working Group on Sarcopenia in Older People (EWGSOP 2) define the ALMI cut-off values for sarcopenia, setting the limit value of low muscle mass at 7 kg/m^2 in men and 5.5 kg/m^2 in women [4].

In DXA, there is a very low dose of exposition radiation (<1 mSv, corresponding to the dose we are exposed to in 1 year for environmental radiation); it has low costs, rapid acquisition times, precision, but also some limitations.

First of all, due to the intrinsic nature of the technique being projective, DXA does not allow the study of a single muscle of interest. Moreover, there may be interferences linked to the hydration state of the patient, in particular in cardiac or nephropathic patients who have water retention problems can occur an overestimation of the lean mass and therefore of the muscle. Finally, it is not a standardized method; the densitometers of the various brands provide different results so when you have to compare values of the same patient from two different devices, it is necessary to perform an in vivo calibration, with the errors that may result.

6.6   Conclusions

In conclusion, there are several techniques for assessing muscle mass, but none meets all the requirements for measuring muscle mass and none is standardized; for this reason, there is still no gold standard.

DXA provides a reliable and reproducible measurement of the muscle mass at low costs and minimal exposure to ionizing radiation, and its results have strong

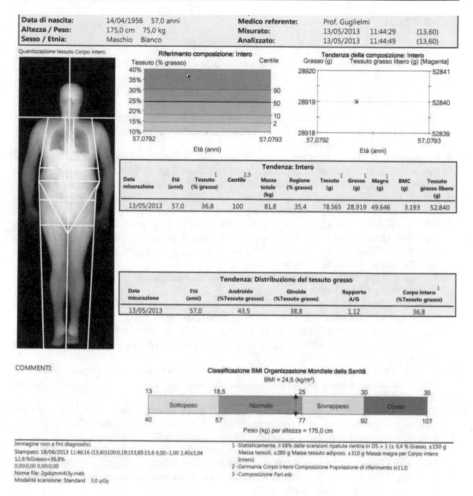

Fig. 6.3 DXA body composition report of a 57 years old male patient. The patient weighs 81.8 kg (180 pounds) ("massa totale" in the report); 28,919 g (63 pounds) are represented by fat mass ("grasso"), 49,646 g (109 pounds) lean mass ("magro"). The total percentage of fat mass is 36.8% ("corpo intero % tessuto grasso"), with a prevalent android distribution. The patient has a BMI = 24.5, a value that falls within the normal range (green line)

correlation with those of CT and MR; moreover, it provides at the same time BC and bone information. For this reason, the EWGSOP guidelines suggest DXA as the first examination to perform for clinical purposes, while CT and MR are limited to research [4].

References

1. Springer J, Springer JI, Anker SD. Muscle wasting and sarcopenia in heart failure and beyond: update 2017. ESC Heart Fail. 2017;4(4):492–8. https://doi.org/10.1002/ehf2.12237.
2. Cui M, Gang X, Wang G, et al. A cross-sectional study: associations between sarcopenia and clinical characteristics of patients with type 2 diabetes. Medicine (Baltimore). 2020;99(2):e18708. https://doi.org/10.1097/MD.0000000000018708.
3. Han P, Kang L, Guo Q, et al. Prevalence and factors associated with sarcopenia in suburb-dwelling older Chinese using the Asian Working Group for sarcopenia definition. J Gerontol A Biol Sci Med Sci. 2016;71:529–35.
4. Cruz-Jentoft AJ, Bahat G, Bauer J, et al. Sarcopenia: revised European consensus on definition and diagnosis [published correction appears in Age Ageing. 2019 Jul 1;48(4):601]. Age Ageing. 2019;48(1):16–31. https://doi.org/10.1093/ageing/afy169.
5. Rizzoli R, et al. Quality of life in sarcopenia and frailty. Calcif Tissue Int. 2013;93:101–20. https://doi.org/10.1007/s00223-013-9758-y.
6. Beaudart C, Rizzoli R, Bruyere O, Reginster JY, Biver E. Sarcopenia: burden and challenges for Public Health. Arch Public Heal. 2014;72:45. https://doi.org/10.1186/2049-3258-72-45.
7. Scherbakov N, Sandek A, Doehner W. Stroke-related sarcopenia: specific characteristics. J Am Med Dir Assoc. 2015;16:272–6.
8. Puthucheary ZA, Rawal J, McPhail M, et al. Acute skeletal muscle wasting in critical illness. JAMA. 2013;310:1591–600.
9. Scott JM, Martin DS, Ploutz-Snyder R, et al. Reliability and validity of panoramic ultrasound for muscle quantification. Ultrasound Med Biol. 2012;38:1656–61.
10. Strasser EM, Draskovits T, Praschak M, Quittan M, Graf A. Association between ultrasound measurements of muscle thickness, pennation angle, echogenicity and skeletal muscle strength in the elderly. Age (Dordr). 2013;35:2377–88.
11. Shen W, Punyanitya M, Wang Z, et al. Total body skeletal muscle and adipose tissue volumes: estimation from a single abdominal cross-sectional image. J Appl Physiol (1985). 2004;97:2333–8.
12. Sherk VD, Thiebaud RS, Chen Z, Karabulut M, Kim SJ, Bemben DA. Associations between pQCT-based fat and muscle area and density and DXA-based total and leg soft tissue mass in healthy women and men. J Musculoskelet Neuronal Interact. 2014;14(4):411–7.
13. Erlandson MC, Lorbergs AL, Mathur S, Cheung AM. Muscle analysis using pQCT, DXA and MRI. Eur J Radiol. 2016;85(8):1505–11. https://doi.org/10.1016/j.ejrad.2016.03.001.
14. Beaudart C, McCloskey E, Bruyere O, et al. Sarcopenia in daily practice: assessment and management. BMC Geriatr. 2016;16:170.
15. Li K, Dortch RD, Welch EB, et al. Multi-parametric MRI characterization of healthy human thigh muscles at 3.0 T - relaxation, magnetization transfer, fat/water, and diffusion tensor imaging. NMR Biomed. 2014;27:1070–84.
16. Boutin RD, Yao L, Canter RJ, Lenchik L. Sarcopenia: current concepts and imaging implications. AJR Am J Roentgenol. 2015;205(3):W255–66. https://doi.org/10.2214/AJR.15.14635.
17. Buckinx F, Landi F, Cesari M, et al. Pitfalls in the measurement of muscle mass: a need for a reference standard. J Cachexia Sarcopenia Muscle. 2018;9(2):269–78. https://doi.org/10.1002/jcsm.12268.
18. Kullberg J, Brandberg J, Angelhed JE, et al. Whole-body adipose tissue analysis: comparison of MRI, CT and dual energy X-ray absorptiometry. Br J Radiol. 2009;82:123–30.

Physical Performance and Muscle Strength Tests: Pros and Cons

7

F. Buckinx and M. Aubertin-Leheudre

7.1 Introduction

Muscle strength and physical performances are evaluated for various conditions and in clinical practice. In geriatric, it is known that older adults with low muscle function are more likely to be dependent in activities of daily living [1]. Therefore, assessing muscle function is essential to prevent these consequences or to rehabilitate it. An international survey found that, among the 255 clinicians, muscle strength and muscle performance are assessed in clinical practice by 54.5% and 71.4% of them, respectively [2]. Moreover, measures of muscle strength and physical performances are also often included in epidemiological studies or clinical trials to monitor, for example, the evolution over time or the change following an intervention in older adults.

From a clinical and epidemiological point of view, identifying individuals at risk is important since poor muscle strength and physical performances, also called sarcopenia, are associated with adverse health outcomes such as falls, hospitalizations, functional decline, loss of autonomy, and mortality [3]. In the literature, a large number of tools are available to assess muscle strength and physical performances, and therefore to diagnose sarcopenia [4]. However, all these tools have advantages and disadvantages. Consequently, clinicians and researchers often struggle to choose the most appropriate and/or validated tool for their needs and for older adults. Briefly, some of these instruments are not available in clinical setting, require

F. Buckinx · M. Aubertin-Leheudre (✉)
Département des Sciences de l'activité physique, Groupe de Recherche en
Activité Physique Adaptée (GRAPA), Université du Québec à Montréal, Montréal, Canada

Centre de Recherche de l'Institut Universitaire de Gériatrie de Montréal (CRIUGM),
Montréal, Canada
e-mail: fanny.buckinx@uliege.be

© Springer Nature Switzerland AG 2021
N. Veronese et al. (eds.), *Sarcopenia*, Practical Issues in Geriatrics,
https://doi.org/10.1007/978-3-030-80038-3_7

highly qualified staff, or are expensive; while more accessible instruments are available for daily practice but their reliability and reproducibility are not always optimal. Therefore, the aim of this chapter is to summarize the pros and cons of the available tests to assess muscle strength and physical function.

7.2 Muscle Strength

Increasingly compelling evidence have highlighted the potential role of muscle function (i.e., strength-power-quality) as a protective factor for health across populations [5]. According to the revised European consensus on sarcopenia, muscle strength is the primary parameter of sarcopenia [6] and is the better predictor of adverse outcomes or physical limitation [7–12]. It is necessary to have objective, reliable, and sensitive tools to assess muscle strength (i.e., upper or lower limb muscle strength) to detect and quantify weakness, to adapt physical exercises to patients' capacity, and to evaluate the effects of intervention [13].

7.2.1 Upper Limb Muscle Strength

In many clinical areas, handgrip strength appears to be the most widely used method for the measurement of overall muscle strength [14]. The international survey published by Bruyere et al. showed that 66.4% of the clinicians (i.e., in the fields of geriatric medicine and rheumatology) used handgrip strength to assess muscle strength in daily practice [2]. Handgrip strength is also used as an indicator of general health [15], nutritional status [16], and has been recently suggested as risk-stratifying method for all-cause death [9]. In addition, good correlation between handgrip strength and lower limb muscle strength is observed [17].

Thus, the use of this measure is not surprising since it is easy to perform, affordable, noninvasive [18], not requiring a highly trained staff [19], highly reliable [20], and very accessible [21]. However, the two main limitations are that (1) only isometric measurement is possible, whereas most daily activities require dynamic muscle contractions and (2) handgrip strength measurement may not overall strength of the body [22].

In addition, a standardized protocol to assess handgrip strength is also recommended in order to make studies comparable to each other [23]. Thus, the protocol should be: (1) tested individual needs to sit in a standard chair with his forearms resting on the armchairs; (2) clinicians or investigators should demonstrate the use of the dynamometer and show how to grip very tightly the hand dynamometer; (3) six handgrip measures should be taken, three with each arm; (4) ideally, encouragements should be given to the patient to invite him to squeeze as hard and as tightly as possible during 3–5 s for each of the six trials and same encouragements between each patient to not induce bias; (5) usually, the highest reading of the six measurements is reported as the final result [24].

Moreover, regarding the handgrip tool, the Jamar dynamometer, or similar hydraulic dynamometer, is the gold standard for this measurement [23]. However, for patients with advanced arthritis, the design of this dynamometer may be a limitation [25]. A pneumatic dynamometer, such as the Martin vigorimeter, may be a good alternative. This flexible pear-shaped vigorimeter is available in three sizes will facilitate the measurement of grip strength in these special cases.

Based on the European Working Group on Sarcopenia in Older People 2 (EWGSOP2), cut-off points for low absolute handgrip strength are <27 kg for men and <16 kg for women [6]. The Foundation for the National Institutes of Health (FNIH) Sarcopenia Study suggested, based on the likelihood of mobility impairment, absolute handgrip strength cut-off points of 26 kg for men and 16 kg for women [26]. Similar values have also been suggested by Dodds et al., who generated grip strength reference values and calculated cut-off points 2.5 standard deviations below the mean from 12 United Kingdom-based epidemiology studies [27].

The minimal clinically important difference in grip strength is critical to interpreting changes in grip strength over time. In the meantime, based on the recent systematic review of Bohannon, absolute changes between 5.0 and 6.5 kg should be considered as meaningful changes in grip strength [28].

7.2.2 Lower Limb Muscle Strength

Lower limb muscle strength (i.e., knee flexors and extensors) is also often studied and used in clinical practice. Lower limb muscle strength is more associated with functional activities than handgrip strength [29–32]. According to Buckinx et al., lower limb muscle strength is also associated with motor skills [29]. The international survey of Bruyere et al. revealed that leg press is used by 24.2% of the clinicians to estimate muscle strength in daily practice. Generally, lower limb muscle strength is measured in isokinetic and/or isometric condition.

The criteria referenced assessment of lower limb muscle strength involves specific dynamometers such as isokinetic devices [33], which proposes a unidirectional analytical motion, performed at a constant angular velocity imposed by the experimenter [34]. This strength is a result from the intervention of a variable resistance, constantly enslaved to the subject's capacity for effort. The isokinetic technique guarantees maximum muscle contraction during the entire exercise, and for each degree of joint movement. The isokinetic strength measure is, therefore, the closest technique to capture a real and physiological muscle contraction. This technique is commonly used in athletes to characterize muscle performance [35] and also to detect bilateral asymmetries or imbalances between agonist and antagonist muscles [36]. This technique has also been found to be useful in clinical practice, for example, in orthopedic patients [37]. However, these devices are often found and used in laboratory-based. In addition, a limitation of these laboratory-based dynamometers is that they are expensive and not handheld, which precludes their use as a clinical device in usual patient assessment and in specific conditions or environments (e.g., at home or in nursing home settings) [38]. The use of these tools may differ depending on the clinical settings or measurement objectives. For example, if it seems worthwhile to recommend assessing grip strength in daily clinical practice, isokinetic therapy has added value in more specific clinical situations (e.g., muscle atrophy). The cut-off values are very variable depending on the population and conditions.

As an alternative to isokinetic devices, portable and low-cost dynamometers seem more appropriate and convenient method to assess muscle strength in clinical and research practice but only if they have been previously validated [33, 38]. In this context, isometric strength method consists in measuring the isometric maximum voluntary strength during contractions performed at constant angular position against resistance. The result is specific to the fixed angular position and reflects the ability of the muscle group to generate a force during isometric contraction (i.e., without variation in overall muscle length). As opposed to dynamic muscle strength, it is therefore considered as a measure of the static muscle strength. A portable dynamometer, even if it is convenient and useful in clinical practice (especially outside medical centers), can induce reproducibility and reliability limitations due to, for example, measurement position (joint angle), measurement site, type of measurement, type of muscle contraction, or movement speed. Standardization of measurement is therefore necessary, and a protocol has been recently proposed [38]. In addition, another bias in the assessment which may affect the result is the skill of the evaluators [39]. Few years ago, Stark and collaborators synthesized the validity of portable dynamometers available in the scientific literature [40]. According to the authors, the reproducibility of portable dynamometers varies from "moderate" to "good." Other portable dynamometers are sometimes used without having been validated. However, it is highly recommended to use tools that have been validated by scientific studies. The measurement of isometric strength has a poor specificity for the evaluation of dynamic strength. In some cases, the clinician cannot be satisfied with an isometric evaluation and must access the dynamic strength (i.e., eccentric and concentric torque). Isometric strength of ten muscle groups has been evaluated, bilaterally (dominant and nondominant), in men and women aged between 50 and 79 years old. Based on these studies, reference values of muscle strength ranged from 66.7 ± 16.0 to 458.4 ± 79.7 N [41, 42]. Buckinx et al. provided also normative values for isometric strength of eight different muscle groups among nursing home residents [43]. Thus, threshold values of relative isometric strength in this specific population were 0.94 N/kg for knee flexors, 1.07 N/kg for knee extensors, 0.77 N/kg for ankle flexors, 0.88 N/kg for ankle extensors, 0.78 N/kg for hip abductor, 0.79 N/kg for hip extensors, 0.99 N/kg for elbow flexors, and 0.71 N/kg for elbow extensors [43].

In clinical practice or in research setting, different validated tests are also used to assess lower limb muscle strength. The most common are:

– **The chair test**: *The 30-s Chair stand test (30s-CST)* was developed by Rikli and Jones [44], and is one of the most commonly used clinical test to assess lower limb muscle function (strength and power) [45]. This test allows to assess functional fitness level [46] and also to monitor training [47, 48] and rehabilitation [49]. This test consists on sit up and get up from a chair as quickly as possible without using arms (i.e., arms crossed over chest), during 30 s and the number of repetitions is recorded. Based on this test, subjects can be classified as having either low physical performance (30s-CST ≤8 rep) or high physical performance (30s-CST >8 rep) [50]. The minimal detectable change is 1.6 repetitions in patient with osteoarthritis [51] and 3 repetitions in Parkinson's patients [52]. Nevertheless, no responsiveness data are available in the general population.

10 sit-to-stand repetition: This test which consists of sit up and get up 10 times from a chair as quickly as possible without using arms (i.e., arms crossed over chest) estimate lower limb functional capacity. This simple clinical measure can also be useful to estimate lower limb muscle power index using the validated Takai equation [53]. To be able to determine the muscle power index, the clinician needs, in addition to the time needed to complete the 10 sit-to-stand repetition (Tsit-stand), to measure the leg length (L; from the head of the femur to the lateral malleolus) using a soft tape measure. The validated Takai equation is: $(L - 0.4^*) \times$ body mass (kg) $\times$ g (9.8 m/s^2) $\times$ 10)/Tsit-stand (*0.4 represents the height of the chair) [53]. Finally, a change of 9–10% is considered clinically significant [54]. This measure was chosen because the strength of the lower limbs is associated with disabilities and functional limitations [55].

5 sit-to-stand repetition: Another alternative of this test consists of recording the amount of time to complete 5 sit-to-stand position [56, 57]. Bohannon demonstrated that individuals can be considered to have worse than average performance when realizing a 5-repetition chair test and having a time exceeding: 11.4 s (60–69 years), 12.6 s (70–79 years), and 14.8 s (80–89 years) [58]. In addition, the cut-off point for the risk of having sarcopenia is 13 s [59]. The Minimal Detectable Change (MDC) time for the test is within 3.6–4.2 s [60] while the Minimal Clinically Important Difference (MCID) is 2.3 s [61].

The advantage of this test is that it is very predicable, but its disadvantage is that it is limited for subjects suffering from moderate to severe mobility limitations. This test has also a restricted capacity to assess a wide variation in ability, which is relevant in older people, since some older adults cannot complete the five attempts and are therefore not assigned a score (i.e., floor effect) [62]. Because of this limitation, the literature recommends the use of the 30-s chair stand test. In addition, this last one is fast, easy to use, quick (i.e., 1–2 min), and therefore feasible in clinical practice. Moreover, only a chair with a straight back without arm rests and a stopwatch is required and highly qualified staff is not required [63]. The reliability of the test is good in healthy older adults [64]. Thus, the 5-chair STS test is a proxy indicator of lower limb muscle speed and power, while the 30-s STS test is a proxy indicator of lower limb endurance (muscular capacity). Both tests are therefore complementary.

- **Leg press/leg extension**: Leg press machine involves subject sitting at an angle that puts his feet against a platform and push away from him by straightening his legs. This test is generally used to quantify maximal muscle strength through the 1RM (1 Repetition Maximum Resistance), wherein the evaluation is carried out at the highest resistance for which the subject can complete the exercise only once. To find the 1RM, the exercise is repeated several times at increasing resistance until failure to complete a single repetition. The range of motion performed during the leg press exercises ranged from 120° to 0° knee flexion, with 0° being understood as a full knee extension [65], except for one study which interpreted 180° as the full knee extension [66].

The minimal detectable change indicates that changes of 0.4 kg can be detected by the leg press 1-RM, which means detectable changes of 1.1% [67]. Because resistance machines such as the leg press only allow movement in a fixed pattern, they are great for non-experimented people or after injuries. They are also useful to isolate a specific muscle. Leg press test presents a high reliability (ICC > 0.94) among community older adults [4]. However, the disadvantage is that these resistance machines do not require the activation or engagement of any of the important stabilizing muscles. More specifically, leg press is performed using closed-chain kinetic effort [68] while the knee extension involves large lower body muscle groups (i.e., the quadriceps, hamstring) [69]. Consequently, the leg press exercise is widely used for strengthening the lower limbs. Currently, a reference range of maximal muscle strength is not yet available.

– **Leg power rig**: This test is generally used to quantify maximal muscle power. In practice, participants were asked to push the pedal down as hard and fast as possible, accelerating a flywheel attached to an A-D converter [70]. Power is recorded for each push until a plateau/decrease was observed. Muscular power among community-dwelling older adults has been reported to range between 1.7 and 8.64 W/kg [71]. Another study showed that mean lower limb muscle power assessed by the Nottingham power rig was 184.9 ± 89.4 W, in older adults [45]. Regarding reliability, mean change remained trivial (1.0–2.5%), typical errors remained small (5.8–8.6%), and ICCs very high (0.94–0.96) [72]. The advantage of assessment has been demonstrated to be safe, sensitive, and reliable in older adults, even in at risk of fracture population (osteoporosis) [70]. The Nottingham power rig has been identified as the "gold standard" assessment of power among older adults. Some disadvantages must also be acknowledged. Measuring muscle power is compromised in clinical settings because it requires complex and sometimes expensive machines, and clinicians need to be trained.

7.2.3 Muscle Strength Indexes

Muscle mass index has long been used as a useful index to evaluate the risks of developing functional impairments in older adults. Nevertheless, the association between functional impairments and muscle strength indexes is even more importantly related [73, 74]. According to Barbat-Artigas et al., the risk of presenting disabilities is at least three times higher in individuals with low muscle strength indexes values compared with individuals with high indexes values [73]. Therefore, there is evidence that muscle strength indexes are useful to evaluate the risks of developing functional impairments [73, 75, 76]. Among these indexes, the lower body muscle strength relative to body weight index seems to be the most relevant [73]. Indeed, the predominant role of lower extremities in performing ADL has previously been emphasized [77]. The advantage of this index is the combination of two measures (i.e., knee extensors muscle strength and body weight) which are easily measurable in the clinical setting.

Moreover, handgrip strength [78, 79] and mostly divided by body weight [80] is considered as a strong clinical predictor of disability and mortality. More importantly, body composition alone (e.g., muscle mass) is of little importance for performing the tasks of daily living (e.g., walking, rising from a chair, or climbing stairs), as long as enough strength is generated to move the entire body [81]. Muscle quality (MQ), defined as the ratio of strength and muscle mass, has been also proposed as a potential clinical index of functional impairments [32, 82]. The limitation of this index is that it neglects body composition, whereas the latter may play a key role in functional performance. In addition, there is no universal consensus definition or assessment method for muscle quality [83]. This is also a complex measure since multiple factors have the potential to influence muscle quality including muscle composition (e.g., architecture, fiber type), metabolism, fat infiltration, fibrosis, and neural activation [83]. Upper body MQ is estimated by dividing the maximum handgrip strength by upper body appendicular lean mass (ALM), with clinical cut-points determined as <5.76 kg/kg for men and <5.47 kg/kg for women [84]. Lower body MQ is defined as the ratio of leg extension strength to leg lean mass, and cut-points of ≤2.11 kg/kg for men and ≤1.56 kg/kg for women have been determined as clinically significant [85, 86].

Muscle strength data are summarized in Table 7.1.

7.3   Physical Performance

Physical performance can be defined as an objective measure of whole body function related with mobility [62]. It is well recognized that poor nutritional status [87], sarcopenia [88], frailty [89], sarcopenic-obesity [90], disability [91], mortality [92], and dementia [93] are health consequences of poor physical performance. Therefore, it is important to assess physical performance among older adults. Based on an international survey, 71.4% of the clinicians measured physical performance in daily practice [2]. More specifically, the most commonly administrated tests were: walking capacity (63.3%), timed up and go test (58.6%) and self-reported physical function (58.1%) [2]. Many tests are described in the literature to measure physical performance of older adults. The advantages and disadvantages of these tests are discussed below and summarized in Table 7.2.

7.3.1   Walking Capacity

Two main types of walking capacity tests exist:

7.3.1.1 The Short-Distance Walking Tests (4-m Distance, 6-m Distance, and 10-m Distance)

These tests measure the overall functional status in older adults [94] and can be used as surrogates for long-distance walking tests. They are also predictive for future care dependence [95], for other adverse health events such as severe mobility

Table 7.1 Muscle strength summary

Test/tool	Illustration	Protocol	Pros and cons	Normative data/cut-off point	Validity data
Upper limb muscle strength					
Hand grip strength		– Tested individual needs to sit in a standard chair with his forearms resting on the armchairs – Clinicians or investigators should demonstrate the use of the dynamometer and show how to grip very tightly the hand dynamometer – Six handgrip measures should be taken, three with each arm – Ideally, encouragements should be given to the patient to invite him to squeeze as hard and as tightly as possible during 3–5 s for each of the six trials and same encouragements between each patient to do not induce bias – Usually, the highest reading of the six measurements is reported as the final result [24]	*Pros* [18–20]: Easy to perform Affordable Noninvasive Not requiring a highly trained staff Highly reliable Very accessible *Cons* [22]: Only isometric measurement is possible Handgrip strength measurement may not overall strength of the body	Men: <27 kg women: <16 kg [6]	*Meaningful change:* 5.0–6.5 kg [28]

Lower limb muscle strength

| Isokinetic strength | | – Unidirectional analytical motion
– Performed at a constant angular velocity imposed by the experimenter [34] | *Pros:*
The closest technique to capture a real and physiological muscle contraction
Useful is clinical practice or to characterize muscle performance
Cons:
Expensive
Not handheld | The cut-off values are very variable depending on the population and conditions. | NA |

(continued)

Table 7.1 (continued)

Test/tool	Illustration	Protocol	Pros and cons	Normative data/cut-off point	Validity data
Isometric strength		– It measures the isometric maximum voluntary strength during contractions performed at constant angular position against resistance – The result is specific to the fixed angular position and reflects the ability of the muscle group to generate a force during isometric contraction (i.e., without variation in overall muscle length)	*Pros:* Convenient Useful in clinical practice (especially outside medical centers) *Cons:* Possible reproducibility and reliability limitations due to, for example, measurement position (joint angle), measurement site, type of measurement, type of muscle contraction, or movement speed The measurement depends on the skill of the evaluators	*General population:* Reference values of 10 muscle strength ranged from 66.7 ± 16.0 to 458.4 ± 79.7 N [41, 42] *Nursing homes setting:* 0.94 N/kg for knee flexors, 1.07 N/kg for knee extensors, 0.77 N/kg for ankle flexors, 0.88 N/kg for ankle extensors, 0.78 N/kg for hip abductor, 0.79 N/kg for hip extensors, 0.99 N/kg for elbow flexors, and 0.71 N/kg for elbow extensors [43]. For ankle extensors, 0.78 N/kg for hip abductor, 0.79 N/kg for hip extensors, 0.99 N/kg for elbow flexors, and 0.71 N/kg for elbow extensors [43]	*Reproducibility:* Varies from "moderate" to "good," according to the portable dynamometers used [40]

| Chair test | The 30-s chair stand test (30s-CST): Consists on sit up and get up from a chair as quickly as possible without using arms (i.e., arms crossed over chest), during 30 s and the number of repetitions is recorded

10 sit-to-stand repetition: Consists on sit up and get up ten times from a chair as quickly as possible without using arms (i.e., arms crossed over chest) estimate lower limb functional capacity. This simple clinical measure can be also useful to estimate lower limb muscle power index using the validated Takai equation [53]. To be able to determine the muscle power index, the clinician needs, in addition to the time needed to complete the 10 sit-to-stand repetition (Tsit-stand), to measure the leg length (L; from the head of the femur to the lateral malleolus) using a soft tape measure. The validated Takai equation is:
$(L - 0.4^*) \times$ body mass (kg) $\times$ g $(9.8 \text{ m/s}^2) \times 10)/$Tsit-stand $(*0.4$ represents the height of the chair) [53]

5 sit-to-stand repetition: Consists of recording the amount of time to complete 5 sit-to-stand position [56, 57] | Pros:
– Very predicable
– Easy to use, quick (i.e., 1–2 min) and therefore feasible in clinical practice
– Few materials are required: Only a chair with a straight back without arm rests and a stopwatch
– Highly qualified staff is not required

Cons:
– Limited for subjects suffering from moderate to severe mobility limitations
– Floor effects | The 30-s chair stand test (30s-CST): Subjects can be classified as having either low physical performance (30s-CST ≤8 rep) or high physical performance (30s-CST >8 rep) [50]

5 sit-to-stand repetition: Individuals can be considered to have worse than average performance when realizing a 5-repetitions chair test and having a time exceeding: 11.4 s (60–69 years), 12.6 s (70–79 years), and 14.8 s (80–89 years) [58]
The cut-off point for the risk of having sarcopenia is 13 s [59] | The 30-s chair stand test (30s-CST): Minimal detectable change: 1.6 repetitions in patient with osteoarthritis [51], 3 repetitions in Parkinson's patients [52]
10 sit-to-stand repetition: Meaningful change: 9–10% is considered clinically significant [54]
5 sit-to-stand repetition: Minimal detectable change: 3.6–4.2 s [60]
Minimal clinically important difference: 2.3 s [61]
Reliability: Is good in healthy older adults [64] |

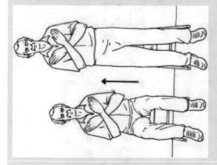

(continued)

Table 7.1 (continued)

Test/tool	Illustration	Protocol	Pros and cons	Normative data/cut-off point	Validity data
Leg press		Leg press machine involves subject sitting at an angle that puts his feet against a platform and push away from him by straightening his legs. This test is generally used to quantify maximal muscle strength through the 1RM (1 repetition maximum resistance), wherein the evaluation is carried out at the highest resistance for which the subject can complete the exercise only once. To find the 1RM, the exercise is repeated several times at increasing resistance until failure to complete a single repetition. The range of motion performed during the leg press exercises ranged from 120° to 0° knee flexion, with 0° being understood as a full knee extension [65], except for one study which interpreted 180° as the full knee extension [66]	*Pros:* – Great for non-experimented people or after injuries – Useful to isolate a specific muscle *Cons:* – Do not require the activation or engagement of any of the important stabilizing muscles (leg press is performed using closed-chain kinetic effort [68] while the knee extension involves large lower-body muscle groups (i.e., the quadriceps, hamstring) [69]) consequently, the leg press exercise is widely used for strengthening the lower limbs	NA	*Minimal detectable change:* A change of 0.4 kg can be detected by the leg press 1-RM, which means detectable changes of 1.1% [67] *Reliability:* High reliability (ICC > 0.94) among community older adults [4]

Leg power rig	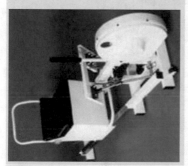 Participants are asked to push the pedal down as hard and fast as possible, accelerating a flywheel attached to an A-D converter [70]. Power is recorded for each push until a plateau/decrease was observed	*Pros:* – Safe – Sensitive and reliable in older adults – "Gold standard" to assess power among older adults *Cons:* – Complex machine – Expensive – Clinicians need to be trained	Muscular power among community-dwelling older adults has been reported ranged between 1.7 and 8.64 W/kg [71] Another study showed that mean lower limb muscle power assessed by the Nottingham power rig was 184.9 ± 89.4 W, in older adults [45]	*Reliability* [72]: *mean change:* (1.0–2.5%) *Typical errors:* (5.8–8.6%) ICCs: (0.94–0.96)

Table 7.2 Physical performance summary

Test/tool	Illustration	Protocol	Pros and cons	Normative data/cut-off point	Validity data
Walking capacity					
Short-distance walking tests		The time needed to cover the entire distance (4 m, 6 m, 10 m) is recorded – Use a static start with timing commencing when the foot touches the floor the first time after the line – Usual or comfortable pace to be used as the standard, with fast pace used as appropriate for specific research questions – Walking protocol to be reported in detail including pace instructions, verbal or other encouragement, and specific timing procedures [100]	*Pros:* – Few time and space are required (easily applicable in routine practice) – No specific material is necessary – No highly qualified human resource is required	*4-m:* Cut-off < 0.8 m/s identifies subjects with poor physical performance [97] *6-m and 10-m:* Cut-off < 1 m/s identifies older adults at high risk of health-related negative events [99]	*Meaningful changes* [98]: – Small change: 0.05 m/s – Substantial change: 0.1 m/s *Reliability* [101]: The 4-m walk distance test has an excellent reliability (ICC = 0.94)

			Pros/Cons	Normative data	Meaningful changes
Long-distance walking tests		*6-min walking test:* Participants are asked to walk as much and fast as possible, without running, during 6 min. In each minute of the test, volunteers received the same standardized encouragement according to the ATS/American College of Chest Physicians recommendations for the 6-min walking test [31]	*Pros:* – Simple – Noninvasive – Low cost *Cons:* – A corridor of at least 20 m is required – At least 15 min for execution	*Normative data:* *6-min walking test* [102]: 400–700 m for healthy adults *400-m walking time* [108]: Sex-specific quartiles: Q1: ≤4.29 min or ≤5.06 min Q2: 4.30– 5.02 min or 5.07–5.44 min Q3: 5.03– 5.44 min or 5.45–6.43 min Q4 ≥ 5.45 min or ≥6.44 min for men and women, respectively	*Meaningful changes:* *6-min walking test* [104]: An improvement of 54 m has been shown to be a clinically important difference *400-m walking time* [109]: – Minimally significant change estimates were 20–30 s – Substantial changes were 50–60 s *Reproducibility* [110]: The walk test had excellent reproducibility
		400-m walking test: Participants received instructions to walk 400 m in a hallway on a 20 m per segment course for 10 laps (40 m per lap) after a 2-min warm-up with standard encouragement given at each lap instructions were to "walk as quickly as you can, without running, at a pace you can maintain" [107]			

(continued)

Table 7.2 (continued)

Test/tool	Illustration	Protocol	Pros and cons	Normative data/cut-off point	Validity data
Lower limb muscle function					
Chair test	*Test described in Table 7.1*				
Alternate step test		Subjects are facing toward a 20-cm height step and instructed to touch the top of it with the right and left foot, alternately, as fast as possible during a 15-s period [116, 117]. At this end, the clinician recorded the number of step counts executed	*Pros:* – Quick (less than 5 min) – Easy to perform – Inexpensive – Few material is required (only access to a step and a stopwatch)	*Normative values:* For step test in age groups between 20 and 79 have been published by isles et al. in 2004 [118]	*Reliability* [116]: Excellent inter- and intra- reliability was observed for the alternate-step test (ICC >0.9)

The unipedal balance test	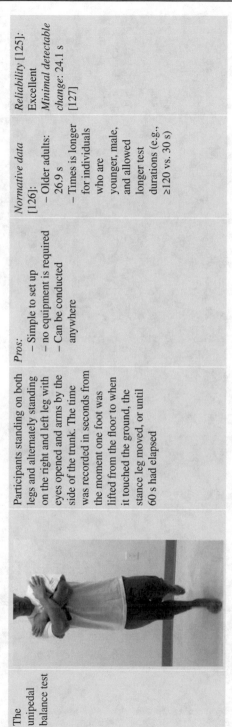	Participants standing on both legs and alternately standing on the right and left leg with eyes opened and arms by the side of the trunk. The time was recorded in seconds from the moment one foot was lifted from the floor to when it touched the ground, the stance leg moved, or until 60 s had elapsed	*Pros:* – Simple to set up – no equipment is required – Can be conducted anywhere	*Normative data* [126]: – Older adults: 26.9 s – Times is longer for individuals who are younger, male, and allowed longer test durations (e.g., ≥120 vs. 30 s)	*Reliability* [125]: Excellent *Minimal detectable change:* 24.1 s [127]

(continued)

Table 7.2 (continued)

Test/tool	Illustration	Protocol	Pros and cons	Normative data/cut-off point	Validity data
The bipedal balance test		It is a part of the SPPB test Subject is asked to hold three increasingly challenging standing positions for 10 s each: (1) a side-by-side position; (2) semi-tandem position (the heel of one foot beside the big toe of the other foot); and (3) tandem position (the heel of one foot in front of and touching the toes of the other foot)	See data of the SPPB test (Table 7.3)		
The Berg Balance Scale		Evaluates functional balance (i.e., static and dynamic) during everyday situations	Pros: – Few equipment are required: Ruler, two standard chairs (one with arm rests, one without), footstool or step, stopwatch or wristwatch, and 15 ft. walkway Cons: – Potential ceiling effects are observed with higher level patients – The scale does not include gait items – The test can take 15–20 min to complete, depending on the level of function and can be demanding to frail population	The maximum score is 56 points A score between 0 and 20 represents balance deficit while a score between 21 and 40 and between 41 and 56 is considered as acceptable balance and good balance, respectively [117]	Meaningful change: A change on the Berg Balance Scale of 4 points is needed if a patient scores within 45–56 initially, 5 points if the score range within 35–44, 6 points if initial score range within 25–34 and, 7 points if the initial score is within 0–24 [131] Reliability: This test is highly reliable between observers and intra-observer

The force platform	It is a plate under which are distributed four dynamometers to measure the three components of force and torque (anterior-posterior, medial-lateral, and vertical) exerted by the body over the platform. The derivation of these forces is shown as a point representing the center of pressure, and the variation of these values through time is the movement of the center of mass and the effect of forces used to maintain balance. The signals are amplified and transmitted to a computer that manages the acquisition of data and can thus be used as an indicator for risk of falls [132]	*Pros:* – Not invasive for patients [134] – Objective measure and no ceiling effects are observed [134] *Cons:* – The equipment is expensive and cumbersome – Training of the staff is required – The results can be affected by emotional status or external factors – It is not so easy and fast to administer [134]	NA	*Reliability:* Moderate to very high in the elderly population [133] *Sensitivity to change:* The tool is also sensitive to change [134]

(continued)

Table 7.2 (continued)

Test/tool	Illustration	Protocol	Pros and cons	Normative data/cut-off point	Validity data
The balance error scoring system (BESS)		The participant is asked to hold different static postures while an evaluator assesses deviations from this desired posture [135]. More specifically, the BESS consists of subjects holding specific stances for 20-s durations with their hands on their hips and eyes closed. The test stances (double leg, single leg, and tandem) are carried out on two surfaces (flat ground and a foam pad). Scoring for the BESS consists of the researcher counting the number of participant errors within each stance [136]	*Pros:* – Portable – Less expensive that force platform – Rapid – Relatively easy to administer *Cons:* – A learning effect is often observed [136]	Iverson et al. have provided normative data for community-dwelling healthy subjects between the ages of 20 and 69 [137]	*Reliability* [138]: A strong test–retest reliability has been identified (ICC = 0.784) *Minimal detectable change* [138]: 6–10 error points

limitation or mortality [96]. Because they require less time and space, these tests are more easily applicable than long-distance walking tests in routine practice. Another advantage is that no specific material is necessary to perform these tests. Moreover, no highly qualified human resource is required. The 4-m walk distance is the most commonly used short-walking test validated in older adults [50, 51]. In practice, the time needed to cover the entire distance is recorded [52], and the cut-off <0.8 m/s identifies subjects with poor physical performance [97]. The 4-m walk speed is responsive since a small change of 0.05 m/s or a substantial change of 0.1 m/s is considered as a clinically meaningful change [98]. For the 6-m and 10-m distances, the cut-off of <1 m/s was chosen to identify older adults at high risk of health-related negative events [99]. A standardized protocol has been defined to assess the 4-m distance walking speed in clinical and in research setting: (1) use a static start with timing commencing when the foot touches the floor the first time after the line; (2) usual or comfortable pace to be used as the standard, with fast pace used as appropriate for specific research questions; (3) walking protocol to be reported in detail including pace instructions, verbal or other encouragement, and specific timing procedures [100]. The 4-m walk distance test has also an excellent reliability (ICC = 0.94) [101].

7.3.1.2 The Long-Distance Walking Tests (400-m Walk Test and 6-min Walk Test)

These tests have the potential to discriminate different categories of risk among older individuals in healthy conditions. In addition to evaluate mobility, these tests also estimate endurance of the subjects [62]. These tests are simple, noninvasive, and low cost. However, the inconvenience is that long-distance walking tests require a corridor of at least 20 m and at least 15 min for execution.

The most common long-distance walking test to assess mobility and aerobic capacity is the 6-min walking test. In practice, participants are asked to walk as much and fast as possible, without running, during 6 min. In each minute of the test, volunteers received the same standardized encouragement according to the ATS/American College of Chest Physicians recommendations for the 6-min walking test [31]. A lower score (reflecting less distance covered in 6 min) indicates worse function. The 6-min walk distance in healthy adults has been reported to range from 400 to 700 m [102]. Moreover, age- and sex-specific reference standards are available and may be helpful for interpreting 6MWT scores for both healthy adults and those with chronic diseases [103]. An improvement of 54 m has been shown to be a clinically important difference [104]. The distance, in meters, is recorded and is also used to estimate aerobic capacity (i.e., VO_2max) according to the following equation: VO_2max (mL·kg^{-1}·min^{-1}): 70.161 + (0.023 × distance [m]) − (0.276 × body weight [kg]) − (6.79 × sex [Men = 0, Women = 1]) − (0.193 × HR [pulse/min]) − (0.191 × age [years]) [38]. The 6-min walk had good test–retest reliability (i.e., ICC between 0.88 and 0.94) in older adults [105]. Test–retest reliability has been reported as high, with an ICC of 0.90 [106].

The time and ability to complete a 400-m walk has been shown to predict adverse events such as mortality, mobility limitation, and disability [107]. In practice, participants received instructions to walk 400-m in a hallway on a 20-m per segment course for 10 laps (40-m per lap) after a 2-min warm-up with standard encouragement given at each lap. Instructions were to "walk as quickly as you can, without running, at a pace you can maintain" [107]. Sex-specific quartiles of 400-m walking time were: Q1: ≤4.29 min or ≤5.06 min; Q2: 4.30–5.02 min or 5.07–5.44 min; Q3: 5.03–5.44 min or 5.45–6.43 min; Q4: ≥5.45 min or ≥6.44 min for men and women, respectively [108]. For this test, minimally significant change estimates were 20–30 s while substantial changes were 50–60 s [109]. Finally, the walk test had excellent reproducibility [110].

During long-distance walk tests, the GAITrite© system can be used. It is a clinical tool for the objective assessment of gait parameters. The walk-way system is embedded with pressure sensors that detect series of foot cycles and allows to estimate temporal and spatial gait parameters through the Gaitrite© software [111]. This objective gait parameter tool has also strong concurrent validity and test–retest reliability [112].

Another tool, the Gait up system, which is a triaxial accelerometer, can also be used to perform motion analysis with high precision outside laboratory. It is composed of two sensors and a software for computer. It has been validated against gold standards in numerous scientific studies on various populations. Dadashi et al. provides normative values for widely used gait parameters in more than 1400 able-bodied adults over the age of 65 [113]. Gait up system allows simple and accurate Gait and analysis in real-world context. The advantages are that it is validated, portable, and affordable.

7.3.2 Lower Limbs Muscle Function

Many tests are described in the literature to measure lower limbs muscle function in older adults. The most widely used in clinical and research settings are described below.

- Chair Test
  Besides measuring lower limbs muscle strength, the chair test, which has been described above, may be one of the most important functional measures of physical capacity [114]. In this sense, the 5-chair STS test is reported to be used by 53.9% of the clinicians in daily practice to assess physical performances [2]. Effectively, the ability to perform the sit-to-stand movement is important to maintaining physical independence. Getting up and sitting in a chair involves activation of lower limb muscles, this is why the sit-to-stand test represents a good alternative for measuring muscle capacity of lower limbs [57, 63].
- Alternate-Step Test
  Going up and down stairs is a commonly performed as activity in daily life and is useful as functional measure in various populations including older adults [115]. This test measures the ability of weight shifting in the forward and upward directions, as well as lower limb muscle power and balance. In practice, subjects

are facing toward a 20-cm height step and instructed to touch the top of it with the right and left foot, alternately, as fast as possible during a 15-s period [116, 117]. At this end, the clinician recorded the number of step counts executed. Normative values for step test in age groups between 20 and 79 have been published by Isles et al. in 2004 [118]. This test is quick (less than 5 min) and easy to perform. This is also an inexpensive test which requires only access to a step and a stopwatch. Excellent inter- and intra-reliability was observed for the alternate-step test (ICC > 0.9) [116]. Finally, the step test is used by 25.1% of the clinicians in daily practice to assess physical performances [2].

7.3.3 Balance

Poor balance is associated with an increased risk of falls among older adults. Effectively, adjusted relative risk estimates for an increased risk of any fall were 1.58 (95% confidence interval = 1.06, 2.35) for self-report of balance problems, 1.58 (95% CI = 1.03, 2.41) for one-leg stance, and 1.46 (95% CI = 1.02, 2.09) for limits of stability [119]. Nevertheless, balance impairment is common among older adults and estimates of its prevalence range between 20 and 50% [120]. More specifically, one-third of community-dwelling older adults over the age of 65 years fall each year; this proportion increases to 50% by the age of 80 years [121].

Postural balance can be estimated subjectively by questionnaires, assessed by clinical examinations but also objectively by means of force platforms. Physical performance tests are based on postural activities and movements which occur in the activities of everyday life and are summarized in this section.

- **The unipedal balance test** in the frontal plane is pertinent to capture the swing phase of bipodal gait [122]. In practice, participants standing on both legs and alternately standing on the right and left leg with eyes opened and arms by the side of the trunk. The time was recorded in seconds from the moment 1 ft. was lifted from the floor to when it touched the ground, the stance leg moved, or until 60 s had elapsed. This test correlated with frailty, peripheral neuropathy, and risk of injurious falls [123, 124]. The unipedal balance test is very popular due to its simplicity. Indeed, advantages of the test are that no equipment is required, it is simple to set up, and it can be conducted almost anywhere. In addition, The reliability of this test is excellent [125]. Normative data for older adults is 26.9 s. Time is longer for individuals who are younger, male, and allowed longer test durations (e.g., ≥120 vs. 30 s) [126]. In addition, minimal detectable change at the 95% confidence level is 24.1 s for this test. More importantly, change in unipedal balance performance should exceed 24.1 s to be considered real change [127]. More precisions have been provided in the paper of Springer et al. presenting normative data for unipedal balance test with closed and open eyes, for males and females [128].
- **The bipodal balance test** is a part of the global Short Physical Performance Battery (SPPB) test and it assesses static balance [92]. Subject is asked to hold

three increasingly challenging standing positions for 10 s each: (1) a side-by-side position; (2) semi-tandem position (the heel of 1 ft. beside the big toe of the other foot); and (3) tandem position (the heel of 1 ft. in front of and touching the toes of the other foot).

- **The berg balance scale** evaluates functional balance (i.e., static and dynamic) during everyday situations using scores to evaluate different populations [117], such as elderly [129], stroke patients [130], and people with severe intellectual and visual disabilities [130]. The maximum score is 56 points, a score between 0 and 20 represents balance deficit while a score between 21 and 40 and between 41 and 56 is considered as acceptable balance and good balance, respectively [117]. In addition, a change on the Berg Balance Scale of 4 points is needed if a patient scores within 45–56 initially, 5 points if the score range within 35–44, 6 points if initial score range within 25–34, and 7 points if the initial score is within 0–24 [131]. This test is highly reliable between observers and intra-observer. Few equipment are required: ruler, two standard chairs (one with arm rests, one without), footstool or step, stopwatch or wristwatch, and 15 ft. walkway. Nevertheless, potential ceiling effects are observed with higher level patients. Another cons is that the scale does not include gait items. Finally, the test can take 15–20 min to complete, depending on the level of function and can be demanding to frail population.

- **The force platform** is a plate under which are distributed four dynamometers to measure the three components of force and torque (anterior-posterior, medial-lateral, and vertical) exerted by the body over the platform. The derivation of these forces is shown as a point representing the center of pressure, and the variation of these values through time is the movement of the center of mass and the effect of forces used to maintain balance. The signals are amplified and transmitted to a computer that manages the acquisition of data and can thus be used as an indicator for risk of falls [132]. The reliability of the balance test using the force platform is moderate to very high in the elderly population [133]. Another pro of this technique is not invasive for patients [134]. In addition, it provides an objective measure and no ceiling effects are observed [134]. The tool is also sensitive to change [134]. Some limitations of force platform must be emphasized: the equipment is expensive and cumbersome, training of the staff is required, the results can be affected by emotional status or external factors, and it is not so easy and fast to administer [134].

- **The balance error scoring system (BESS):** Static balance is sometimes assessed using BESS, which is an easily administered, static balance assessment for sideline use. The participant is asked to hold different static postures while an evaluator assesses deviations from this desired posture [135]. More specifically, the BESS consists of subjects holding specific stances for 20-s durations with their hands on their hips and eyes closed. The test stances (double leg, single leg, and tandem) are carried out on two surfaces (flat ground and a foam pad). Scoring for the BESS consists of the researcher counting the number of participant errors within each stance [136]. The maximum total number of errors for any single condition is 10. Thus, lower BESS scores are associated with better postural control. Iverson et al. have provided normative data for community-dwelling healthy subjects between the ages of 20 and 69 [137]. The cons of the BESS is that the learning effect is often observed in studies involving the BESS [136]. However, it is more portable and less expensive than force platform, it is a rapid, relatively easy-to-administer. Then, a strong test-retest reliability has been identified (ICC = 0.784) with a MDC (minimal detectable change) of 6–10 error points [138].

7.4   Global Functional Capacity

The SPPB evaluates lower extremity functional performance using timed measures of balance test, walking speed, and chair stand test. Both the global score and its individual elements may be analyzed separately in different clinical or research settings. Effectively, the score of each of the three tests ranges from 0 to 4, where 4 indicates the best result and 0 the worst result. Therefore, a summary score ranging from 0 (worst performers) to 12 (best performers) is calculated. Cut-off point of ≤8 points has been showed to be associated with mobility-related disability and is used for the diagnosis of sarcopenia [95]. More precisely, a score ranged between 0 and 6 is associated with poor performance, a score ranged between 7 and 9 is associated with intermediary performance while a score above 9 indicates high performance [95]. The relative risks of mobility-related disability for those with scores of 4–6 ranged from 2.9 to 4.9, and the relative risk of disability for those with scores of 7–9 ranged from 1.5 to 2.1, with similar consistent results for ADL disability [95].

More specifically, for the balance test, the subject is asked to hold three increasingly challenging standing positions for 10 s each: (1) a side-by-side position; (2) semi-tandem position (the heel of 1 ft. beside the big toe of the other foot); and (3) tandem position (the heel of 1 ft. in front of and touching the toes of the other foot). For the walking speed test, the subject is asked to walk at his usual pace over a 4-m course. The use of walking aids (cane, walker, or other walking aid) is allowed if necessary, but no assistance by another person can be provided. The time (in seconds) needed to complete the entire distance is recorded. Finally, for the repeated chair stands test, a straight-backed chair is used. The subjects are placed with its back against a wall. The subject is asked to stand from a sitting position and to sit down without using their arms (arms folded across the chest), five consecutive times. The time to complete this task is recorded. These independent tests have been described more in details above.

The test is applicable in research and in clinics as well as in GPs offices but small training is required, which may limit its use. The time of administration is around 10 min, and few equipment are needed: a 4-m track, ground marks, a chronometer, and straight-backed chair. Moreover, the reproducibility and the reliability of the SPPB are excellent [139, 140]. The SPPB is also responsive to clinically meaningful changes [140]: 0.5 points indicate a small change (i.e., not at individual-level) and 1 point indicates a substantial change [98]. However, a disadvantage is that ceiling effects can be observed for high functioning and very fit older adults (who will score 12 points) while floor effects can be observed for very low functioning adults [62].

The **Tinetti test or performance oriented mobility assessment (POMA)** is an easily administered task-oriented test that measures an older adult's gait and balance abilities. This is the oldest clinical balance assessment tool and one of the widest used among older people [141]. It consists of two subtests: a balance test (9 items scored on 16 points) and a gait test (7 items scored on 12 points). A total score <19 points indicates severe risk, a score between 19 and 24 points indicates moderate risk, and a score of more than 24 points indicates low risk of falls [142]. On the basis of the MDC(95) values, a change in POMA scores at the individual level should be at least 5 points and that those at the group level should be at least 0.8 point to be considered reliable [143]. It simple and easy with a completion time of around 10 min. Few equipment are needed: hard armless chair, stopwatch or wristwatch, and 15 ft. walkway. In addition, the test presents a good inter-rater reliability and a good sensitivity (93% of fallers were identified) [144, 145]. The disadvantages of the Tinetti test are: a poor specificity (only 11% of non-fallers were identified), ceiling effect, and no identification of the type of balance problem [146, 147].

This section is summarized in Table 7.3.

Table 7.3 Global functional capacity summary

Test/tool	Illustration	Protocol	Pros and cons	Normative data/cut-off point	Validity data
SPPB test	Side by side Semi tandem Tandem Usual gait Speed 1m Sit to Stand	Evaluates lower extremity functional performance using timed measures of balance test, walking speed, and chair stand test More specifically, for the **balance test**, the subject is asked to hold three increasingly challenging standing positions for 10 s each: (1) a side-by-side position; (2) semi-tandem position (the heel of one foot beside the big toe of the other foot); and (3) tandem position (the heel of one foot in front of and touching the toes of the other foot) For the **walking speed test**, the subject is asked to walk at his usual pace over a 4-m course. The use of walking aids (cane, walker, or other walking aid) is allowed if necessary, but no assistance by another person can be provided. The time (in seconds) needed to complete the entire distance is recorded Finally, for the **repeated chair stands test**, a straight-backed chair is used. The subjects are placed with its back against a wall. The subject is asked to stand from a sitting position and to sit down without using their arms (arms folded across the chest), five consecutive times. The time to complete this task is recorded	*Pros:* – Applicable in research and in clinics – The time of administration is around 10 min and few equipment are needed: a 4-m track, ground marks, a chronometer, and straight-backed chair *Cons:* – Small training is required, which may limit its use – Ceiling effects can be observed for high functioning and very fit older adults (who will score 12 points) while floor effects can be observed for very low functioning adults [62]	A score range between 0 and 6 (/12) is associated with poor performance, a score ranged between 7 and 9 is associated with intermediary performance while a score above 9 indicates high performance [95]	*Reproducibility and reliability:* Are excellent [139, 140] *Meaningful change* [140]: 0.5 points indicate a small change (i.e., not at individual-level), 1 point indicates a substantial change [98]

(continued)

Table 7.3 (continued)

Test/tool	Illustration	Protocol	Pros and cons	Normative data/cut-off point	Validity data
Tinetti test or POMA	Feet Together, Semi Tandem, Full Tandem	It consists of two subtests: a balance test (9 items scored on 16 points) and a gait test (7 items scored on 12 points)	*Pros:* – Simple test – Completion time of around 10 min – Few equipment are needed: Hard armless chair, stopwatch or wristwatch, and 15 ft. walkway *Cons:* – Ceiling effect – No identification of the type of balance problem [146, 147]	A total score < 19 points indicates severe risk, a score between 19 and 24 points indicates moderate risk, and a score of more than 24 points indicates low risk of falls [142]	*Minimal detectable change:* A change, at the individual level, should be at least 5 points and that those at the group level should be at least 0.8 point to be considered reliable [143] The test presents a good inter-rater *reliability* and a good *sensitivity* (93% of fallers were identified) but a poor *specificity* (only 11% of non-fallers were identified) [144, 145]

7.5 Conclusion

Limited muscle strength and/or physical performance results in physical limitations which are important predictors of adverse health outcomes (e.g., care dependence, falls, fractures, hospitalization, and even death). Moreover, the diagnosis of sarcopenia requires the presence of both low muscle mass and low muscle function, which can be defined by low muscle strength or low physical performance. It is therefore essential to assess accurately muscle strength and physical performance in an aging population, and clinicians are encouraged to routinely assess these parameters. Indeed, measurements of muscle strength and function are facilitated by their noninvasiveness and their effective limited time for application. However, many tools are referenced in the literature to assess muscle strength and physical performance. Since some of these instruments are less validated than others, a greater awareness among practitioners of the importance of using a fully validated tool is essential. In fact, the choice of the methods used depends on several criteria, such as accessibility, cost, specificity, and performance of the tool.

References

1. Janssen I, Heymsfield SB, Ross R. Low relative skeletal muscle mass (sarcopenia) in older persons is associated with functional impairment and physical disability. J Am Geriatr Soc. 2002;50(5):889–96.
2. O Bruyère CB, Reginster J-Y, Buckinx F, Schoene D, Hirani V, Cooper C, Kanis JA, Rizzoli R, McCloskey E, Cederholm T, Cruz-Jentoft A, Freiberger E. Assessment of muscle mass, muscle strength and physical performance in clinical practice: an international survey. Eur Geriatric Med. 2016;7(3):243–6.
3. Beaudart C, et al. Health outcomes of sarcopenia: a systematic review and meta-analysis. PLoS One. 2017;12(1):e0169548.
4. Mijnarends DM, et al. Validity and reliability of tools to measure muscle mass, strength, and physical performance in community-dwelling older people: a systematic review. J Am Med Dir Assoc. 2013;14(3):170–8.
5. Peterson MD, Krishnan C. Growth charts for muscular strength capacity with quantile regression. Am J Prev Med. 2015;49(6):935–8.
6. Cruz-Jentoft AJ, et al. Sarcopenia: revised European consensus on definition and diagnosis. Age Ageing. 2019;48:16–31.
7. Schaap LA, et al. Associations of sarcopenia definitions, and their components, with the incidence of recurrent falling and fractures: the longitudinal aging study Amsterdam. J Gerontol A Biol Sci Med Sci. 2018;73(9):1199–204.
8. Ibrahim K, et al. A feasibility study of implementing grip strength measurement into routine hospital practice (GRImP): study protocol. Pilot Feasibility Stud. 2016;2:27.
9. Leong DP, et al. Prognostic value of grip strength: findings from the Prospective Urban Rural Epidemiology (PURE) study. Lancet. 2015;386(9990):266–73.
10. Schaap LA, Koster A, Visser M. Adiposity, muscle mass, and muscle strength in relation to functional decline in older persons. Epidemiol Rev. 2013;35:51–65.
11. Barbat-Artigas S, et al. Relationship between dynapenia and cardiorespiratory functions in healthy postmenopausal women: novel clinical criteria. Menopause. 2011;18(4):400–5.
12. Dulac MC, Carvalho LP, Aubertin-Leheudre M. Functional capacity depends on lower limb muscle strength rather than on abdominal obesity in active postmenopausal women. Menopause. 2018;25(2):176–81.

13. Morris MG, et al. Relationships between muscle fatigue characteristics and markers of endurance performance. J Sports Sci Med. 2008;7(4):431–6.
14. Wind AE, et al. Is grip strength a predictor for total muscle strength in healthy children, adolescents, and young adults? Eur J Pediatr. 2010;169(3):281–7.
15. Bohannon RW. Hand-grip dynamometry predicts future outcomes in aging adults. J Geriatr Phys Ther. 2008;31(1):3–10.
16. Norman K, et al. Hand grip strength: outcome predictor and marker of nutritional status. Clin Nutr. 2011;30(2):135–42.
17. Stevens PJ, et al. Is grip strength a good marker of physical performance among community-dwelling older people? J Nutr Health Aging. 2012;16(9):769–74.
18. Taekema DG, et al. Handgrip strength as a predictor of functional, psychological and social health. A prospective population-based study among the oldest old. Age Ageing. 2010;39(3):331–7.
19. Ploegmakers JJ, et al. Grip strength is strongly associated with height, weight and gender in childhood: a cross sectional study of 2241 children and adolescents providing reference values. J Physiother. 2013;59(4):255–61.
20. Hamilton GF, McDonald C, Chenier TC. Measurement of grip strength: validity and reliability of the sphygmomanometer and jamar grip dynamometer. J Orthop Sports Phys Ther. 1992;16(5):215–9.
21. Mathiowetz V. Comparison of Rolyan and Jamar dynamometers for measuring grip strength. Occup Ther Int. 2002;9(3):201–9.
22. Buckley C, Stokes M, Samuel D. Muscle strength, functional endurance, and health-related quality of life in active older female golfers. Aging Clin Exp Res. 2018;30(7):811–8.
23. Roberts HC, et al. A review of the measurement of grip strength in clinical and epidemiological studies: towards a standardised approach. Age Ageing. 2011;40(4):423–9.
24. Waak K, Zaremba S, Eikermann M. Muscle strength measurement in the intensive care unit: not everything that can be counted counts. J Crit Care. 2013;28(1):96–8.
25. Bean JF, et al. The relationship between leg power and physical performance in mobility-limited older people. J Am Geriatr Soc. 2002;50(3):461–7.
26. Studenski SA, et al. The FNIH sarcopenia project: rationale, study description, conference recommendations, and final estimates. J Gerontol A Biol Sci Med Sci. 2014;69(5):547–58.
27. Dodds RM, et al. Grip strength across the life course: normative data from twelve British studies. PLoS One. 2014;9(12):e113637.
28. Bohannon RW. Minimal clinically important difference for grip strength: a systematic review. J Phys Ther Sci. 2019;31(1):75–8.
29. Buckinx F, et al. Relationship between isometric strength of six lower limb muscle groups and motor skills among nursing home residents. J Frailty Aging. 2015;4(4):184–7.
30. Harris-Love MO, et al. The influence of upper and lower extremity strength on performance-based sarcopenia assessment tests. J Funct Morphol Kinesiol. 2018;3(4):53.
31. Barbat-Artigas S, et al. Muscle quantity is not synonymous with muscle quality. J Am Med Dir Assoc. 2013;14(11):852.e1–7.
32. Barbat-Artigas S, et al. How to assess functional status: a new muscle quality index. J Nutr Health Aging. 2012;16(1):67–77.
33. Mentiplay BF, et al. Assessment of lower limb muscle strength and power using hand-held and fixed dynamometry: a reliability and validity study. PLoS One. 2015;10(10):e0140822.
34. Croisier JL, Crielaard JM. Isokinetic exercise and sports injuries. Rev Med Liege. 2001;56(5):360–8.
35. Amaral GM, et al. Muscular performance characterization in athletes: a new perspective on isokinetic variables. Braz J Phys Ther. 2014;18(6):521–9.
36. Croisier JL, et al. Strength imbalances and prevention of hamstring injury in professional soccer players: a prospective study. Am J Sports Med. 2008;36(8):1469–75.
37. Almekinders LC, Oman J. Isokinetic muscle testing: is it clinically useful? J Am Acad Orthop Surg. 1994;2(4):221–5.

38. Buckinx F, et al. Reliability of muscle strength measures obtained with a hand-held dynamometer in an elderly population. Clin Physiol Funct Imaging. 2017;37(3):332–40.
39. Keating JL, Matyas TA. The influence of subject and test design on dynamometric measurements of extremity muscles. Phys Ther. 1996;76(8):866–89.
40. Stark T, et al. Hand-held dynamometry correlation with the gold standard isokinetic dynamometry: a systematic review. PM R. 2011;3(5):472–9.
41. Andrews AW, Thomas MW, Bohannon RW. Normative values for isometric muscle force measurements obtained with hand-held dynamometers. Phys Ther. 1996;76(3):248–59.
42. Bohannon RW. Reference values for extremity muscle strength obtained by hand-held dynamometry from adults aged 20 to 79 years. Arch Phys Med Rehabil. 1997;78(1):26–32.
43. Buckinx F, et al. Normative data for isometric strength of 8 different muscle groups and their usefulness as a predictor of loss of autonomy among physically active nursing home residents: the SENIOR cohort. J Musculoskelet Neuronal Interact. 2019;19(3):258–65.
44. Rikli RE, Jones CJ. Development and validation of criterion-referenced clinically relevant fitness standards for maintaining physical independence in later years. Gerontologist. 2013;53(2):255–67.
45. Alcazar J, et al. Relation between leg extension power and 30-s sit-to-stand muscle power in older adults: validation and translation to functional performance. Sci Rep. 2020;10(1):16337.
46. Okamoto N, et al. Increasing the number of steps walked each day improves physical fitness in Japanese community-dwelling adults. Int J Sports Med. 2010;31(4):277–82.
47. Sáez Sáez De Villarreal E, et al. Effect of plyometric training on chair-rise, jumping and sprinting performance in three age groups of women. J Sports Med Phys Fitness. 2010;50(2):166–73.
48. Mato L, et al. Centella asiatica improves physical performance and health-related quality of life in healthy elderly volunteer. Evid Based Complement Alternat Med. 2011;2011:579467.
49. Nyland J, et al. Self-reported chair-rise ability relates to stair-climbing readiness of total knee arthroplasty patients: a pilot study. J Rehabil Res Dev. 2007;44(5):751–9.
50. Bruun IH, et al. Validity and responsiveness to change of the 30-second chair-stand test in older adults admitted to an emergency department. J Geriatr Phys Ther. 2019;42(4):265–74.
51. Wright AA, et al. A comparison of 3 methodological approaches to defining major clinically important improvement of 4 performance measures in patients with hip osteoarthritis. J Orthop Sports Phys Ther. 2011;41(5):319–27.
52. Petersen C, et al. Reliability and minimal detectable change for sit-to-stand tests and the functional gait assessment for individuals with Parkinson disease. J Geriatr Phys Ther. 2017;40(4):223–6.
53. Takai Y, et al. Sit-to-stand test to evaluate knee extensor muscle size and strength in the elderly: a novel approach. J Physiol Anthropol. 2009;28(3):123–8.
54. Kirn DR, et al. What is a clinically meaningful improvement in leg-extensor power for mobility-limited older adults? J Gerontol A Biol Sci Med Sci. 2016;71(5):632–6.
55. Puthoff ML, Nielsen DH. Relationships among impairments in lower-extremity strength and power, functional limitations, and disability in older adults. Phys Ther. 2007;87(10):1334–47.
56. Goldberg A, et al. The five-times-sit-to-stand test: validity, reliability and detectable change in older females. Aging Clin Exp Res. 2012;24(4):339–44.
57. Bohannon RW, et al. Sit-to-stand test: performance and determinants across the age-span. Isokinet Exerc Sci. 2010;18(4):235–40.
58. Bohannon RW. Reference values for the five-repetition sit-to-stand test: a descriptive meta-analysis of data from elders. Percept Mot Skills. 2006;103(1):215–22.
59. Pinheiro PA, et al. "Chair Stand Test" as simple tool for sarcopenia screening in elderly women. J Nutr Health Aging. 2016;20(1):56–9.
60. Schaubert KL, Bohannon RW. Reliability and validity of three strength measures obtained from community-dwelling elderly persons. J Strength Cond Res. 2005;19(3):717–20.
61. Meretta BM, et al. The five times sit to stand test: responsiveness to change and concurrent validity in adults undergoing vestibular rehabilitation. J Vestib Res. 2006;16(4-5):233–43.

62. Beaudart C, et al. Assessment of muscle function and physical performance in daily clinical practice : a position paper endorsed by the European Society for Clinical and Economic Aspects of Osteoporosis, Osteoarthritis and Musculoskeletal Diseases (ESCEO). Calcif Tissue Int. 2019;105(1):1–14.
63. Zanini A, et al. The one repetition maximum test and the sit-to-stand test in the assessment of a specific pulmonary rehabilitation program on peripheral muscle strength in COPD patients. Int J Chron Obstruct Pulmon Dis. 2015;10:2423–30.
64. Jones CJ, Rikli RE, Beam WC. A 30-s chair-stand test as a measure of lower body strength in community-residing older adults. Res Q Exerc Sport. 1999;70(2):113–9.
65. Martín-Fuentes I, Oliva-Lozano JM, Muyor JM. Evaluation of the lower limb muscles' electromyographic activity during the leg press exercise and its variants: a systematic review. Int J Environ Res Public Health. 2020;17(13):4626.
66. Walker S, et al. Kinetic and electromyographic analysis of single repetition constant and variable resistance leg press actions. J Electromyogr Kinesiol. 2011;21(2):262–9.
67. Barbalho M, et al. High 1RM tests reproducibility and validity are not dependent on training experience, muscle group tested or strength level in older women. Sports (Basel). 2018;6(4):171.
68. Ivey FM, et al. Strength training for skeletal muscle endurance after stroke. J Stroke Cerebrovasc Dis. 2017;26(4):787–94.
69. Da Silva EM, et al. Analysis of muscle activation during different leg press exercises at submaximum effort levels. J Strength Cond Res. 2008;22(4):1059–65.
70. Skelton DA, Kennedy J, Rutherford OM. Explosive power and asymmetry in leg muscle function in frequent fallers and non-fallers aged over 65. Age Ageing. 2002;31(2): 119–25.
71. Gray M, Paulson S. Developing a measure of muscular power during a functional task for older adults. BMC Geriatr. 2014;14:145.
72. Hurst C, et al. Short- and long-term reliability of leg extensor power measurement in middle-aged and older adults. J Sports Sci. 2018;36(9):970–7.
73. Barbat-Artigas S, et al. Clinical relevance of different muscle strength indexes and functional impairment in women aged 75 years and older. J Gerontol A Biol Sci Med Sci. 2013;68(7):811–9.
74. Barbat-Artigas S, et al. Exploring the role of muscle mass, obesity, and age in the relationship between muscle quality and physical function. J Am Med Dir Assoc. 2014;15(4): 303.e13–20.
75. Ploutz-Snyder LL, et al. Functionally relevant thresholds of quadriceps femoris strength. J Gerontol A Biol Sci Med Sci. 2002;57(4):B144–52.
76. Manini TM, et al. Knee extension strength cutpoints for maintaining mobility. J Am Geriatr Soc. 2007;55(3):451–7.
77. Reid KF, et al. Lower extremity muscle mass predicts functional performance in mobility-limited elders. J Nutr Health Aging. 2008;12(7):493–8.
78. Al Snih S, et al. Handgrip strength and mortality in older Mexican Americans. J Am Geriatr Soc. 2002;50(7):1250–6.
79. Al Snih S, et al. Hand grip strength and incident ADL disability in elderly Mexican Americans over a seven-year period. Aging Clin Exp Res. 2004;16(6):481–6.
80. Dulac M, et al. Is handgrip strength normalized to body weight a useful tool to identify dynapenia and functional incapacity in post-menopausal women? Braz J Phys Ther. 2016;20(6):510–6.
81. Buckinx F, Aubertin-Leheudre M. Relevance to assess and preserve muscle strength in aging field. Prog Neuropsychopharmacol Biol Psychiatry. 2019;94:109663.
82. Clark BC, Manini TM. Sarcopenia =/= dynapenia. J Gerontol A Biol Sci Med Sci. 2008;63(8):829–34.
83. McGregor RA, Cameron-Smith D, Poppitt SD. It is not just muscle mass: a review of muscle quality, composition and metabolism during ageing as determinants of muscle function and mobility in later life. Longev Healthspan. 2014;3(1):9.

84. Cooper R, et al. Body mass index from age 15 years onwards and muscle mass, strength, and quality in early old age: findings from the MRC National Survey of Health and Development. J Gerontol A Biol Sci Med Sci. 2014;69(10):1253–9.
85. Hairi NN, et al. Loss of muscle strength, mass (sarcopenia), and quality (specific force) and its relationship with functional limitation and physical disability: the Concord Health and Ageing in Men Project. J Am Geriatr Soc. 2010;58(11):2055–62.
86. Lees MJ, et al. Muscle quality as a complementary prognostic tool in conjunction with sarcopenia assessment in younger and older individuals. Eur J Appl Physiol. 2019;119(5):1171–81.
87. Penninx BW, et al. Anemia is associated with disability and decreased physical performance and muscle strength in the elderly. J Am Geriatr Soc. 2004;52(5):719–24.
88. Janssen I. Influence of sarcopenia on the development of physical disability: the Cardiovascular Health Study. J Am Geriatr Soc. 2006;54(1):56–62.
89. Landi F, et al. Calf circumference, frailty and physical performance among older adults living in the community. Clin Nutr. 2014;33(3):539–44.
90. Rolland Y, et al. Difficulties with physical function associated with obesity, sarcopenia, and sarcopenic-obesity in community-dwelling elderly women: the EPIDOS (EPIDemiologie de l'OSteoporose) Study. Am J Clin Nutr. 2009;89(6):1895–900.
91. Guralnik JM, et al. Lower-extremity function in persons over the age of 70 years as a predictor of subsequent disability. N Engl J Med. 1995;332(9):556–61.
92. Guralnik JM, et al. A short physical performance battery assessing lower extremity function: association with self-reported disability and prediction of mortality and nursing home admission. J Gerontol. 1994;49(2):M85–94.
93. Wang L, et al. Performance-based physical function and future dementia in older people. Arch Intern Med. 2006;166(10):1115–20.
94. Rolland YM, et al. Reliability of the 400-m usual-pace walk test as an assessment of mobility limitation in older adults. J Am Geriatr Soc. 2004;52(6):972–6.
95. Guralnik JM, et al. Lower extremity function and subsequent disability: consistency across studies, predictive models, and value of gait speed alone compared with the short physical performance battery. J Gerontol A Biol Sci Med Sci. 2000;55(4):M221–31.
96. Abellan van Kan G, et al. Gait speed at usual pace as a predictor of adverse outcomes in community-dwelling older people an International Academy on Nutrition and Aging (IANA) Task Force. J Nutr Health Aging. 2009;13(10):881–9.
97. Lauretani F, et al. Age-associated changes in skeletal muscles and their effect on mobility: an operational diagnosis of sarcopenia. J Appl Physiol (1985). 2003;95(5):1851–60.
98. Perera S, et al. Meaningful change and responsiveness in common physical performance measures in older adults. J Am Geriatr Soc. 2006;54(5):743–9.
99. Cesari M, et al. Added value of physical performance measures in predicting adverse health-related events: results from the Health, Aging And Body Composition Study. J Am Geriatr Soc. 2009;57(2):251–9.
100. Graham JE, et al. Assessing walking speed in clinical research: a systematic review. J Eval Clin Pract. 2008;14(4):552–62.
101. Unver B, et al. Reliability of 4-meter and 10-meter walk tests after lower extremity surgery. Disabil Rehabil. 2017;39(25):2572–6.
102. Enright PL. The six-minute walk test. Respir Care. 2003;48(8):783–5.
103. Casanova C, et al. The 6-min walk distance in healthy subjects: reference standards from seven countries. Eur Respir J. 2011;37(1):150–6.
104. Redelmeier DA, et al. Interpreting small differences in functional status: the Six Minute Walk test in chronic lung disease patients. Am J Respir Crit Care Med. 1997;155(4):1278–82.
105. Jones RRJ. The reliability and validity of a 6-Minute Walk Test as a measure of physical endurance in older adults. J Aging Phys Act. 1998;6(4):363–75.
106. Demers C, et al. Reliability, validity, and responsiveness of the six-minute walk test in patients with heart failure. Am Heart J. 2001;142(4):698–703.
107. Newman AB, et al. Association of long-distance corridor walk performance with mortality, cardiovascular disease, mobility limitation, and disability. JAMA. 2006;295(17):2018–26.

108. Vestergaard S, et al. Characteristics of 400-meter walk test performance and subsequent mortality in older adults. Rejuvenation Res. 2009;12(3):177–84.
109. Kwon S, et al. What is a meaningful change in physical performance? Findings from a clinical trial in older adults (the LIFE-P study). J Nutr Health Aging. 2009;13(6):538–44.
110. Pettee Gabriel KK, et al. Test-retest reliability and validity of the 400-meter walk test in healthy, middle-aged women. J Phys Act Health. 2010;7(5):649–57.
111. Youdas JW, et al. Agreement between the GAITRite walkway system and a stopwatch-footfall count method for measurement of temporal and spatial gait parameters. Arch Phys Med Rehabil. 2006;87(12):1648–52.
112. Bilney B, Morris M, Webster K. Concurrent related validity of the GAITRite walkway system for quantification of the spatial and temporal parameters of gait. Gait Posture. 2003;17(1):68–74.
113. Dadashi F, et al. Gait and foot clearance parameters obtained using shoe-worn inertial sensors in a large-population sample of older adults. Sensors (Basel). 2013;14(1):443–57.
114. McCarthy EK, et al. Repeated chair stands as a measure of lower limb strength in sexagenarian women. J Gerontol A Biol Sci Med Sci. 2004;59(11):1207–12.
115. Bean JF, et al. Is stair climb power a clinically relevant measure of leg power impairments in at-risk older adults? Arch Phys Med Rehabil. 2007;88(5):604–9.
116. Chung MM, et al. Reliability and validity of Alternate Step Test times in subjects with chronic stroke. J Rehabil Med. 2014;46(10):969–74.
117. Berg KO, et al. Measuring balance in the elderly: validation of an instrument. Can J Public Health. 1992;83(Suppl 2):S7–11.
118. Isles RC, et al. Normal values of balance tests in women aged 20-80. J Am Geriatr Soc. 2004;52(8):1367–72.
119. Muir SW, et al. Balance impairment as a risk factor for falls in community-dwelling older adults who are high functioning: a prospective study. Phys Ther. 2010;90(3):338–47.
120. Rubenstein LZ, Josephson KR. The epidemiology of falls and syncope. Clin Geriatr Med. 2002;18(2):141–58.
121. Orces CH. Prevalence and determinants of falls among older adults in Ecuador: an analysis of the SABE I survey. Curr Gerontol Geriatr Res. 2013;2013:495468.
122. Nnodim JO, Yung RL. Balance and its clinical assessment in older adults - a review. J Geriatr Med Gerontol. 2015;1(1):003.
123. Drusini AG, et al. One-leg standing balance and functional status in an elderly community-dwelling population in northeast Italy. Aging Clin Exp Res. 2002;14(1):42–6.
124. Hurvitz EA, Richardson JK, Werner RA. Unipedal stance testing in the assessment of peripheral neuropathy. Arch Phys Med Rehabil. 2001;82(2):198–204.
125. Ponce-González JG, et al. A reliable unipedal stance test for the assessment of balance using a force platform. J Sports Med Phys Fitness. 2014;54(1):108–17.
126. Bohannon RW, Tudini F. Unipedal balance test for older adults: a systematic review and meta-analysis of studies providing normative data. Physiotherapy. 2018;104(4):376–82.
127. Goldberg A, Casby A, Wasielewski M. Minimum detectable change for single-leg-stance-time in older adults. Gait Posture. 2011;33(4):737–9.
128. Springer BA, et al. Normative values for the unipedal stance test with eyes open and closed. J Geriatr Phys Ther. 2007;30(1):8–15.
129. Steffen TM, Hacker TA, Mollinger L. Age- and gender-related test performance in community-dwelling elderly people: Six-Minute Walk Test, Berg Balance Scale, Timed Up & Go Test, and gait speeds. Phys Ther. 2002;82(2):128–37.
130. Blum L, Korner-Bitensky N. Usefulness of the Berg Balance Scale in stroke rehabilitation: a systematic review. Phys Ther. 2008;88(5):559–66.
131. Donoghue D, Stokes EK. How much change is true change? The minimum detectable change of the Berg Balance Scale in elderly people. J Rehabil Med. 2009;41(5):343–6.
132. Piirtola M, Era P. Force platform measurements as predictors of falls among older people - a review. Gerontology. 2006;52(1):1–16.

133. Moghadam M, et al. Reliability of center of pressure measures of postural stability in healthy older adults: effects of postural task difficulty and cognitive load. Gait Posture. 2011;33(4):651–5.
134. Prosperini L, Pozzilli C. The clinical relevance of force platform measures in multiple sclerosis: a review. Mult Scler Int. 2013;2013:756564.
135. Bell DR, et al. Systematic review of the balance error scoring system. Sports Health. 2011;3(3):287–95.
136. Campolettano ET, Gellner RA, Rowson S. Assessing static and dynamic postural control in a healthy population. Biomed Sci Instrum. 2018;54(1):24–31.
137. Iverson GL, Kaarto ML, Koehle MS. Normative data for the balance error scoring system: implications for brain injury evaluations. Brain Inj. 2008;22(2):147–52.
138. Amin D, Coleman J, Herrington L. The test-retest reliability and minimal detectable change of the balance error scoring system. J Sports Sci. 2014;2:200–7.
139. Freire AN, et al. Validity and reliability of the short physical performance battery in two diverse older adult populations in Quebec and Brazil. J Aging Health. 2012;24(5):863–78.
140. Ostir GV, et al. Reliability and sensitivity to change assessed for a summary measure of lower body function: results from the Women's Health and Aging Study. J Clin Epidemiol. 2002;55(9):916–21.
141. Perell KL, et al. Fall risk assessment measures: an analytic review. J Gerontol A Biol Sci Med Sci. 2001;56(12):M761–6.
142. Tinetti ME. Performance-oriented assessment of mobility problems in elderly patients. J Am Geriatr Soc. 1986;34(2):119–26.
143. Faber MJ, Bosscher RJ, van Wieringen PC. Clinimetric properties of the performance-oriented mobility assessment. Phys Ther. 2006;86(7):944–54.
144. Maki BE, Holliday PJ, Topper AK. A prospective study of postural balance and risk of falling in an ambulatory and independent elderly population. J Gerontol. 1994;49(2):M72–84.
145. Topper AK, Maki BE, Holliday PJ. Are activity-based assessments of balance and gait in the elderly predictive of risk of falling and/or type of fall? J Am Geriatr Soc. 1993;41(5):479–87.
146. Yelnik A, Bonan I. Clinical tools for assessing balance disorders. Neurophysiol Clin. 2008;38(6):439–45.
147. Mancini M, Horak FB. The relevance of clinical balance assessment tools to differentiate balance deficits. Eur J Phys Rehabil Med. 2010;46(2):239–48.

Is Sarcopenia a Condition, a Disorder, a Disease, or a True Geriatric Syndrome?

8

Jean-Pierre Michel, Fiona Ecarnot, and Christophe Graf

"After a long history of near neglect, unimaginative structure, and factious development, health terminologies are in an era of unprecedented importance, sophistication, and international collaboration/implications"
G CHUTE [1]

With the emergence of precision [2] and high-definition medicine [3], the interrogative title of this chapter seems obvious. However, it reflects the current state of the art regarding sarcopenia, as a recent literature review has proven [4]. Sarcopenia has been indifferently labeled as a "condition," [5–7] "disorder," [8] "disease," [9] "syndrome," [10, 11] or "geriatric syndrome" [12, 13] in the most recent international scientific papers.

The confusion surrounding sarcopenia is exacerbated by the appearance of combinations of physiopathological mechanisms, giving rise to terms such as "sarcopenic obesity" [14] and more recently "osteosarcopenia" [15, 16].

The explanation of the imprecision in nomenclature is undoubtedly linked to the short history of the concept of sarcopenia, which was first elaborated in the 1990s by Rosenberg, and defined as a loss of muscle mass and muscle function, related to important changes in body composition during illness or age [17]. Since

J.-P. Michel (✉)
University of Geneva, Geneva, Switzerland
e-mail: jean-pierre.michel@unige.ch

F. Ecarnot
Department of Cardiology, University Hospital Besancon, Besancon, France

EA3920, University of Burgundy Franche-Comté, Besancon, France

C. Graf
University of Geneva, Geneva, Switzerland

University Hospital of Geneva, University of Geneva, Geneva, Switzerland
e-mail: christophe.graf@hcuge.ch

© Springer Nature Switzerland AG 2021
N. Veronese et al. (eds.), *Sarcopenia*, Practical Issues in Geriatrics,
https://doi.org/10.1007/978-3-030-80038-3_8

then, numerous authors have discussed, completed, or radically changed its definition and scope, proposing other terms, such as "dynapenia" (loss of muscle power) [18] or "keratopenia" (loss of muscle force) [5]. Recently, discussions have mostly focused on improved understanding of the physiopathology, early recognition of risk factors, an integrative approach to clinical presentations, complications and preventive treatment, and the reversibility of the loss of skeletal muscle mass and function. However, the major issue in this ever-changing context is the search for the best clinical diagnostic criteria. After the first attempt by the European Working Group on Sarcopenia in Older Adults (EWGSOP) [19], numerous international initiatives have been set up to establish other criteria, more suited to their own populations, including (but not limited to): the International Working Group on Sarcopenia (IWGS) [20], the Foundation for the National Institutes of Health (FNIH) project [21], and the Asian Working Group on Sarcopenia (AWDS) [12]. This continuous evolution of the diagnostic criteria has modified the prevalence and incidence of sarcopenia. Indeed, in parallel to the search for the most appropriate set of diagnostic criteria, pharmacological and non-pharmacological interventions have been developed, but are beyond the scope of this chapter.

It is crucial to celebrate the most important achievement to come out of the international involvement of the scientific community, with the recognition of sarcopenia as a "disease" in 2016, and its inclusion in the ICD-10-CM (M62.84 code for sarcopenia) [9]. Yet, the official integration of sarcopenia into the ICD-10 as a "disease" only served to increase the uncertainty regarding the correct labeling of sarcopenia. To come full circle, therefore, we can see that the question raised by the title of this chapter is still relevant. To answer it, a short recap is warranted of the meaning of terms such as clinical condition, medical disorder, disease, syndrome, and geriatric syndrome, before deciding which term is the best fit for the concept of sarcopenia.

8.1   Is Sarcopenia a "Clinical Condition"?

The term "clinical condition" corresponds to any disease, illness, or injury as well as any physiologic, mental or psychological organ, or functional disturbances, which exceeds the normal range. Several criteria are used to describe medical conditions as "serious and complex." These could include the severity of the condition (life threatening or degree of impairment or disability), and the level of need in terms of comprehensive care management (frequent monitoring, interdisciplinary teamwork, implication of caregivers). The term "medical condition" is often used in official documents (medical boards, professional insurance, and government classifications).

Sarcopenia could be included in the very wide and imprecise definition "clinical condition," with neither specific meaning nor valuable information on its prevalence, physiopathology, diagnostic criteria, management, and functional outcomes.

8.2   Is Sarcopenia a "Disorder"?

The term *disorder* is often considered more value-neutral and less stigmatizing than the term *disease* and is therefore a preferred terminology in some circumstances, primarily to identify physical disorders that are not caused by infectious organisms, such as metabolic disorders. It is also used to describe a disruption to the normal or regular functions in the body (or part thereof) occurring as the result of a disease. A clinical disorder disturbs a person's thinking, feeling, and general daily functioning. For example, a disorder resulting from cardiovascular disease could be arrhythmia or breathlessness.

In mental health, the term mental disorder is used as a means of acknowledging the complex interaction of biological, social, and psychological factors at play in psychiatric conditions. A mental disorder affects thinking, feeling, mood, and behavior and may be occasional or long-lasting (chronic).

Can this equivocal definition of a disorder be applied to describe sarcopenia? Yes, indeed it could, because sarcopenia alters gait speed, increases mobility disorders, and remodels a person's ability to perform daily activities. However, labeling sarcopenia as a disorder is wide and imprecise, affirming that sarcopenia compounds inability in physical functioning, yet without acknowledging its epidemiology, complex risk factors, intricate physiopathological interactions, and outcomes.

8.3   Is Sarcopenia a Disease?

The word "disease" apparently first appeared in the fourteenth century as a derivative of the old French "desaise," meaning "lack of ease or convenience" ("des-" expressing reversal and "aise" meaning "ease"). In the sixteenth and seventeenth centuries, deaths started to be distinguished by medieval causes (scurvy, leprosy, and plague). Currently, disease is defined as a clinical entity that is medically diagnosed by a physician. Disease has an unequivocal etiology and pathogenesis, as well as a classical or attenuated clinical presentation, which may either be a single symptom or clinical sign, or a well-known combination of clinical signs. The disease construct may be developed on one or more types of bases:

- An anatomical base (e.g., aortic or mitral insufficiency).
- A physiological or metabolic base (e.g., hypercholesterolemia, diabetes, malabsorption, vasculitis).
- An etiological base (e.g., infectious diseases: HIV, influenza, pneumococcal pneumonia).
- Or a combination of one or more of these bases (myocardial infarction, stroke, prostate cancer).

Diseases do not generally have discrete boundaries, and clinical judgment is required to determine the thresholds for diagnoses. Being diagnosed with a disease only benefits the patient if the diagnosis assists in understanding current symptoms or the risk of future clinically important events, and/or if the patient can benefit from specific treatment.

The disease definition, for instance, is the only one that is universally recognized. Diseases are generally more frequent at a given stage of the life course; for example, genetic disease can become clinically apparent at any stage of the life course, even very late [22]. Measles is frequent in early life, while tuberculosis and varicella/ herpes zoster occur in early life, but also in old age.

Considering the different criteria of the current definition of a disease, it is logical to consider that sarcopenia could be labeled as a disease that predominates in the late stage of life. Indeed, it corresponds to a specific medical diagnosis with different grades of severity (from pre-sarcopenia to severe sarcopenia or sarcopenia with disability). However, the "disease" definition does not encompass the high prevalence, shared risk factors, multiple etiologies, and the absence of specific treatment. Moreover, sarcopenia cannot be considered as a standalone disease, independent of the aging process [23].

8.4   Is Sarcopenia a "Syndrome" or a "Geriatric Syndrome"?

Derived from the Greek "syn" (meaning together) and "drom-" (meaning to run) or "concurrence" (proposed by the Greek physician Galen), and translated into English in 1541, a syndrome is a set of symptoms and clinical signs that are not correlated and not fixed, and whose combination, more frequent than it would be by chance alone, constitutes a clinical entity.

Various types of syndromes can be distinguished, such as:

- Those with an evident pathogenesis (Cushing's syndrome).
- Those with evident etiology, but with unclear or as yet unknown pathogenesis (e.g., Marfan syndrome).
- A combination of symptoms grouped together, without current evidence of etiology or pathogenesis (e.g., chronic fatigue syndrome).

In the cases mentioned above, the cure of the evident etiology or pathogenesis makes it possible to cure the syndrome. After controlling the specific morbid process (for example, cortisol excess), the multiple phenotypes of the syndrome (e.g., moon facies, buffalo neck, truncal obesity, proximal muscle weakness, skin thinning and bruisability, as well as osteoporosis) tend to disappear or at least sharply decrease [24].

Prior to the publication of the landmark paper by Inouye [25], the term "geriatric syndrome" was commonly used to capture clinical conditions in older persons that do not fit into discrete disease categories, but was already recognized as being an "ill-defined concept" [24]. In their report on the clinical, research, and policy implications of "geriatric syndrome" as a core geriatric concept, Inouye et al. reviewed the risk factors for five frequent geriatric conditions (delirium, falls, functional decline, incontinence, and pressure ulcers). For each of these clinical conditions, the authors found the following common characteristics:

- High prevalence of the clinical issue.
- Shared risk factors (older age, impaired cognition, mobility disorders and inability in daily functioning).
- Multifactorial and cross-organ components.
- Association with another morbidity.
- Poor outcomes (disability, dependence, nursing home placement, and ultimately death).

This unifying concept made it possible to add further entities to the initial five, including anorexia of aging [26] and frailty [27], but also sarcopenia [19], sarcopenic obesity [14], osteosarcopenia [16], and locomotive syndrome [28].

The specific phenomenology of all these geriatric syndromes is caused by a variety of multimorbid processes, which complicate the treatment approach. For example, typical delirium can be linked to bladder retention, constipation, dehydration, fever, infections, drugs, and more. The reversal of the delirium will occur only after controlling its unique or combined causes. This illustrates the complexity of geriatric medicine and the need for a holistic approach in this population. Comprehensive geriatric assessment helps to detect these syndromes accurately and may positively influence prognosis in terms of such outcomes as hospitalization, institutionalization, and even mortality, although cost-effectiveness data remain sparse.

8.5   The Confirmation That Sarcopenia Must be Considered as a Geriatric Syndrome

Following the acclaimed 2007 definition of the geriatric syndrome [25], it is important to underline once again how the different facets of sarcopenia make it possible to integrate sarcopenia into this category.

8.5.1   High Prevalence of Sarcopenia

In a systematic review of the prevalence of sarcopenia in the world based on general population estimates and totalling over 58,000 individuals, overall prevalence was estimated at 10% (95% CI: 8–12%) in men and 10% (95% CI: 8–13%) in women, respectively [29]. In a recent paper, Martone et al. [30] applied the second version of the EWGSOP diagnostic criteria [8] to a community-dwelling population of 11,253 adults aged from 18 to 98 years (mean age: 55.6 years), including 56% women. The authors found 8.6% of patients to be sarcopenic. The prevalence of sarcopenia increases with age, sedentary lifestyle, unhealthy diet, diabetes, and impairment on the 400 m walk test [30].

Another interesting paper recently published by Van Ancum et al. [31] compared the prevalence of sarcopenia in 2256 participants, including community-dwelling older adults, geriatric outpatients, and patients admitted to acute and subacute inpatient wards, according to the 2010 and 2019 EWGSOP diagnostic criteria [8, 31, 32]. Prevalence changed in relation with the modified cut-offs for handgrip strength (30 to 27 kg in men and 20 to 16 kg in women). As expected, the prevalence of sarcopenic patients decreased sharply in males using the more recent criteria (EWGSOP-2) instead of the initial version (EWGSOP) (falling from 31.9 to 12%), whereas no significant difference was noticed in women (prevalence increased slightly from 4.9 to 6.1%) [31].

Regardless of whether the modifications to the diagnostic criteria for sarcopenia were justified or not, and regardless of the conflicting results that arise from the different definitions, it remains undisputed that sarcopenia is highly prevalent in the aged population.

8.5.2 Shared Risk Factors

Among the common features defined by Inouye et al., increasing age is one of the main risk factors for sarcopenia [30, 33], along with sedentary lifestyle and malnutrition [34, 35]. Mobility disorders and inability in the activities of daily living can be considered both as risks for and consequences of sarcopenia [36].

8.5.3 Multifactorial and Cross-Organ Components of Sarcopenia

The aging of the muscle leads to reduction in muscle size, with a reduction in the fibers expressing type II (fast) myosin heavy chain, a decline of the number and function of satellite cells (type II fibers), decrements in elasticity of the whole muscle as well as in single fibers, a decrease in muscle capillary density, and loss of the number and function of mitochondria. Moreover, fragmentation of the sarcoplasmic reticulum impairs calcium release and muscle activation [37, 38].

On top of these age-related changes to the muscle composition and function, hormonal modifications also partially explain the protein imbalance, which combines with increased oxidative stress and inflammaging to accelerate the sarcopenia process [39, 40].

8.5.4 Association with Another Morbidity

Apart from the classical association of sarcopenia and diabetes, it should be underlined that numerous links with the skeletal muscle have recently been brought to light. The "bone muscle unit," [41] "muscle brain cross talk," [42] and "gut muscle axis" [43] are opening new avenues of thought, research, and maybe even treatment for sarcopenia.

8.5.5   Poor Outcomes of Sarcopenia

A meta-analysis of 33 studies totalling 45,926 individuals concluded that sarcopenia was associated with a significantly higher risk of falls (with an OR of 1.89; 95%CI 1.33–2.68 in prospective studies, $p < 0.001$) and fractures (OR in prospective studies 1.71; 95% CI 1.44–2.03, $p = 0.011$), compared to non-sarcopenic individuals [44]. These data are in line with previous reports indicating that sarcopenia is associated with a 50% increase in hospital admission, a 20-day increase in the length of hospital stay, and a 34%–58% increase in hospital care costs, leading to a greater risk of dependency, loss of quality of life, and a 3.7-fold increase in mortality [45–48].

8.6   Conclusion

The history of sarcopenia has accelerated greatly since its first pathophysiological and clinical definition in the late 1990s. Sarcopenia has now become one of the most intensely investigated topics among the scientific community working in the field of aging. Its current denomination as a "clinical condition" or "disorder" in the scientific literature is imprecise and inconsistent. However, the intensity of multidomain research into aging muscle dysfunction, clinical consequences, and preventable outcomes led to the inclusion of sarcopenia in the International Classification of Disease in 2016 under the official label of "disease." Nevertheless, this term does not capture the full spectrum of the functional interactions of the skeletal muscle with the other parts of the body. As noted by Casati et al. [23], "sarcopenia cannot be considered as a standalone disease, independent of the ageing process." Rather, the characteristics sarcopenia fit better with Inouye's 2007 definition of "geriatric syndrome" [25].

Acknowledgments   The authors report no conflict of interest.

References

1. Chute CG. Clinical classification and terminology: some history and current observations. J Am Med Inform Assoc. 2000;7:298–303.
2. Precision Medicine Coalition. The personalized medicine report 2017: opportunity, challenges, and the future. 2017. http://www.personalizedmedicinecoalition.org/Userfiles/PMC-Corporate/file/The-Personalized-Medicine-Report1.pdf. Accessed 25 Jan 2021.
3. Torkamani A, Andersen KG, Steinhubl SR, Topol EJ. High-definition medicine. Cell. 2017;170:828–43.
4. Lenchik L, Boutin RD. Sarcopenia: beyond muscle atrophy and into the new frontiers of opportunistic imaging, precision medicine, and machine learning. Semin Musculoskelet Radiol. 2018;22:307–22.
5. Fuggle N, Shaw S, Dennison E, Cooper C. Sarcopenia. Best Pract Res Clin Rheumatol. 2017;31:218–42.
6. Polyzos SA, Margioris AN. Sarcopenic obesity. Hormones (Athens). 2018;17:321–31.

7. Papadopoulou SK. Sarcopenia: a contemporary health problem among older adult populations. Nutrients. 2020;12:1293.
8. Cruz-Jentoft AJ, Bahat G, Bauer J, Boirie Y, Bruyere O, Cederholm T, Cooper C, Landi F, Rolland Y, Sayer AA, Schneider SM, Sieber CC, Topinkova E, Vandewoude M, Visser M, Zamboni M, Writing Group for the European Working Group on sarcopenia in older P, the extended Group for E. Sarcopenia: revised European consensus on definition and diagnosis. Age Ageing. 2019;48:601.
9. Anker SD, Morley JE, von Haehling S. Welcome to the ICD-10 code for sarcopenia. J Cachexia Sarcopenia Muscle. 2016;7:512–4.
10. Bravo-Jose P, Moreno E, Espert M, Romeu M, Martinez P, Navarro C. Prevalence of sarcopenia and associated factors in institutionalised older adult patients. Clin Nutr ESPEN. 2018;27:113–9.
11. Koliaki C, Liatis S, Kokkinos A. Obesity and cardiovascular disease: revisiting an old relationship. Metabolism. 2019;92:98–107.
12. Chen LK, Liu LK, Woo J, Assantachai P, Auyeung TW, Bahyah KS, Chou MY, Chen LY, Hsu PS, Krairit O, Lee JS, Lee WJ, Lee Y, Liang CK, Limpawattana P, Lin CS, Peng LN, Satake S, Suzuki T, Won CW, Wu CH, Wu SN, Zhang T, Zeng P, Akishita M, Arai H. Sarcopenia in Asia: consensus report of the Asian working Group for Sarcopenia. J Am Med Dir Assoc. 2014;15:95–101.
13. Bayraktar E, Tasar PT, Binici DN, Karasahin O, Timur O, Sahin S. Relationship between sarcopenia and mortality in elderly inpatients. Eur J Med. 2020;52:29–33.
14. Batsis JA, Villareal DT. Sarcopenic obesity in older adults: aetiology, epidemiology and treatment strategies. Nat Rev Endocrinol. 2018;14:513–37.
15. Hirschfeld HP, Kinsella R, Duque G. Osteosarcopenia: where bone, muscle, and fat collide. Osteoporos Int. 2017;28:2781–90.
16. Hassan EB, Duque G. Osteosarcopenia: a new geriatric syndrome. Aust Fam Physician. 2017;46:849–53.
17. Rosenberg IH. Sarcopenia: origins and clinical relevance. J Nutr. 1997;127:990S–1S.
18. Clark BC, Manini TM. What is dynapenia? Nutrition. 2012;28:495–503.
19. Cruz-Jentoft AJ, Landi F, Topinkova E, Michel JP. Understanding sarcopenia as a geriatric syndrome. Curr Opin Clin Nutr Metab Care. 2010;13:1–7.
20. Fielding RA, Vellas B, Evans WJ, Bhasin S, Morley JE, Newman AB, Abellan van Kan G, Andrieu S, Bauer J, Breuille D, Cederholm T, Chandler J, De Meynard C, Donini L, Harris T, Kannt A, Keime Guibert F, Onder G, Papanicolaou D, Rolland Y, Rooks D, Sieber C, Souhami E, Verlaan S, Zamboni M. Sarcopenia: an undiagnosed condition in older adults. Current consensus definition: prevalence, etiology, and consequences. International Working Group on sarcopenia. J Am Med Dir Assoc. 2011;12:249–56.
21. Studenski SA, Peters KW, Alley DE, Cawthon PM, McLean RR, Harris TB, Ferrucci L, Guralnik JM, Fragala MS, Kenny AM, Kiel DP, Kritchevsky SB, Shardell MD, Dam TT, Vassileva MT. The FNIH sarcopenia project: rationale, study description, conference recommendations, and final estimates. J Gerontol A Biol Sci Med Sci. 2014;69:547–58.
22. Rockwood K, Stadnyk K, MacKnight C, McDowell I, Hebert R, Hogan DB. A brief clinical instrument to classify frailty in elderly people. Lancet. 1999;353:205–6.
23. Casati M, Costa AS, Capitanio D, Ponzoni L, Ferri E, Agostini S, Lori E. The biological foundations of sarcopenia: established and promising markers. Front Med (Lausanne). 2019;6:184.
24. Flacker JM. What is a geriatric syndrome anyway? J Am Geriatr Soc. 2003;51:574–6.
25. Inouye SK, Studenski S, Tinetti ME, Kuchel GA. Geriatric syndromes: clinical, research, and policy implications of a core geriatric concept. J Am Geriatr Soc. 2007;55:780–91.
26. Landi F, Picca A, Calvani R, Marzetti E. Anorexia of aging: assessment and management. Clin Geriatr Med. 2017;33:315–23.
27. Xue QL. The frailty syndrome: definition and natural history. Clin Geriatr Med. 2011;27:1–15.

28. Nakamura K. Locomotive syndrome: disability-free life expectancy and locomotive organ health in a "super-aged" society. J Orthop Sci. 2009;14:1–2.
29. Shafiee G, Keshtkar A, Soltani A, Ahadi Z, Larijani B, Heshmat R. Prevalence of sarcopenia in the world: a systematic review and meta-analysis of general population studies. J Diabetes Metab Disord. 2017;16:21.
30. Martone AM, Marzetti E, Salini S, Zazzara MB, Santoro L, Tosato M, Picca A, Calvani R, Landi F. Sarcopenia identified according to the EWGSOP2 definition in community-living people: prevalence and clinical features. J Am Med Dir Assoc. 2020;21:1470–4.
31. Van Ancum JM, Alcazar J, Meskers CGM, Nielsen BR, Suetta C, Maier AB. Impact of using the updated EWGSOP2 definition in diagnosing sarcopenia: a clinical perspective. Arch Gerontol Geriatr. 2020;90:104125.
32. Cruz-Jentoft AJ, Baeyens JP, Bauer JM, Boirie Y, Cederholm T, Landi F, Martin FC, Michel JP, Rolland Y, Schneider SM, Topinkova E, Vandewoude M, Zamboni M, European Working Group on Sarcopenia in Older P. Sarcopenia: European consensus on definition and diagnosis: report of the European working group on sarcopenia in older people. Age Ageing. 2010;39:412–23.
33. Cruz-Jentoft AJ, Sayer AA. Sarcopenia. Lancet. 2019;393:2636–46.
34. Robinson SM, Reginster JY, Rizzoli R, Shaw SC, Kanis JA, Bautmans I, Bischoff-Ferrari H, Bruyere O, Cesari M, Dawson-Hughes B, Fielding RA, Kaufman JM, Landi F, Malafarina V, Rolland Y, van Loon LJ, Vellas B, Visser M, Cooper C, Group EW. Does nutrition play a role in the prevention and management of sarcopenia? Clin Nutr. 2018;37:1121–32.
35. Welch AA. Nutritional influences on age-related skeletal muscle loss. Proc Nutr Soc. 2014;73:16–33.
36. Billot M, Calvani R, Urtamo A, Sanchez-Sanchez JL, Ciccolari-Micaldi C, Chang M, Roller-Wirnsberger R, Wirnsberger G, Sinclair A, Vaquero-Pinto N, Jyvakorpi S, Ohman H, Strandberg T, Schols J, Schols A, Smeets N, Topinkova E, Michalkova H, Bonfigli AR, Lattanzio F, Rodriguez-Manas L, Coelho-Junior H, Broccatelli M, Delia ME, Biscotti D, Marzetti E, Freiberger E. Preserving mobility in older adults with physical frailty and sarcopenia: opportunities, challenges, and recommendations for physical activity interventions. Clin Interv Aging. 2020;15:1675–90.
37. Frontera WR, Ochala J. Skeletal muscle: a brief review of structure and function. Calcif Tissue Int. 2015;96:183–95.
38. Joanisse S, Nederveen JP, Snijders T, McKay BR, Parise G. Skeletal muscle regeneration, repair and remodelling in aging: the importance of muscle stem cells and vascularization. Gerontology. 2017;63:91–100.
39. Vitale G, Cesari M, Mari D. Aging of the endocrine system and its potential impact on sarcopenia. Eur J Intern Med. 2016;35:10–5.
40. Guadalupe-Grau A, Carnicero JA, Losa-Reyna J, Tresguerres J, Gomez-Cabrera MD, Castillo C, Alfaro-Acha A, Rosado-Artalejo C, Rodriguez-Manas L, Garcia-Garcia FJ. Endocrinology of aging from a muscle function point of view: results from the Toledo study for healthy aging. J Am Med Dir Assoc. 2017;18:234–9.
41. Tagliaferri C, Wittrant Y, Davicco MJ, Walrand S, Coxam V. Muscle and bone, two interconnected tissues. Ageing Res Rev. 2015;21:55–70.
42. Delezie J, Handschin C. Endocrine crosstalk between skeletal muscle and the brain. Front Neurol. 2018;9:698.
43. Grosicki GJ, Fielding RA, Lustgarten MS. Gut microbiota contribute to age-related changes in skeletal muscle size, composition, and function: biological basis for a gut-muscle Axis. Calcif Tissue Int. 2018;102:433–42.
44. Yeung SSY, Reijnierse EM, Pham VK, Trappenburg MC, Lim WK, Meskers CGM, Maier AB. Sarcopenia and its association with falls and fractures in older adults: a systematic review and meta-analysis. J Cachexia Sarcopenia Muscle. 2019;10:485–500.

45. Beaudart C, Zaaria M, Pasleau F, Reginster JY, Bruyere O. Health outcomes of sarcopenia: a systematic review and Meta-analysis. PLoS One. 2017;12:e0169548.
46. Beaudart C, Locquet M, Reginster JY, Delandsheere L, Petermans J, Bruyere O. Quality of life in sarcopenia measured with the SarQoL(R): impact of the use of different diagnosis definitions. Aging Clin Exp Res. 2018;30:307–13.
47. Sousa AS, Guerra RS, Fonseca I, Pichel F, Amaral TF. Sarcopenia and length of hospital stay. Eur J Clin Nutr. 2016;70:595–601.
48. Sousa AS, Guerra RS, Fonseca I, Pichel F, Ferreira S, Amaral TF. Financial impact of sarcopenia on hospitalization costs. Eur J Clin Nutr. 2016;70:1046–51.

Sarcopenia in Other Settings: Primary Care, Cardiovascular Disease, Surgery

9

L. Bracchitta, A. Minuzzo, M. Solari, Fiona Ecarnot, and J. Demurtas

9.1   Introduction

Sarcopenia is defined as a progressive syndrome that reduces whole-body muscle mass, muscle strength, and muscle function [1]. It is increasingly recognized as a correlate of ageing and is associated with increased probability of adverse outcomes including falls, fractures, frailty, and mortality [2–4]. In older adults in particular, the function and strength of muscles may be reduced or weakened due to the advancement of age, affecting the ability to remain active, underscoring the need to assess this condition in daily practice. Sarcopenia has multifactorial origins, involving lifestyle habits, disease triggers, and age-dependent biological changes (e.g., chronic inflammation, mitochondrial abnormalities, loss of neuromuscular junctions, reduced satellite cell numbers, hormonal alterations). Moreover, sarcopenia carries a high personal, social, and economic burden when untreated. However, the

L. Bracchitta
Primary Care Department, Local Health Authority ATS Città Metropolitana di Milano, Milan, Italy

A. Minuzzo
General Surgery Unit, USL Toscana Nord-Ovest, Piombino, Italy

M. Solari
Department of Cardiology, Misericordia Hospital, Grosseto, Italy

F. Ecarnot
Department of Cardiology, University Hospital Besancon, Besancon, France

EA3920, University of Burgundy Franche-Comté, Besancon, France

J. Demurtas (✉)
Primary Care Department USL Toscana Sud-Est, Grosseto, Italy

Clinical and Experimental Medicine PhD Program, University of Modena and Reggio Emilia, Modena, Italy
e-mail: jacopo.demurtas@unimore.it

© Springer Nature Switzerland AG 2021
N. Veronese et al. (eds.), *Sarcopenia*, Practical Issues in Geriatrics,
https://doi.org/10.1007/978-3-030-80038-3_9

complexities of determining which variables to measure, how to measure them, which cut-off points may best guide diagnosis and treatment, and how to best evaluate effects of therapeutic interventions, have resulted in sarcopenia remaining a long neglected and undertreated condition [5].

In this chapter, we will discuss the strategies to detect sarcopenia and its impact in different settings, namely primary care, cardiovascular disease, and surgery.

9.2 Sarcopenia in Primary Care

The existence of several definitions of sarcopenia, the time constraints related to assessing various features of sarcopenia, and the lack of access to specialized equipment, may render the evaluation of sarcopenia challenging in the primary care context. In this regard, a recent consensus defined the role of the primary care physician in sarcopenia as that of identifying patients who are at risk of sarcopenia and referring them to specialists in the field [6]. To this end, primary care physicians should consider possible sarcopenia in older individuals (e.g., ≥65 years) with signs or symptoms suggestive of the condition. Several rapid and inexpensive methods can be employed in primary care to detect patients in need of specialist referral for suspected sarcopenia, and the most common of these methods are outlined below.

9.2.1 Screening and Evaluation

9.2.1.1 The Red Flag Method
In every consultation or health assessment, warning signs or "red flags" alerting to the possible presence of sarcopenia or pre-sarcopenia may be detected by the primary care physician (Table 9.1). Notably, signs of declining muscle mass or general

Table 9.1 Red Flag Method

	Red flags[a]
Clinician's observation	General weakness of the subject
	Visual identification of loss of muscle mass
	Low walking speed
Subject's presenting features	Weight loss
	Loss of muscle strength (arms or legs)
	General weakness
	Fatigue
	Falls
	Impaired mobility
	Loss of energy
	Difficulties performing physical activity or activities of daily living
Clinician's assessment	Nutrition
	Body weight
	Physical activity

[a]Red flags identified by review and published in a consensus paper by Beaudart et al. [6]

weakness may be detected or investigated, as physical signs of sarcopenia. The physician should also inquire about symptoms such as loss of weight, loss of muscle strength, loss of energy, or falls. In parallel, patients should be questioned about their level of physical activity, as reduced activity or sedentary behavior may also alert to the possible onset of sarcopenia. Finally, a rapid assessment of the risk of nutrition should also be performed, for example, using the Mini Nutritional Assessment [7]. The presence of any one or more red flags should prompt the primary care physician to refer the patient for specialist evaluation for suspected sarcopenia.

9.2.1.2 The SARC-F Questionnaire

The SARC-F questionnaire was developed by Malmstrom et al. as a means for primary care providers to rapidly screen for sarcopenia during a standard consultation [8, 9]. The SARC-F questionnaire comprises five components, namely strength, assistance with walking, rising from a chair, climbing stairs, and falls. Each item is score 0 to 2 points, yielding a total score ranging from 0 to 10. Malmstrom et al. suggest that a score of 4 or more is predictive of sarcopenia and poor outcomes [9]. This cut-off should thus be a trigger for more detailed assessment of sarcopenia through specialist referral.

A prospective study of 4000 community-living Chinese men and women aged 65 years and older by Woo et al. compared the SARC-F against three consensus definitions of sarcopenia from Europe, Asia, and an international group, notably in terms of the ability of all four measures to predict 4-year physical limitation [10]. They found that the SARC-F questionnaire had excellent specificity but poor sensitivity for sarcopenia classification. Nevertheless, the SARC-F remains one of the best available tools for use in primary care for the diagnosis of sarcopenia.

9.2.2 Management of Sarcopenia in Primary Care

9.2.2.1 Physical Activity

As regards physical activity, there is currently no standardized physical intervention that can be recommended to enhance muscle strength. However, a general practitioner may advice the patient to engage in aerobic and resistance exercise that have been shown to improve muscle mass and strength in older adults with sarcopenia [11]. A recent meta-analysis of 22 studies totaling 1041 individuals (81% female, mean age 60 to 86 years) investigated the effects of exercise programs consisting of 30 to 80 min of training, with 1 to 5 training sessions weekly for 6 to 36 weeks [12]. The authors reported a significant improvement in muscle strength but not muscle mass following exercise treatment. For exercise interventions, the EWGSOP and IWGS Report of the International Sarcopenia Initiative suggests that supervised resistance exercise or composite exercise programs may be recommended for frail or sedentary community-dwelling individuals and that a minimum duration of at least 3 months (and probably longer) is necessary to achieve a notable benefit in relevant clinical parameters (muscle strength and physical performance) [13]. In addition, they advise that increased physical activity in daily life be recommended.

9.2.2.2 Nutrition

Regarding nutrition, similar to physical activity, there are currently no consensual recommendations regarding nutritional intake or supplementation in individuals with sarcopenia. Results of randomized trials of nutritional supplementation are inconsistent, but there is a growing body of evidence indicating that maintaining adequate levels of protein intake in older age is important to preserve muscle mass and strength [6, 14–16]. The European Society for Clinical Nutrition and Metabolism (ESPEN) recommends protein consumption of over 1 g/kg/day (up to 1.5 g/kg/day) for older adults in order to delay the increased risk of sarcopenia [17]. However, older people often have lower nutrient intake than recommended, especially protein [18], for various reasons including lack of appetite or low income, and may avoid meat due to difficulties in chewing or swallowing [14–16]. This in turn can lead to a failure to achieve the recommended protein intake, which is associated with an increased risk of developing severe sarcopenia [14]. A meta-analysis of 30 randomized controlled trials totaling 5615 individuals (mean age: 61 years) reported a small but significant positive effect of vitamin D supplementation on global muscle strength [19]. In summary, based on available evidence, primary care physicians should investigate overall calorie intake and, if possible, protein intake in older individuals. Prescription of nutritional supplements may be useful in patients at risk of insufficient protein or dietary intake [6].

9.3   Sarcopenia and Cardiovascular Diseases

Metabolic and cardiovascular risks are also closely related to aging, and cardiovascular diseases (CVDs) are an important worldwide cause of disability and mortality. Although the pathways have not yet been completely elucidated, numerous studies have shown an association between sarcopenia and cardiovascular complications [20, 21].

9.3.1   Heart Failure

Chronic heart failure (CHF) is a common condition in old age, and its prevalence doubles approximately every 10 years in men, and every 7 years in women beyond the age of 55 years [22]. With improvements in therapy and population ageing, the number of persons with heart failure is likely to continue rising in the coming decades.

Sarcopenia is closely related to chronic heart failure (CHF), and its prevalence is higher in older patients with than in those without CHF. Sarcopenia occurs in 30–50% of patients with heart failure with reduced ejection fraction (<40%) (HFrEF) [23], and prevalence is higher in people aged <80 years [24], at about 20% more than in the healthy population [23]. Sarcopenia can account for the loss of

1–2% of skeletal muscle per year [25]. Heart failure could compound this patho-physiological process, impairing muscle strength and function. Indeed, CHF and sarcopenia are intricately linked in a vicious circle, where the former may cause the latter through common pathways, including inflammation, hormonal changes, physical inactivity, low ventricular ejection fraction, malnutrition, and oxidative stress [20]. Conversely, sarcopenia may contribute to the development or aggrava-tion of heart failure through reduced muscle mass, declining muscle strength, lack of physical activity, and endothelial dysfunction.

Unfortunately, there are limited treatment options for sarcopenia in CHF, and strategies are mainly limited to resistance exercise [26–28], possibly also in combi-nation with nutritional supplements, aimed at increasing the intake of protein, in particular [29]. In CHF, exercise training has been shown to prevent the progressive loss of exercise capacity by antagonizing peripheral skeletal muscle wasting and by promoting left ventricular reverse remodeling, consequently improving ejection fraction [30]. This effect can slow the transition from cardiac dysfunction to (chronic) heart failure by counteracting the increased catabolic state [31].

Of note, the skeletal and myocardial muscles are histologically similar, so the systemic pathways that cause sarcopenia may influence myocardial mass, strength, and function [32]. Sarcopenia is characterized by the atrophy of type II muscle fibers and apoptosis with progressive reduction of organelles, such as mitochondria dysfunction and progressive denervation and reinnervation resulting in the loss of motor units [33]. Angiotensin II may lead to apoptosis, ubiquitin-proteasome sys-tem activation, continuous sympathetic nerve activity, and excessive oxidative stress by modifying the insulin-like growth factor-1 signal. This may cause mitochondrial damage, muscle protein degradation, and decreased appetite, eventually leading to muscle wasting [34]. Secondly, the infiltration of fat and connective tissue is another important element of reduced muscle mass. As adipose tissue is constantly depos-ited between muscle fibers, the number of muscle satellite cells continues to decrease, and muscle function declines further [35]. In addition, sarcopenia can also weaken left ventricular mass through some common pathways, including muscle tissue remodeling, complications (e.g., frailty and CHF), low nutritional intake, and lack of activity. Finally, skeletal muscle can secrete several substances that have protective and anti-inflammatory paracrine or endocrine effects on myocardial tis-sue such as Akt protein kinase B [36, 37]. However, recent evidence from sarcope-nic patients suggests that pathological abnormalities in skeletal muscular tissue could reduce the protective effects of cardiac protective factors [35].

The most important therapy for CHF patients is a maximal tolerated dose of ACE inhibitors and beta-blockers, with the addition of mineralocorticoid-receptor antagonists if the patient remains symptomatic. There is robust scientific evidence in favor of the beneficial effects of these drugs on symptom relief and prognosis, with results that both ESC and AHA/ACC guidelines for the management of heart failure strongly recommend [38–40]. Moreover, there are also some data showing a potential reduction in muscle wasting [41, 42]. Data from the SOLVD trial showed that patients receiving enalapril had a reduced risk of muscle wasting compared to the placebo group [41], but this was a cross-sectional study and prospective validation is warranted. A small, prospective study examined muscle wasting in 27 CHF patients with and without cachexia undergoing beta-blockade with carvedilol or long-acting metoprolol. After 6 months of follow-up, subjects with baseline cachexia demonstrated significantly greater weight gain (+5.2 ± 9.6 vs. +0.8 ± 5.0 kg, $p = 0.027$), a greater increase in plasma leptin levels, and a greater decrease in plasma norepinephrine levels when compared with noncachectic subjects [42]. However, the effects on body weight were likely due to the increase in fat mass. There are no available data on other CHF drugs. Promising new drugs such as sacubitril/valsartan are now being progressively administered in increasing numbers of HF patients, with consistent efficacy across a range of subgroups including age, sex, HR etiology, comorbidities, EF, and estimated cardiovascular risk [43]. These drugs might indirectly impede sarcopenia, but to date, data are lacking to substantiate this hypothesis.

9.3.2 Coronary Artery Disease

There is paucity of data regarding the frequency and prognostic value of sarcopenia in patients with ischemic heart disease, with only few studies published to date. A study from China reported that the prevalence of sarcopenia was 22.6% (defined by the Asian working group definition [44]) among patients with coronary heart disease [45]. In a multicenter pooled registry of 1086 older patients (≥65 years) undergoing percutaneous coronary intervention (PCI) with drug-eluting stent implantation, sarcopenia, as assessed by the ratio of serum creatinine to serum cystatin C (or sarcopenia index, SI), was found to be an independent predictor of major adverse cardiovascular events (hazard ratio (HR) 2.2, 95% confidence interval (CI) 1.6–3.1, $p < 0.001$) [46]. In another study of 9394 consecutive patients aged ≥65 years undergoing PCI from 2000 to 2011, compared with patients with normal body mass index (BMI), those with low BMI had significantly increased all-cause mortality (HR 1.4, 95% CI 1.1–1.7), related to both cardiovascular (HR 1.4, 95% CI 1.0–1.8) and noncardiovascular causes (HR 1.4, 95% CI 1.06–1.9) [47]. However, it should be noted that in this study, the authors evaluated only BMI and not sarcopenia per se.

9.3.3 Transcatheter Aortic Valve Replacement

Several meta-analyses have investigated the prognostic value of sarcopenia (or components thereof) in the setting of transcatheter aortic valve replacement (TAVR). In a meta-analysis of six studies including 1237 TAVR patients with available 1- to 2-year follow-up, psoas-muscle area was associated with significantly higher mortality ($p < 0.0001$) in both men and women [48]. In another meta-analysis of studies reporting CT-derived skeletal muscle area (SMA) and survival outcomes, Soud et al. identified eight studies totaling 1881 patients (mean age 81.8 ± 12 years,

55.9% men) that evaluated the incidence of early (≤30 days) and late all-cause mortality (>30 days) post TAVR [49]. They reported that higher SMA was associated with lower long-term mortality [odds ratio (OR) 0.49, 95% CI 0.28–0.83, $p = 0.049$], but not with early mortality [49]. Finally, Bertschi et al. performed a meta-analysis of 18 observational studies enrolling a total of 9513 patients that assessed skeletal muscle mass, muscle quality, and muscle function as measures for sarcopenia in patients undergoing TAVR [50]. They investigated the effects of sarcopenia on mortality at ≥1 year, length of hospital stay, and functional decline. Among seven studies that measured the prevalence of sarcopenia, five found it to be a significant predictor of mortality at 1 year or beyond, while several studies in the meta-analysis also found muscle mass to be a significant predictor of mortality at ≥1 year [50]. Of note, these authors found no study in the literature that measured the effect of nutritional and/or exercise interventions on sarcopenia in patients undergoing TAVR.

9.3.4   Atrial Fibrillation

Few studies have investigated the association between sarcopenia and atrial fibrillation, but available studies report an approximately fivefold increase in the risk of atrial fibrillation (OR 5.68 [1.34–24.12], $P = 0.019$) in patients with concomitant sarcopenia and overweight/obesity [51]. In another study of 596 patients with non-valvular atrial fibrillation and a mean age of 84.9 ± 5.2 years, 295 (49.5%) presented sarcopenia, which was significantly associated with mortality (HR: 1.77; 95%CI: 1.27–2.48) [52].

9.3.5   Peripheral Artery Disease (PAD)

PAD is an age-related condition affecting up to 20% of older adults [53, 54]. It results in decreased blood flow to the lower limbs due to atherosclerosis, and patients with PAD may experience exertional leg symptoms including intermittent claudication, resting pain, and ulcers [54]. The prevalence of sarcopenia in community-dwelling males with PAD ranges from 2 to 13% in various publications. Smoliner et al. found a prevalence of 15.2% in hospitalized patients from acute geriatric wards with a mean age of 82.8 ± 5.9 years [55], while Landi et al. reported a prevalence of 32.8% in a population of 122 nursing-home residents in Italy [56]. In another study of the same cohort, Landi et al. reported that residents with sarcopenia were more likely to die compared to those without sarcopenia (HR 2.34; 95% CI 1.04–5.24), after adjustment for age, gender, cerebrovascular diseases, osteoarthritis, chronic obstructive pulmonary disease, activity of daily living impairment, and body mass index [57]. According to a study by Addison et al., sarcopenia was more prevalent in patients with PAD than in matched non-PAD controls (23.8% vs. 2.4%; $p < 0.05$) [58]. Furthermore, the authors reported a lower 6-min walk distance in those with both PAD and sarcopenia compared to those with only PAD, indicating a possible increased risk for accelerated loss of mobility in individuals with both conditions [58].

9.4   Sarcopenia and Surgery

The prevalence of sarcopenia in surgical patients varies widely, with lower rates in hepatocellular (40.3%–54.1%) and colorectal cancer (38.9%–47.7%), but higher rates in gastric (43–79%) and esophageal cancer (14%–80%) [59, 60]. It is also frequently reported in patients undergoing surgery for benign pathologies, such as inflammatory bowel disease (12%–21%) [61], and in speciality surgeries, such as cardiac surgery (27%) [62], orthopedics (41%) [63], and vascular surgery (41%) [64].

The causes of sarcopenia in the surgical patient are complex and are frequently the sum of a paraphysiologic aging process with other diseases. Consequently, sarcopenia can have multifactorial causes, including reduced appetite (increase of tumor necrosis factor, etc.), malnutrition and reduction of protein intake (on a dysphagic, malabsorbent basis), and increase in the use of proteins linked to the underlying disease (cancer, inflammatory bowel disease, cirrhosis, etc.). Furthermore, the surgery itself can impact the patient by compounding a state of frailty or sarcopenia [65].

The need for major surgery in a sarcopenic patients places them at an increased risk of several complications [66] and higher postoperative mortality [67–69]. Sarcopenia was also found to be an independent predictor of postoperative mortality in the context of emergency surgery [70]. Consequently, sarcopenic patients represent a particularly costly patient demographic [71]. Given that sarcopenia may be remediable, efforts to attenuate the costs associated with major surgery should focus on targeted preoperative interventions to optimize these high-risk patients and prepare them to undergo surgery [72]. To this end, it is therefore necessary to recognize the sarcopenic patient, or the potentially sarcopenic patient, in order to evaluate the risk, and balance the risk against the benefit of the surgical procedure. Finally, it is essential to identify surgical patients at risk of, or with existing sarcopenia, in order to implement activities aimed at improving the sarcopenic condition or actively preventing its development or aggravation.

9.4.1   Preoperative Assessment of Sarcopenia

Careful selection of the surgical patient is essential in daily clinical practice and is one of the most challenging areas of surgical management. It is particularly important in geriatric surgical patients in whom preoperative evaluation makes it possible to assign them to a specific risk class. In recent years, sarcopenia has been studied as a risk parameter in the evaluation of the fragile patient and for the evaluation of surgical risk, but the role of sarcopenia in preoperative risk stratification remains unclear.

Some studies have reported better stratification of complication risk when sarcopenia is taken into consideration in gastrointestinal surgical oncology [73], gastric cancer [74], hepatobiliary malignancy [75], and colorectal cancer [76]. In esophageal cancer, the value of considering sarcopenia is debated, with contrasting evidence [77–79]. Similar results have been reported also for urological oncologic surgery [80], gynecological surgery [81, 82], and orthopedic surgery [83], while worse long-term outcomes after thoracic surgery have been reported [84]. Due to the heterogeneity of data published, further studies are needed to better evaluate the role of sarcopenia as a risk factor in surgical patients [85].

According to the recent consensus conference on sarcopenia [86], every patient aged over 65 years should be screened prior to surgery, with evaluation of muscle strength, muscle quantity, and physical performance. However, due to the various definitions available and the variety of cut-off values in use, sarcopenia is notoriously difficult to evaluate on a clinical level or through the classic anthropometric parameters (BMI, etc.), and frequently used nutritional scores [87] are not accurate, especially in the early stages of the syndrome. Moreover, most of the clinical and surgical stratification scores in elderly and/or frail patients do not include an assessment of sarcopenia. As suggested above for primary care, suitable methods for performing a rapid assessment of sarcopenia during a standard consultation include the use of the gait speed test [88] or the SARC-F questionnaire [89]. These tests can be included in the initial surgical multidimensional assessment and could be integrated into more widely known multidimensional instruments (ASA, frailty scores, etc.). In patients with abnormal screening results, these initial evaluations can prompt the use of second-level diagnostic tests as suggested by the algorithm of EWGSOP guidelines [1]. For surgical patients, the frequently available CT or MRI images make radiological measurement of muscular compartments [87] (such as psoas muscle mass) more feasible and more easily available compared to DXA [86]. Moreover, it has been shown that muscular evaluation by imaging is a strong predictive prognostic factor of postoperative complications [85], even if there is considerable variance in the cut-off values reported for these diagnostic exams [90]. Potentially useful new methods for the diagnosis of sarcopenia have been proposed such as ultrasound evaluation [91], but more evidence is needed to increase its applicability.

In order to integrate sarcopenia into the assessment of frailty in surgical patients, Buettner et al. developed a 28-point preoperative frailty risk model capable of stratifying patients based on 1-year mortality risk [92]. This score was developed on a sample of patients undergoing abdominal surgery and was found to be more accurate than the frailty index (C-statistic = 0.55) and ECOG score (C-statistic = 0.57). Further studies are needed to develop and validate multidimensional indices that integrate sarcopenia as a risk factor for the development of postoperative complications and mortality [85].

9.4.2 Prehabilitation and Sarcopenia

The success of a surgical intervention is not limited to the technical act alone but requires restoring the patient's physical and psychological balance as close as possible to the preoperative state [93]. This objective can be obtained by close cooperation across all the phases of the surgical activity in a multidisciplinary fashion.

Preoperative sarcopenia is widely known to be one of the risk factors predicting poor postoperative outcomes (sarcopenia, frailty, malnutrition, impaired exercise tolerance). Due to the interdependence of the causal factors of sarcopenia, a multidisciplinary approach must be applied in the surgical patient, with a multidimensional approach during all the perioperative phases (pre, intra, postoperative). In particular, sarcopenic patients must be managed before surgery to correct, as far as possible, the nutritional state, and to optimize muscle mass and physical function [94] as much as possible according to the patient's general state.

In recent decades, the concept of prehabilitation has been developed [95] to describe a multimodal program based on three fundamental pillars: physical exercise, nutritional optimization, and psychological well-being [93] with the aim of improving surgical outcomes. Prehabilitation is especially appropriate in the time interval after neoadjuvant treatment before surgery [96], but is potentially applicable in all surgical cases.

Prehabilitation strategies have been applied in elderly [97] and fragile patients [98]. They can be also useful in sarcopenic patients, although there is a lack of evidence of the benefit of such a strategy in these subgroups of patients. The waiting time prior to the surgical procedure can be used profitably to implement multifactorial optimization of the patient's physical state and increase functional reserve through multiple activities and actions. Various models following this principle have been developed, which provide for an initial assessment with screening tools and initial information that can be proposed to all surgical patients [99, 100]. No clear evidence of the superiority of any specific program over the others has emerged. Further degrees of implementation can be offered based on the characteristics and needs of individual patients under the supervision of an integrated professional team [101]. The various activities of the prehabilitation program must be tailored on the patient, taking into account the general characteristics, comorbidities, and functional capacity of each individual patient.

To date, data on the effects of prehabilitation are conflicting. It is generally accepted that prehabilitation before surgery results in a more rapid return to baseline functional capacity after surgery [102]. As a consequence of the short waiting period frequently available between diagnosis and surgery, it is necessary to implement a program that encompasses multifaceted action targeting the various factors to obtain the best results [93]. Particular attention must be paid to the evaluation of nutritional status. Patients in whom there is an identified risk of malnutrition, or documented malnutrition, must undergo a dietary intervention to correct nutritional deficiencies, restore energy deficit, improve functional performance, avoid weight loss, and preserve the intestinal microbiome. Preoperative nutritional conditioning must be personalized and prescribed by dedicated professionals taking into account the patient's comorbidities. The basic principles of this approach are reported in the ESPEN guidelines on the perioperative treatment of sarcopenia. A norm-calorie diet with a protein intake of 1.2 g/kg is recommended [103]. In general, the enteral route should be preferred, but when this is not possible, different means of administering nutrients (parenteral route, etc.) may be considered. When patients have a normal diet, it is often insufficient to meet their energy needs, so it is recommended that patients receive oral dietary supplements (ONS) in the preoperative period, regardless of their nutritional status [104]. There is good evidence to support ONS in the perioperative period. A meta-analysis of nine studies [105] found that nutritional supplementation prior to surgery was associated with a 35% reduction in total complications ($p < 0.001$). In parallel with the correction of nutritional status, it is important to stimulate physical activity. Performing regular strength, aerobic exercise [106–109], and physical conditioning has been shown to be effective in positively modifying cardiorespiratory function, reducing weight [108], and improving physical performance [99], particularly in elderly patients. Based on these findings, presurgical exercise programs should include both strength and aerobic training [106–109] and some stretching exercises [110, 111]. Aerobic and muscular strength training in elderly patients increases endurance capacity [112], reduces weight gain [108], improves muscle strength [113], reduces fall risk [114], and increases range of motion in a number of joints [108].

In recent years, there has been increasing interest in the utility of physical activity programs for the treatment of sarcopenia, with or without additional nutritional supplementation [115, 116]. Published meta-analyses have evaluated the impact of physical activity programs on sarcopenic patients preoperatively and have yielded conflicting results. A recent meta-analysis of physical exercise before major surgery [117] evaluated prehabilitation in various subgroups of surgical interventions (hepatic, colorectal, gastroesophageal, major abdominal surgery) in a total of 442 patients. Across the various randomized controlled trials included in the meta-analysis, there was wide variability in terms of the type of surgery, the duration of prehabilitation (7–49 days), the type of prehabilitation program, and the outcomes assessed. However, better results were observed following the application of prehabilitation in terms of overall postoperative morbidity (OR 0.52; $p = 0.01$) and pulmonary complications (OR = 0.20; $p = 0.001$). Despite these encouraging results, in clinical practice, prehabilitation with targeted exercise programs is not always feasible, not only due to the patient's general state of health but often due to organizational constraints and a lack of available human resources.

9.4.3   Enhanced Recovery After Surgery (ERAS)

The Enhanced Recovery After Surgery (ERAS) program was developed to optimize and standardize the post-surgery pathway, with the goal of reducing postoperative stress, and enabling rapid recovery and early discharge. Based largely on the fast-track surgery theory devised by Kehlet in 2000 [118], the ERAS program has been progressively developed on the basis of evidence-based medicine and applied in general surgery and other specialized surgical branches. Unlike prehabilitation, ERAS interventions focus more on hospital care and the postoperative period, applying a series of interventions that are implemented starting from hospitalization and progressively applied in all surgical phases (intraoperative, postoperative) until discharge. The ERAS approach is based on fundamental pillars, such as the reduction of preoperative fasting, optimization of hemoglobin values, reduction of surgical trauma (use of minimally invasive surgery, intraoperative normothermia, reduction of the number of drains), improved intraoperative and postoperative anesthetic management, mobilization early and physiotherapy incentives, and resumption of normal nutrition to reduce catabolism and hypofunction syndrome. It requires multidimensional activity involving many healthcare professionals (nurses, physiotherapists, dieticians, anesthetists, surgeons, etc.) who take care of the patient in a multidimensional way aimed at improving surgical outcomes. This has been shown to be feasible by multiple studies and scientifically consolidated by reports and a Cochrane systematic review demonstrating the ability of the ERAS program to reduce postoperative morbidity, reduce length of hospital stay, and improve patient satisfaction [119–122].

In recent years, evidence has emerged regarding the usefulness of the ERAS approach in the elderly patient (>70 years old) undergoing colorectal surgery, not only confirming the classic postoperative outcomes but also demonstrating a lower rate of anastomotic dehiscence and a high compliance with the protocol (70%) [123]. There has been some evidence demonstrating the efficacy of ERAS in improving outcomes in sarcopenic patients, particularly in association with laparoscopic colorectal resection [124]. On the contrary, the application of the ERAS protocol and an intensive postoperative nutrition after esophagectomy did not show benefits in terms of improving sarcopenia [125]. Consequently, the application of the ERAS approach is not currently supported by strong evidence in terms of correction of sarcopenia. Further studies are needed to investigate whether there is any specific benefit to be yielded on sarcopenia outcomes by the use of the ERAS approach.

9.5 Conclusion

In summary, sarcopenia is a frequent finding in patients across a range of medical disciplines and settings. It may compound the severity of comorbidities and expose the patient to a higher risk of complications, morbidity, and mortality In primary care, it is essential to screen for salient features of sarcopenia using validated tools that are rapid and easy to implement during a standard consultation, such as the red flag method or the SARC-F questionnaire. Physical activity and nutritional supplementation are the cornerstones of management of sarcopenia in primary care, but detection of patients with sarcopenia or at risk thereof should also prompt referral for specialist evaluation. In cardiovascular disease, sarcopenia may be brought on by conditions that share common pathophysiological pathways, such as heart failure. Conversely, sarcopenia may contribute to the development or aggravation of heart failure, through reduced muscle mass and lack of physical activity. Here again, physical activity may yield benefits both on sarcopenia and physical function. In heart failure patients in particular, maximal tolerated medical therapy must be maintained. Sarcopenia has been shown to be associated with higher post-procedural mortality in patients undergoing transcatheter aortic valve replacement and may also have a negative prognostic effect in atrial fibrillation, coronary artery disease, and peripheral artery disease. In surgical patients, sarcopenia is highly prevalent and places them at increased risk of postoperative complications and mortality. Approaches such as prehabilitation and enhanced recovery after surgery may help to reduce surgical stress response, optimize physiologic function, and facilitate recovery.

References

1. Cruz-Jentoft AJ, Bahat G, Bauer J, Boirie Y, Bruyere O, Cederholm T, et al. Sarcopenia: revised European consensus on definition and diagnosis. Age Ageing. 2019;48:16–31. PubMed PMID: 30312372; PubMed Central PMCID: PMCPMC6322506. https://doi.org/10.1093/ageing/afy169.
2. Fried TR, Bradley EH, Williams CS, Tinetti ME. Functional disability and health care expenditures for older persons. Arch Intern Med. 2001;161:2602–7. https://doi.org/10.1001/archinte.161.21.2602.
3. Clegg A, Young J, Iliffe S, Rikkert MO, Rockwood K. Frailty in elderly people. Lancet. 2013;381:752–62. PubMed PMID: 23395245; PubMed Central PMCID: PMCPMC4098658. https://doi.org/10.1016/S0140-6736(12)62167-9.
4. Veronese N, Demurtas J, Soysal P, Smith L, Torbahn G, Schoene D, et al. Sarcopenia and health-related outcomes: an umbrella review of observational studies. Eur Geriatr Med. 2019;10:853–62. https://doi.org/10.1007/s41999-019-00233-w.
5. Han A, Bokshan SL, Marcaccio SE, DePasse JM, Daniels AH. Diagnostic criteria and clinical outcomes in sarcopenia research: a literature review. J Clin Med. 2018;7:70. PubMed PMID: 29642478; PubMed Central PMCID: PMCPMC5920444. https://doi.org/10.3390/jcm7040070.
6. Beaudart C, McCloskey E, Bruyere O, Cesari M, Rolland Y, Rizzoli R, et al. Sarcopenia in daily practice: assessment and management. BMC Geriatr. 2016;16:170. PubMed PMID: 27716195; PubMed Central PMCID: PMCPMC5052976. https://doi.org/10.1186/s12877-016-0349-4.
7. Rubenstein LZ, Harker JO, Salva A, Guigoz Y, Vellas B. Screening for undernutrition in geriatric practice: developing the short-form mini-nutritional assessment (MNA-SF). J Gerontol A Biol Sci Med Sci. 2001;56:M366–72. https://doi.org/10.1093/gerona/56.6.m366.
8. Malmstrom TK, Miller DK, Simonsick EM, Ferrucci L, Morley JE. SARC-F: a symptom score to predict persons with sarcopenia at risk for poor functional outcomes. J Cachexia Sarcopenia Muscle. 2016;7:28–36. PubMed PMID: 27066316; PubMed Central PMCID: PMCPMC4799853. https://doi.org/10.1002/jcsm.12048.
9. Malmstrom TK, Morley JE. SARC-F: a simple questionnaire to rapidly diagnose sarcopenia. J Am Med Dir Assoc. 2013;14:531–2. https://doi.org/10.1016/j.jamda.2013.05.018.
10. Woo J, Leung J, Morley JE. Validating the SARC-F: a suitable community screening tool for sarcopenia? J Am Med Dir Assoc. 2014;15:630–4. https://doi.org/10.1016/j.jamda.2014.04.021.
11. Li Z, Cui M, Yu K, Zhang X, Li C, Nie X, et al. Effects of nutrition supplementation and physical exercise on muscle mass, muscle strength and fat mass among sarcopenic elderly: a randomized controlled trial. Appl Physiol Nutr Metab. 2020; https://doi.org/10.1139/apnm-2020-0643.

12. Bao W, Sun Y, Zhang T, Zou L, Wu X, Wang D, et al. Exercise programs for muscle mass, muscle strength and physical performance in older adults with sarcopenia: a systematic review and meta-analysis. Aging Dis. 2020;11:863–73. PubMed PMID: 32765951; PubMed Central PMCID: PMCPMC7390512. https://doi.org/10.14336/AD.2019.1012.

13. Cruz-Jentoft AJ, Landi F, Schneider SM, Zuniga C, Arai H, Boirie Y, et al. Prevalence of and interventions for sarcopenia in ageing adults: a systematic review. Report of the International Sarcopenia Initiative (EWGSOP and IWGS). Age Ageing. 2014;43:748–59. PubMed PMID: 25241753; PubMed Central PMCID: PMCPMC4204661. https://doi.org/10.1093/ageing/afu115.

14. Beaudart C, Sanchez-Rodriguez D, Locquet M, Reginster JY, Lengele L, Bruyere O. Malnutrition as a strong predictor of the onset of sarcopenia. Nutrients. 2019;11:2883. PubMed PMID: 31783482; PubMed Central PMCID: PMCPMC6950107. https://doi.org/10.3390/nu11122883.

15. Abiri B, Vafa M. The role of nutrition in attenuating age-related skeletal muscle atrophy. Adv Exp Med Biol. 2020;1260:297–318. https://doi.org/10.1007/978-3-030-42667-5_12.

16. Paproski JJ, Finello GC, Murillo A, Mandel E. The importance of protein intake and strength exercises for older adults. JAAPA. 2019;32:32–6. https://doi.org/10.1097/01.JAA.0000586328.11996.c0.

17. Deutz NE, Bauer JM, Barazzoni R, Biolo G, Boirie Y, Bosy-Westphal A, et al. Protein intake and exercise for optimal muscle function with aging: recommendations from the ESPEN Expert Group. Clin Nutr. 2014;33:929–36. PubMed PMID: 24814383; PubMed Central PMCID: PMCPMC4208946. https://doi.org/10.1016/j.clnu.2014.04.007.

18. Deer RR, Volpi E. Protein intake and muscle function in older adults. Curr Opin Clin Nutr Metab Care. 2015;18:248–53. PubMed PMID: 25807346; PubMed Central PMCID: PMCPMC4394186. https://doi.org/10.1097/MCO.0000000000000162.

19. Beaudart C, Buckinx F, Rabenda V, Gillain S, Cavalier E, Slomian J, et al. The effects of vitamin D on skeletal muscle strength, muscle mass, and muscle power: a systematic review and meta-analysis of randomized controlled trials. J Clin Endocrinol Metab. 2014;99:4336–45. https://doi.org/10.1210/jc.2014-1742.

20. Yin J, Lu X, Qian Z, Xu W, Zhou X. New insights into the pathogenesis and treatment of sarcopenia in chronic heart failure. Theranostics. 2019;9:4019–29. PubMed PMID: 31281529; PubMed Central PMCID: PMCPMC6592172. https://doi.org/10.7150/thno.33000.

21. Lai S, Muscaritoli M, Andreozzi P, Sgreccia A, De Leo S, Mazzaferro S, et al. Sarcopenia and cardiovascular risk indices in patients with chronic kidney disease on conservative and replacement therapy. Nutrition. 2019;62:108–14. https://doi.org/10.1016/j.nut.2018.12.005.

22. Springer J, Springer JI, Anker SD. Muscle wasting and sarcopenia in heart failure and beyond: update 2017. ESC Heart Fail. 2017;4:492–8. PubMed PMID: 29154428; PubMed Central PMCID: PMCPMC5695190. https://doi.org/10.1002/ehf2.12237.

23. Fulster S, Tacke M, Sandek A, Ebner N, Tschope C, Doehner W, et al. Muscle wasting in patients with chronic heart failure: results from the studies investigating co-morbidities aggravating heart failure (SICA-HF). Eur Heart J. 2013;34:512–9. https://doi.org/10.1093/eurheartj/ehs381.

24. Morley JE, Anker SD, von Haehling S. Prevalence, incidence, and clinical impact of sarcopenia: facts, numbers, and epidemiology-update 2014. J Cachexia Sarcopenia Muscle. 2014;5:253–9. PubMed PMID: 25425503; PubMed Central PMCID: PMCPMC4248415. https://doi.org/10.1007/s13539-014-0161-y.

25. Doherty TJ. Invited review: aging and sarcopenia. J Appl Physiol (1985). 2003;95:1717–27. https://doi.org/10.1152/japplphysiol.00347.2003.

26. Landi F, Marzetti E, Martone AM, Bernabei R, Onder G. Exercise as a remedy for sarcopenia. Curr Opin Clin Nutr Metab Care. 2014;17:25–31. https://doi.org/10.1097/MCO.0000000000000018.

27. Ebner N, Sliziuk V, Scherbakov N, Sandek A. Muscle wasting in ageing and chronic illness. ESC Heart Fail. 2015;2:58–68. PubMed PMID: 28834653; PubMed Central PMCID: PMCPMC6410534. https://doi.org/10.1002/ehf2.12033.

28. Phu S, Boersma D, Duque G. Exercise and sarcopenia. J Clin Densitom. 2015;18:488–92. https://doi.org/10.1016/j.jocd.2015.04.011.
29. Santarpia L, Contaldo F, Pasanisi F. Dietary protein content for an optimal diet: a clinical view. J Cachexia Sarcopenia Muscle. 2017;8:345–8. PubMed PMID: 28444858; PubMed Central PMCID: PMCPMC5476844. https://doi.org/10.1002/jcsm.12176.
30. Gielen S, Laughlin MH, O'Conner C, Duncker DJ. Exercise training in patients with heart disease: review of beneficial effects and clinical recommendations. Prog Cardiovasc Dis. 2015;57:347–55. https://doi.org/10.1016/j.pcad.2014.10.001.
31. Souza RW, Piedade WP, Soares LC, Souza PA, Aguiar AF, Vechetti-Junior IJ, et al. Aerobic exercise training prevents heart failure-induced skeletal muscle atrophy by anti-catabolic, but not anabolic actions. PLoS One. 2014;9:e110020. PubMed PMID: 25330387; PubMed Central PMCID: PMCPMC4201522. https://doi.org/10.1371/journal.pone.0110020.
32. Wang M, Hu S, Zhang F, Liu J, Mao Y. Correlation between sarcopenia and left ventricular myocardial mass in chronic heart failure patients. Aging Med (Milton). 2020;3:138–41. PubMed PMID: 32666029; PubMed Central PMCID: PMCPMC7338701. https://doi.org/10.1002/agm2.12111.
33. Rolland Y, Czerwinski S, Abellan Van Kan G, Morley JE, Cesari M, Onder G, et al. Sarcopenia: its assessment, etiology, pathogenesis, consequences and future perspectives. J Nutr Health Aging. 2008;12:433–50. PubMed PMID: 18615225; PubMed Central PMCID: PMCPMC3988678. https://doi.org/10.1007/BF02982704.
34. Dos Santos MR, Saitoh M, Ebner N, Valentova M, Konishi M, Ishida J, et al. Sarcopenia and endothelial function in patients with chronic heart failure: results from the studies investigating comorbidities aggravating heart failure (SICA-HF). J Am Med Dir Assoc. 2017;18:240–5. https://doi.org/10.1016/j.jamda.2016.09.006.
35. Keng BMH, Gao F, Teo LLY, Lim WS, Tan RS, Ruan W, et al. Associations between skeletal muscle and myocardium in aging: a syndrome of "Cardio-Sarcopenia"? J Am Geriatr Soc. 2019;67:2568–73. PubMed PMID: 31418823; PubMed Central PMCID: PMCPMC6898740. https://doi.org/10.1111/jgs.16132.
36. Curcio F, Testa G, Liguori I, Papillo M, Flocco V, Panicara V, et al. Sarcopenia and heart failure. Nutrients. 2020;12:211. PubMed PMID: 31947528; PubMed Central PMCID: PMCPMC7019352. https://doi.org/10.3390/nu12010211.
37. Oshima Y, Ouchi N, Sato K, Izumiya Y, Pimentel DR, Walsh K. Follistatin-like 1 is an Akt-regulated cardioprotective factor that is secreted by the heart. Circulation. 2008;117:3099–108. PubMed PMID: 18519848; PubMed Central PMCID: PMCPMC2679251. https://doi.org/10.1161/CIRCULATIONAHA.108.767673.
38. Ponikowski P, Voors AA, Anker SD, Bueno H, Cleland JGF, Coats AJS, et al. 2016 ESC guidelines for the diagnosis and treatment of acute and chronic heart failure: the task force for the diagnosis and treatment of acute and chronic heart failure of the European Society of Cardiology (ESC)developed with the special contribution of the heart failure association (HFA) of the ESC. Eur Heart J. 2016;37:2129–200. https://doi.org/10.1093/eurheartj/ehw128.
39. Yancy CW, Jessup M, Bozkurt B, Butler J, Casey DE Jr, Colvin MM, et al. 2017 ACC/AHA/HFSA focused update of the 2013 ACCF/AHA guideline for the Management of Heart Failure: a report of the American College of Cardiology/American Heart Association task force on clinical practice guidelines and the Heart Failure Society of America. J Am Coll Cardiol. 2017;70:776–803. https://doi.org/10.1016/j.jacc.2017.04.025.
40. Yancy CW, Jessup M, Bozkurt B, Butler J, Casey DE Jr, Drazner MH, et al. 2013 ACCF/AHA guideline for the management of heart failure: a report of the American College of Cardiology Foundation/American Heart Association task force on practice guidelines. J Am Coll Cardiol. 2013;62:e147–239. https://doi.org/10.1016/j.jacc.2013.05.019.
41. Anker SD, Negassa A, Coats AJ, Afzal R, Poole-Wilson PA, Cohn JN, et al. Prognostic importance of weight loss in chronic heart failure and the effect of treatment with angiotensin-converting-enzyme inhibitors: an observational study. Lancet. 2003;361:1077–83. https://doi.org/10.1016/S0140-6736(03)12892-9.

42. Hryniewicz K, Androne AS, Hudaihed A, Katz SD. Partial reversal of cachexia by beta-adrenergic receptor blocker therapy in patients with chronic heart failure. J Card Fail. 2003;9:464–8. https://doi.org/10.1016/s1071-9164(03)00582-7.
43. Volpe M, Bauersachs J, Bayes-Genis A, Butler J, Cohen-Solal A, Gallo G, et al. Sacubitril/valsartan for the management of heart failure: a perspective viewpoint on current evidence. Int J Cardiol. 2021;327:138–45. https://doi.org/10.1016/j.ijcard.2020.11.071.
44. Chen LK, Liu LK, Woo J, Assantachai P, Auyeung TW, Bahyah KS, et al. Sarcopenia in Asia: consensus report of the Asian working Group for Sarcopenia. J Am Med Dir Assoc. 2014;15:95–101. https://doi.org/10.1016/j.jamda.2013.11.025.
45. Zhang N, Zhu WL, Liu XH, Chen W, Zhu ML, Kang L, et al. Prevalence and prognostic implications of sarcopenia in older patients with coronary heart disease. J Geriatr Cardiol. 2019;16:756–63. PubMed PMID: 31700515; PubMed Central PMCID: PMCPMC6828602. https://doi.org/10.11909/j.issn.1671-5411.2019.10.002.
46. Lee HS, Park KW, Kang J, Ki YJ, Chang M, Han JK, et al. Sarcopenia index as a predictor of clinical outcomes in older patients with coronary artery disease. J Clin Med. 2020;9:3121. PubMed PMID: 32992530; PubMed Central PMCID: PMCPMC7600792. https://doi.org/10.3390/jcm9103121.
47. Goel K, Gulati R, Reeder GS, Lennon RJ, Lewis BR, Behfar A, et al. Low body mass index, serum creatinine, and cause of death in patients undergoing percutaneous coronary intervention. J Am Heart Assoc. 2016;5:e003633. PubMed PMID: 27799234; PubMed Central PMCID: PMCPMC5210329.
48. Takagi H, Hari Y, Kawai N, Ando T, Group A. Meta-analysis of the prognostic value of psoas-muscle area on mortality in patients undergoing Transcatheter aortic valve implantation. Am J Cardiol. 2018;122:1394–400. https://doi.org/10.1016/j.amjcard.2018.06.049.
49. Soud M, Alahdab F, Ho G, Kuku KO, Cejudo-Tejeda M, Hideo-Kajita A, et al. Usefulness of skeletal muscle area detected by computed tomography to predict mortality in patients undergoing transcatheter aortic valve replacement: a meta-analysis study. Int J Cardiovasc Imaging. 2019;35:1141–7. https://doi.org/10.1007/s10554-019-01582-0.
50. Bertschi D, Kiss CM, Schoenenberger AW, Stuck AE, Kressig RW. Sarcopenia in patients undergoing transcatheter aortic valve implantation (TAVI): a systematic review of the literature. J Nutr Health Aging. 2021;25:64–70. https://doi.org/10.1007/s12603-020-1448-7.
51. Xia MF, Chen LY, Wu L, Ma H, Li XM, Li Q, et al. Sarcopenia, sarcopenic overweight/obesity and risk of cardiovascular disease and cardiac arrhythmia: a cross-sectional study. Clin Nutr. 2021;40(2):571–80. https://doi.org/10.1016/j.clnu.2020.06.003.
52. Requena Calleja MA, Arenas Miquelez A, Diez-Manglano J, Gullon A, Pose A, Formiga F, et al. Sarcopenia, frailty, cognitive impairment and mortality in elderly patients with non-valvular atrial fibrillation. Rev Clin Esp. 2019;219:424–32. https://doi.org/10.1016/j.rce.2019.04.001.
53. Collins TC, Petersen NJ, Suarez-Almazor M, Ashton CM. The prevalence of peripheral arterial disease in a racially diverse population. Arch Intern Med. 2003;163:1469–74. https://doi.org/10.1001/archinte.163.12.1469.
54. Writing Group M, Mozaffarian D, Benjamin EJ, Go AS, Arnett DK, Blaha MJ, et al. Heart disease and stroke statistics-2016 update: a report from the American Heart Association. Circulation. 2016;133:e38–360. https://doi.org/10.1161/CIR.0000000000000350.
55. Smoliner C, Sieber CC, Wirth R. Prevalence of sarcopenia in geriatric hospitalized patients. J Am Med Dir Assoc. 2014;15:267–72. https://doi.org/10.1016/j.jamda.2013.11.027.
56. Landi F, Liperoti R, Fusco D, Mastropaolo S, Quattrociocchi D, Proia A, et al. Prevalence and risk factors of sarcopenia among nursing home older residents. J Gerontol A Biol Sci Med Sci. 2012;67:48–55. https://doi.org/10.1093/gerona/glr035.
57. Landi F, Liperoti R, Fusco D, Mastropaolo S, Quattrociocchi D, Proia A, et al. Sarcopenia and mortality among older nursing home residents. J Am Med Dir Assoc. 2012;13:121–6. https://doi.org/10.1016/j.jamda.2011.07.004.
58. Addison O, Prior SJ, Kundi R, Serra MC, Katzel LI, Gardner AW, et al. Sarcopenia in peripheral arterial disease: prevalence and effect on functional status. Arch Phys Med Rehabil.

2018;99:623–8. PubMed PMID: 29138051; PubMed Central PMCID: PMCPMC5871593. https://doi.org/10.1016/j.apmr.2017.10.017.

59. Levolger S, van Vugt JL, de Bruin RW, JN IJ. Systematic review of sarcopenia in patients operated on for gastrointestinal and hepatopancreatobiliary malignancies. Br J Surg. 2015;102:1448–58. https://doi.org/10.1002/bjs.9893.

60. Wang PY, Xu LD, Chen XK, Xu L, Yu YK, Zhang RX, et al. Sarcopenia and short-term outcomes after esophagectomy: a meta-analysis. Ann Surg Oncol. 2020;27:3041–51. https://doi.org/10.1245/s10434-020-08236-9.

61. Bryant RV, Ooi S, Schultz CG, Goess C, Grafton R, Hughes J, et al. Low muscle mass and sarcopenia: common and predictive of osteopenia in inflammatory bowel disease. Aliment Pharmacol Ther. 2015;41:895–906. https://doi.org/10.1111/apt.13156.

62. Teng CH, Chen SY, Wei YC, Hsu RB, Chi NH, Wang SS, et al. Effects of sarcopenia on functional improvement over the first year after cardiac surgery: a cohort study. Eur J Cardiovasc Nurs. 2019;18:309–17. https://doi.org/10.1177/1474515118822964.

63. Bokshan SL, DePasse JM, Daniels AH. Sarcopenia in orthopedic surgery. Orthopedics. 2016;39:e295–300. https://doi.org/10.3928/01477447-20160222-02.

64. Heard R, Black D, Ramsay G, Scott N, Hildebrand D. The prevalence of sarcopaenia in a vascular surgical patient cohort and its impact on outcome. Surgeon. 2018;16:325–32. https://doi.org/10.1016/j.surge.2018.03.001.

65. Takahashi S, Maeta M, Mizusawa K, Kaneko T, Naka T, Ashida K, et al. Long-term postoperative analysis of nutritional status after limited gastrectomy for early gastric cancer. Hepatogastroenterology. 1998;45:889–94.

66. Sandini M, Pinotti E, Persico I, Picone D, Bellelli G, Gianotti L. Systematic review and meta-analysis of frailty as a predictor of morbidity and mortality after major abdominal surgery. BJS Open. 2017;1:128–37. PubMed PMID: 29951615; PubMed Central PMCID: PMCPMC5989941. https://doi.org/10.1002/bjs5.22.

67. Kim YK, Yi SR, Lee YH, Kwon J, Jang SI, Park SH. Effect of sarcopenia on postoperative mortality in osteoporotic hip fracture patients. J Bone Metab. 2018;25:227–33. PubMed PMID: 30574467; PubMed Central PMCID: PMCPMC6288605. https://doi.org/10.11005/jbm.2018.25.4.227.

68. Landi F, Liperoti R, Russo A, Giovannini S, Tosato M, Capoluongo E, et al. Sarcopenia as a risk factor for falls in elderly individuals: results from the ilSIRENTE study. Clin Nutr. 2012;31:652–8. https://doi.org/10.1016/j.clnu.2012.02.007.

69. Englesbe MJ, Patel SP, He K, Lynch RJ, Schaubel DE, Harbaugh C, et al. Sarcopenia and mortality after liver transplantation. J Am Coll Surg. 2010;211:271–8. PubMed PMID: 20670867; PubMed Central PMCID: PMCPMC2914324. https://doi.org/10.1016/j.jamcollsurg.2010.03.039.

70. Hajibandeh S, Hajibandeh S, Jarvis R, Bhogal T, Dalmia S. Meta-analysis of the effect of sarcopenia in predicting postoperative mortality in emergency and elective abdominal surgery. Surgeon. 2019;17:370–80. https://doi.org/10.1016/j.surge.2018.09.003.

71. Beaudart C, Zaaria M, Pasleau F, Reginster JY, Bruyere O. Health outcomes of sarcopenia: a systematic review and meta-analysis. PLoS One. 2017;12:e0169548. PubMed PMID: 28095426; PubMed Central PMCID: PMCPMC5240970. https://doi.org/10.1371/journal.pone.0169548.

72. Sheetz KH, Waits SA, Terjimanian MN, Sullivan J, Campbell DA, Wang SC, et al. Cost of major surgery in the sarcopenic patient. J Am Coll Surg. 2013;217:813–8. PubMed PMID: 24119996; PubMed Central PMCID: PMCPMC3809011. https://doi.org/10.1016/j.jamcollsurg.2013.04.042.

73. Simonsen C, de Heer P, Bjerre ED, Suetta C, Hojman P, Pedersen BK, et al. Sarcopenia and postoperative complication risk in gastrointestinal surgical oncology: a meta-analysis. Ann Surg. 2018;268:58–69. https://doi.org/10.1097/SLA.0000000000002679.

74. Yang Z, Zhou X, Ma B, Xing Y, Jiang X, Wang Z. Predictive value of preoperative sarcopenia in patients with gastric cancer: a meta-analysis and systematic review. J Gastrointest Surg. 2018;22:1890–902. https://doi.org/10.1007/s11605-018-3856-0.

75. Cao Q, Xiong Y, Zhong Z, Ye Q. Computed tomography-assessed sarcopenia indexes predict major complications following surgery for hepatopancreatobiliary malignancy: a meta-analysis. Ann Nutr Metab. 2019;74:24–34. https://doi.org/10.1159/000494887.
76. Huang DD, Wang SL, Zhuang CL, Zheng BS, Lu JX, Chen FF, et al. Sarcopenia, as defined by low muscle mass, strength and physical performance, predicts complications after surgery for colorectal cancer. Colorectal Dis. 2015;17:O256–64. https://doi.org/10.1111/codi.13067.
77. Elliott JA, Doyle SL, Murphy CF, King S, Guinan EM, Beddy P, et al. Sarcopenia: prevalence, and impact on operative and oncologic outcomes in the multimodal management of locally advanced esophageal cancer. Ann Surg. 2017;266:822–30. https://doi.org/10.1097/SLA.0000000000002398.
78. Schizas D, Frountzas M, Lidoriki I, Spartalis E, Toutouzas K, Dimitroulis D, et al. Sarcopenia does not affect postoperative complication rates in oesophageal cancer surgery: a systematic review and meta-analysis. Ann R Coll Surg Engl. 2020;102:120–32. PubMed PMID: 31508983; PubMed Central PMCID: PMCPMC6996429. https://doi.org/10.1308/rcsann.2019.0113.
79. Deng HY, Zha P, Peng L, Hou L, Huang KL, Li XY. Preoperative sarcopenia is a predictor of poor prognosis of esophageal cancer after esophagectomy: a comprehensive systematic review and meta-analysis. Dis Esophagus. 2019;32:doy115. https://doi.org/10.1093/dote/doy115.
80. Guo Z, Gu C, Gan S, Li Y, Xiang S, Gong L, et al. Sarcopenia as a predictor of postoperative outcomes after urologic oncology surgery: a systematic review and meta-analysis. Urol Oncol. 2020;38:560–73. https://doi.org/10.1016/j.urolonc.2020.02.014.
81. Allanson ER, Peng Y, Choi A, Hayes S, Janda M, Obermair A. A systematic review and meta-analysis of sarcopenia as a prognostic factor in gynecological malignancy. Int J Gynecol Cancer. 2020;30:1791–7. https://doi.org/10.1136/ijgc-2020-001678.
82. Ubachs J, Ziemons J, Minis-Rutten IJG, Kruitwagen R, Kleijnen J, Lambrechts S, et al. Sarcopenia and ovarian cancer survival: a systematic review and meta-analysis. J Cachexia Sarcopenia Muscle. 2019;10:1165–74. PubMed PMID: 31389674; PubMed Central PMCID: PMCPMC6903439. https://doi.org/10.1002/jcsm.12468.
83. Yoshimura Y, Wakabayashi H, Yamada M, Kim H, Harada A, Arai H. Interventions for treating sarcopenia: a systematic review and meta-analysis of randomized controlled studies. J Am Med Dir Assoc. 2017;18:553 e1–e16. https://doi.org/10.1016/j.jamda.2017.03.019.
84. Shinohara S, Otsuki R, Kobayashi K, Sugaya M, Matsuo M, Nakagawa M. Impact of sarcopenia on surgical outcomes in non-small cell lung cancer. Ann Surg Oncol. 2020;27:2427–35. https://doi.org/10.1245/s10434-020-08224-z.
85. Weerink LBM, van der Hoorn A, van Leeuwen BL, de Bock GH. Low skeletal muscle mass and postoperative morbidity in surgical oncology: a systematic review and meta-analysis. J Cachexia Sarcopenia Muscle. 2020;11:636–49. PubMed PMID: 32125769; PubMed Central PMCID: PMCPMC7296274. https://doi.org/10.1002/jcsm.12529.
86. Dent E, Morley JE, Cruz-Jentoft AJ, Arai H, Kritchevsky SB, Guralnik J, et al. International clinical practice guidelines for sarcopenia (ICFSR): screening, diagnosis and management. J Nutr Health Aging. 2018;22:1148–61. https://doi.org/10.1007/s12603-018-1139-9.
87. Holubar SD, Soop M. Perioperative optimization of patient nutritional status. In: Ljungqvist O, Francis N, Urman R, editors. Enhanced recovery after surgery. Cham: Springer; 2020.
88. Peel NM, Kuys SS, Klein K. Gait speed as a measure in geriatric assessment in clinical settings: a systematic review. J Gerontol A Biol Sci Med Sci. 2013;68:39–46. https://doi.org/10.1093/gerona/gls174.
89. Ida S, Kaneko R, Murata K. SARC-F for screening of sarcopenia among older adults: a meta-analysis of screening test accuracy. J Am Med Dir Assoc. 2018;19:685–9. https://doi.org/10.1016/j.jamda.2018.04.001.
90. Bahat G, Tufan A, Tufan F, Kilic C, Akpinar TS, Kose M, et al. Cut-off points to identify sarcopenia according to European working group on sarcopenia in older people (EWGSOP) definition. Clin Nutr. 2016;35:1557–63. https://doi.org/10.1016/j.clnu.2016.02.002.

91. Ivanoski S, Vasilevska NV. Future ultrasou nd biomarkers for sarcopenia: elastography, contrast-enhanced ultrasound, and speed of sound ultrasound imaging. Semin Musculoskelet Radiol. 2020;24:194–200. https://doi.org/10.1055/s-0040-1701630.

92. Buettner S, Wagner D, Kim Y, Margonis GA, Makary MA, Wilson A, et al. Inclusion of sarcopenia outperforms the modified frailty index in predicting 1-year mortality among 1,326 patients undergoing gastrointestinal surgery for a malignant indication. J Am Coll Surg. 2016;222:397–407 e2. https://doi.org/10.1016/j.jamcollsurg.2015.12.020.

93. Scheede-Bergdahl C, Minnella EM, Carli F. Multi-modal prehabilitation: addressing the why, when, what, how, who and where next? Anaesthesia. 2019;74(Suppl 1):20–6. https://doi.org/10.1111/anae.14505.

94. Hill A, Arora RC, Engelman DT, Stoppe C. Preoperative treatment of malnutrition and sarcopenia in cardiac surgery: new frontiers. Crit Care Clin. 2020;36:593–616. https://doi.org/10.1016/j.ccc.2020.06.002.

95. Carli F, Gillis C, Scheede-Bergdahl C. Promoting a culture of prehabilitation for the surgical cancer patient. Acta Oncol. 2017;56:128–33. https://doi.org/10.108 0/0284186X.2016.1266081.

96. Weimann A. Is there a rationale for perioperative nutrition therapy in the times of ERAS? Innov Surg Sci. 2019;4:152–7. https://doi.org/10.1515/iss-2019-0012.

97. Bruns ER, van den Heuvel B, Buskens CJ, van Duijvendijk P, Festen S, Wassenaar EB, et al. The effects of physical prehabilitation in elderly patients undergoing colorectal surgery: a systematic review. Colorectal Dis. 2016;18:O267–77. https://doi.org/10.1111/codi.13429.

98. Milder DA, Pillinger NL, Kam PCA. The role of prehabilitation in frail surgical patients: a systematic review. Acta Anaesthesiol Scand. 2018;62:1356–66. https://doi.org/10.1111/aas.13239.

99. Carli F, Zavorsky GS. Optimizing functional exercise capacity in the elderly surgical population. Curr Opin Clin Nutr Metab Care. 2005;8:23–32. https://doi.org/10.1097/00075197-200501000-00005.

100. Barberan-Garcia A, Ubre M, Roca J, Lacy AM, Burgos F, Risco R, et al. Personalised prehabilitation in high-risk patients undergoing elective major abdominal surgery: a randomized blinded controlled trial. Ann Surg. 2018;267:50–6. https://doi.org/10.1097/SLA.0000000000002293.

101. Durand MJ, Beckert AK, Peterson CY, Ludwig KA, Ridolfi TJ, Lauer KK, et al. You are only as frail as your arteries: prehabilitation of elderly surgical patients. Curr Anesthesiol Rep. 2019;9:380–6. https://doi.org/10.1007/s40140-019-00357-6.

102. Howard R, Yin YS, McCandless L, Wang S, Englesbe M, Machado-Aranda D. Taking control of your surgery: impact of a prehabilitation program on major abdominal surgery. J Am Coll Surg. 2019;228:72–80. PubMed PMID: 30359831; PubMed Central PMCID: PMCPMC6309718. https://doi.org/10.1016/j.jamcollsurg.2018.09.018.

103. Lobo DN, Gianotti L, Adiamah A, Barazzoni R, Deutz NEP, Dhatariya K, et al. Perioperative nutrition: recommendations from the ESPEN expert group. Clin Nutr. 2020;39:3211–27. https://doi.org/10.1016/j.clnu.2020.03.038.

104. Weimann A, Braga M, Carli F, Higashiguchi T, Hubner M, Klek S, et al. ESPEN guideline: clinical nutrition in surgery. Clin Nutr. 2017;36:623–50. https://doi.org/10.1016/j.clnu.2017.02.013.

105. Elia M, Normand C, Norman K, Laviano A. A systematic review of the cost and cost effectiveness of using standard oral nutritional supplements in the hospital setting. Clin Nutr. 2016;35:370–80. https://doi.org/10.1016/j.clnu.2015.05.010.

106. Pierson LM, Herbert WG, Norton HJ, Kiebzak GM, Griffith P, Fedor JM, et al. Effects of combined aerobic and resistance training versus aerobic training alone in cardiac rehabilitation. J Cardiopulm Rehabil. 2001;21:101–10. https://doi.org/10.1097/00008483-200103000-00007.

107. Carvalho J, Mota J, Soares JM. Strength training vs. aerobic training: cardiovascular tolerance in elderly adults. Rev Port Cardiol. 2003;22:1315–30.

108. Fatouros IG, Taxildaris K, Tokmakidis SP, Kalapotharakos V, Aggelousis N, Athanasopoulos S, et al. The effects of strength training, cardiovascular training and their

combination on flexibility of inactive older adults. Int J Sports Med. 2002;23:112–9. https://doi.org/10.1055/s-2002-20130.

109. Mayo JJ, Kravitz L. A review of the acute cardiovascular responses to resistance exercise of healthy young and older adults. J Strength Cond Res. 1999;13:90–6. PubMed PMID: 00124278-199902000-00016.

110. Topp R, Ditmyer M, King K, Doherty K, Hornyak J III. The effect of bed rest and potential of prehabilitation on patients in the intensive care unit. AACN Clin Issues. 2002;13:263–76. https://doi.org/10.1097/00044067-200205000-00011.

111. Ditmyer MM, Topp R, Pifer M. Prehabilitation in preparation for orthopaedic surgery. Orthop Nurs. 2002;21:43–51; quiz 2–4. https://doi.org/10.1097/00006416-200209000-00008.

112. Izquierdo M, Hakkinen K, Ibanez J, Anton A, Garrues M, Ruesta M, et al. Effects of strength training on submaximal and maximal endurance performance capacity in middle-aged and older men. J Strength Cond Res. 2003;17:129–39. https://doi.org/10.1519/1533-4287(2003)017<0129:eostos>2.0.co;2.

113. Kalapotharakos VI, Michalopoulou M, Godolias G, Tokmakidis SP, Malliou PV, Gourgoulis V. The effects of high- and moderate-resistance training on muscle function in the elderly. J Aging Phys Act. 2004;12:131–43. https://doi.org/10.1123/japa.12.2.131.

114. Liu-Ambrose T, Khan KM, Eng JJ, Janssen PA, Lord SR, McKay HA. Resistance and agility training reduce fall risk in women aged 75 to 85 with low bone mass: a 6-month randomized, controlled trial. J Am Geriatr Soc. 2004;52:657–65. PubMed PMID: 15086643; PubMed Central PMCID: PMCPMC3344816. https://doi.org/10.1111/j.1532-5415.2004.52200.x.

115. Wynter-Blyth V, Moorthy K. Prehabilitation: preparing patients for surgery. BMJ. 2017;358:j3702. https://doi.org/10.1136/bmj.j3702.

116. Denison HJ, Cooper C, Sayer AA, Robinson SM. Prevention and optimal management of sarcopenia: a review of combined exercise and nutrition interventions to improve muscle outcomes in older people. Clin Interv Aging. 2015;10:859–69. PubMed PMID: 25999704; PubMed Central PMCID: PMCPMC4435046. https://doi.org/10.2147/CIA.S55842.

117. Heger P, Probst P, Wiskemann J, Steindorf K, Diener MK, Mihaljevic AL. A systematic review and meta-analysis of physical exercise prehabilitation in major abdominal surgery (PROSPERO 2017 CRD42017080366). J Gastrointest Surg. 2020;24:1375–85. https://doi.org/10.1007/s11605-019-04287-w.

118. Kehlet H. Fast-track surgery—an update on physiological care principles to enhance recovery. Langenbecks Arch Surg. 2011;396:585–90. https://doi.org/10.1007/s00423-011-0790-y.

119. Vlug MS, Wind J, Hollmann MW, Ubbink DT, Cense HA, Engel AF, et al. Laparoscopy in combination with fast track multimodal management is the best perioperative strategy in patients undergoing colonic surgery: a randomized clinical trial (LAFA-study). Ann Surg. 2011;254:868–75. https://doi.org/10.1097/SLA.0b013e31821fd1ce.

120. Spanjersberg WR, Reurings J, Keus F, van Laarhoven CJ. Fast track surgery versus conventional recovery strategies for colorectal surgery. Cochrane Database Syst Rev. 2011:CD007635. https://doi.org/10.1002/14651858.CD007635.pub2.

121. Lau CS, Chamberlain RS. Enhanced recovery after surgery programs improve patient outcomes and recovery: a meta-analysis. World J Surg. 2017;41:899–913. https://doi.org/10.1007/s00268-016-3807-4.

122. Greco M, Capretti G, Beretta L, Gemma M, Pecorelli N, Braga M. Enhanced recovery program in colorectal surgery: a meta-analysis of randomized controlled trials. World J Surg. 2014;38:1531–41. https://doi.org/10.1007/s00268-013-2416-8.

123. Ostermann S, Morel P, Chale JJ, Bucher P, Konrad B, Meier RPH, et al. Randomized controlled trial of enhanced recovery program dedicated to elderly patients after colorectal surgery. Dis Colon Rectum. 2019;62:1105–16. https://doi.org/10.1097/DCR.0000000000001442.

124. Pedziwiatr M, Pisarska M, Major P, Grochowska A, Matlok M, Przeczek K, et al. Laparoscopic colorectal cancer surgery combined with enhanced recovery after surgery

protocol (ERAS) reduces the negative impact of sarcopenia on short-term outcomes. Eur J Surg Oncol. 2016;42:779–87. https://doi.org/10.1016/j.ejso.2016.03.037.
125. Ni Bhuachalla E, Cushen S, Murphy T, Ryan A. Changes in nutritional status after minimally invasive oesophagectomy with an enhanced recovery after surgery (ERAS) programme & aggressive nutritional intervention; results of a prospective investigation. Proc Nutr Soc. 2015;74:E212. Epub 09/11. https://doi.org/10.1017/S0029665115002542.

Acute Sarcopenia: Definition and Actual Issues

10

Carly Welch

10.1 Acute Sarcopenia: The Last Remaining Acute Organ Insufficiency

The revised European Working Group on Sarcopenia in Older People 2 (EWGSOP2) definition distinguishes acute and chronic sarcopenia [1]. Acute sarcopenia is defined as declines in muscle quantity/quality and/or function leading to incident sarcopenia within 6 months, normally following a stressor event [1]. As has been described, sarcopenia can be considered as muscle insufficiency [2]; this can be either acute or chronic. Acute sarcopenia should be considered as acute organ insufficiency, akin to acute organ dysfunction elsewhere (e.g., acute kidney injury, delirium) [3]. Unfortunately, changes in muscle quantity/quality and function are currently not routinely measured in clinical practice. It is not known how acute sarcopenia relates to longer term outcomes. Deteriorations in muscle quantity, quality, and function experienced following a stressor event may be partially recoverable, but may increase the risk of chronic sarcopenia over time (Fig. 10.1) [3].

Acute sarcopenia, in line with chronic sarcopenia, is currently defined by the demonstration of muscle function (normally handgrip strength) and muscle quantity/quality more than two standard deviations (SDs) below the mean of a young healthy reference population [1]. However, this diagnosis will only encompass the

C. Welch (✉)
Institute of Inflammation and Ageing, College of Medical and Dental Sciences, University of Birmingham, Birmingham, UK

Medical Research Council - Versus Arthritis Centre for Musculoskeletal Ageing Research, University of Birmingham and University of Nottingham, Birmingham, UK

Department of Geriatric Medicine, University Hospitals Birmingham NHS Trust, Birmingham, UK
e-mail: c.welch@bham.ac.uk

© Springer Nature Switzerland AG 2021
N. Veronese et al. (eds.), *Sarcopenia*, Practical Issues in Geriatrics,
https://doi.org/10.1007/978-3-030-80038-3_10

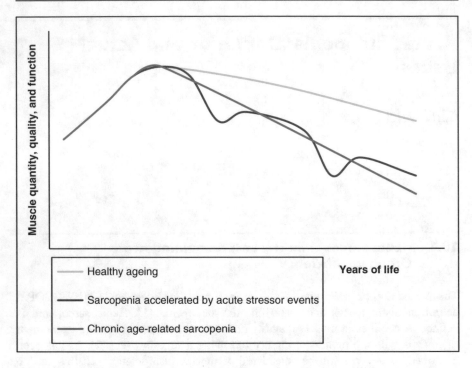

Fig. 10.1 Hypothesised trajectories of acute and chronic sarcopenia (adapted from previously published figure [3]). Deteriorations in muscle quantity, quality, and function may be partially recoverable but may be associated with an acceleration in chronic sarcopenia over time

most extreme cases where the muscle has already reached the point of insufficiency. Indeed, it is recognised that in individuals with previously normal muscle quantity/ quality or function, declines that do not acutely meet criteria for sarcopenia may still be highly significant for the individual [3]. In these cases, an acute percentage decline may be significant and warrant treatment. At present, no consensus cut-off for a percentage decline or dynamic change in muscle quantity/quality or function has been agreed. Older adults are considered most at risk; however, it is increasingly recognised that sarcopenia can occur at any age, particularly in the presence of organ dysfunction elsewhere [4]. Acute sarcopenia may affect younger individuals with underlying morbidity or in the presence of critical illness.

10.2 Mechanisms and Drivers of Acute Sarcopenia

The precise mechanisms involved in the development of acute sarcopenia and biological and clinical risk factors remain undetermined [3]. Figure 10.2 demonstrates how proposed mechanisms and drivers interact. Determining factors that are most predictive of risk of acute sarcopenia will enable targeted interventions towards prevention, as well as treatment. Acute sarcopenia is hypothesised to be caused by

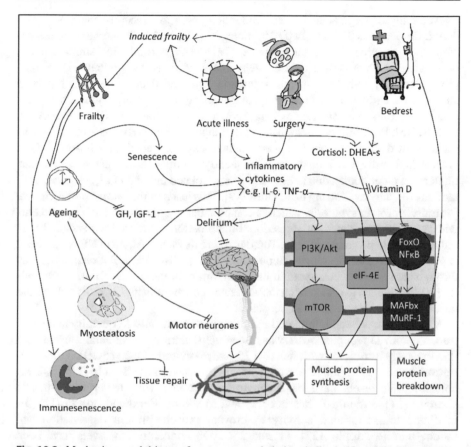

Fig. 10.2 Mechanisms and drivers of acute sarcopenia in hospitalised older adults. Acute sarcopenia is considered to be precipitated by a combination of heightened inflammation and bedrest, on a background of age-associated vulnerability. This leads to an imbalance in muscle protein synthesis and degradation. Inhibited pathways are shown by transverse double lines, and upregulated pathways are shown by arrows. *GH* growth hormone, *IGF-1* insulin-like growth factor 1, *IL-6* Interleukin 6, *TNF-α* tumour necrosis factor alpha, *DHEA-s* Dehydroepiandrosterone sulphate

a combination of reduced physical activity, increased inflammatory surge, and anabolic resistance (blunted muscle protein synthesis with expected protein intake) [3]. Hospitalisation is frequently associated with periods of bedrest. Studies involving healthy volunteers have demonstrated that bedrest is associated with declines in muscle quantity, strength, and aerobic performance and that this effect is exacerbated by age [5, 6]. Bedrest has been shown to lead to reduced muscle protein synthesis via altered expression of muscle-specific E3 ubiquitin protein ligases Muscle Atrophy F-box (MAFbx) and Muscle RING Finger protein-1 (MuRF-1) [7], increased insulin resistance [8], and reduced oxidation of saturated dietary fat [9] in healthy younger adults. However, it is not known how muscle "senses" bedrest to precipitate these effects [10].

Acute illness (e.g., acute bacterial infection and, most recently, the global pandemic Coronavirus 2019, COVID-19, infection [11]) and major surgery are associated with systemic inflammatory response [12] and endocrinological stress response (e.g., increased cortisol, decreased dehydroepiandrosterone sulphate (DHEA-s)) [13]. Medically induced hypercortisolaemia (hydrocortisone injection) has been shown to exacerbate loss of muscle quantity during bedrest [14], and synthetic glucocorticoid (dexamethasone) has been shown to upregulate MuRF-1 and MAFbx tenfold [15]. Preliminary research suggested that baseline DHEA-s levels may correlate with declines in physical performance experienced during hospitalisation [16]. Additionally, nutritional intake frequently declines during acute illness, particularly in older adults, due to age- and illness-related anorexia [17], physical limitations [18], and swallowing difficulties [19]. This leads to ineffective protein intake for muscle protein synthesis, which is compounded by higher protein requirements with acute illness-related inflammation. Inflammation associated with acute illness reduces muscle protein synthesis. Tumour Necrosis Factor Alpha (TNF-α) has been shown to decrease messenger ribonucleic acid (mRNA) translational efficiency through alterations in eukaryotic translation initiation factor 4E (eIF-4E) availability [20]. This leads to a state of anabolic resistance whereby higher protein doses are needed to stimulate an adequate response.

Vitamin D has been implicated in the regulation of muscle quantity and function. Vitamin D receptor mRNA has been demonstrated in skeletal muscle, and this inversely correlates with inactive 25-hydroxyvitamin D3 (25OHD3) concentration levels [21]. Active serum 1,25-dihydroxyvitamin D3 (1α,25(OH)2D3) concentration levels have been shown to correlate with lower limb muscle strength [21]. Vitamin D has been shown to inhibit Forkhead box O (FoxO)-mediated transcriptional activity to prevent muscle protein degradation and induce muscle atrophy [22]. Plasma 25OHD3 concentration levels have been shown to decline following elective surgery, with this change correlating with inflammation [23]. Therefore, vitamin D deficiency or insufficiency may contribute towards the development of acute sarcopenia following surgery or acute illness.

Ageing is associated with cellular senescence; a process whereby cells stop dividing [24]. Senescence is considered to be protective against cancer by preventing uncontrolled cell division and replication [24]. However, senescent cells have been shown to be metabolically active and contribute to production of inflammatory mediators (e.g., TNF-α, Interleukin-6, IL-6) [25]. Senescence-associated inflammation may drive sarcopenia via activation of Nuclear Factor Kappa-light-chain-enhancer of activated B cells (NFκB) and FoxO in muscle by pro-inflammatory cytokines [26]. Activation of NFκB and FoxO is considered to lead to increased muscle protein degradation via activation of MAFbx and MuRF-1 [15, 27]. Secretion of growth hormone (GH) and insulin-like growth factor-1 (IGF-1) declines with age after approximately 60 years of age; the "somatopause" which has also been demonstrated in other mammals [28]. IGF-1 stimulates muscle protein synthesis via stimulation of the mammalian/mechanistic target of rapamycin (mTOR) via the phosphatidylinositol-3-kinase (PI3K)/alpha serine/threonine-protein kinase (Akt) pathway, thus reduced IGF-1 secretion with age leads to reduced muscle protein synthesis [29].

Additionally, the number of motor neurones has been shown to decline with age [30]. However, mechanisms of this are unclear; this may relate to feedback from already dysfunctional muscle, impaired signalling from the central nervous system, local degeneration, or a combination of all of these factors [31]. Additionally, prevalence of myosteatosis (intra- and intermuscular fat infiltration) increases with age [32], leading to reduced muscle quality and impaired physical performance [33]. The mechanisms that drive myosteatosis with ageing are unclear. It has been proposed that this may be driven by the differentiation of satellite cells (pluripotent muscle "stem" cells involved in muscle regeneration) into adipocytes, or increased fatty acid transport, uptake, and storage [34]. Adipose tissue itself secretes proinflammatory cytokines [35], which further induces muscle protein degradation.

Ageing and frailty, the syndrome of increased likelihood of reduced resolution of homeostasis following a stressor event [36], are associated with immunesenescence [37]. Impairments in the immune response can lead to impairments in muscle metabolism. Following injury, immune cells are recruited into muscles in order to initiate pathogen clearance and tissue repair [38]. Frailty is associated with impaired migration of neutrophils and other immune cells meaning this process may be impaired [39], potentially increasing the risk of acute sarcopenia in this vulnerable population. Acute illness may also lead to a state of "induced frailty," which is associated with systemic inflammation and catabolism [40], thus compounding the development of acute sarcopenia.

Frail older adults are also at increased risk of development of delirium during acute illness and hospitalisation [41]. Delirium is an acute severe neuropsychiatric condition, which is increasingly recognised to be associated with systemic inflammation [42]. Combined with the cognitive effects of delirium which may directly impact upon the initiation of motor control, this may also be associated with increased risk of acute sarcopenia. Although acute declines in muscle quantity, quality, or function may be experienced during acute illness at any age, it is this interplay between ageing, immunesenescence, and acute illness factors that makes older adults most vulnerable.

Conversely, there is increasing evidence that older adults with chronic sarcopenia and severely reduced muscle quantity experience minimal further declines in muscle quantity during periods of immobility and acute illness. Bedrest studies have involved participants who were far younger and fitter than the typical population of older adults admitted to hospital within developed countries; these studies did not involve participants with frailty or chronic sarcopenia [5, 6]. This "end-stage" of muscle organ dysfunction may lead to blunting of responsiveness of communication between the muscle and immune system. In the presence of pronounced chronic sarcopenia, the muscle may no longer respond and react to systemic inflammation. This is important as this group of individuals may require a different focus of treatment to prevent further loss of function. Increased understanding will ensure that clinicians can appropriately prognosticate for their patients and that the information patients are given is correct and of relevance to them.

10.3   Overlap with Other Clinical Syndromes

Acute sarcopenia can be considered part of a spectrum of acute muscle wasting disorders. Intensive Care Unit-Acquired Weakness (ICU-AW) is a recognised complication following admission to critical care. Similarly to acute sarcopenia, it is considered to arise due to a combination of prolonged bedrest and acute surge in systemic inflammation. Following the COVID-19 pandemic, many patients who were previously fit with normal muscle quantity and function who survived admission to critical care with COVID-19 infection were found to develop profound skeletal muscle atrophy and required intense targeted multidisciplinary rehabilitation [11]. The longer term effects of ICU-AW on these patients remain unknown.

Another overlapping syndrome with acute sarcopenia is that of "induced frailty" [40], as described in the previous section. Similar to sarcopenia, frailty can be considered a dynamic process. A patient who was previously fit and robust may become more dependent and vulnerable as a result of acute illness, and a patient who was previously mildly frail may become moderately or even severely frail [43]. Importantly, however, this process is potentially reversible [44]. Nonetheless, this state will increase the risk of adverse outcomes if they should develop a second acute illness and may increase their risk of frailty in the future, even after they have recovered.

"Deconditioning" is another term that has been widely used in the medical literature. However, there is no one recognised definition for this term [45]. Rather it is an all-encompassing term that is not organ-specific, but implies a worsening in the overall health state of the individual, related to illness, bedrest, or restrictive caregiving. It encompasses the development of any or all of pressure ulcers, urinary incontinence, demotivation, falls related to instability and balance disorders, as well as declines in muscle strength [46]. Declines in muscle strength in the context of deconditioning may relate to fatigue, lack of motivation, or acute sarcopenia.

10.4   Diagnosis of Acute Sarcopenia in Clinical Settings

Handgrip strength is recommended for initial assessment for sarcopenia by EWGSOP2, with low muscle quantity or quality being only confirmatory [1]. However, this definition was developed with a focus on chronic sarcopenia. In the context of acute illness, handgrip strength may be affected by fatigue, impairments in consciousness, and effort [47]. This may mean that handgrip strength actually increases during the course of illness, representing a recovery from illness fatigue rather than a recovery of muscle function. In addition, acute changes in muscle quantity and quality may occur rapidly, with longer term impacts on muscle function [3]. Therefore, measurement of muscle quantity or quality may be especially important in the assessment of acute sarcopenia compared to chronic sarcopenia. Computed tomography (CT), magnetic resonance imaging (MRI), or dual-energy X-ray absorptiometry (DXA) are recommended for gold standard quantification of muscle quantification by EWGSOP2 [1]. However, none of these tests can be performed at the bedside, and all have limitations when performed serially (e.g., due to the risk of ionising radiation, physical/psychological burden to patients).

Bioelectrical impedance analysis (BIA) has been used for the assessment of chronic sarcopenia, but measurements may be affected by fluid balance [48]. Ultrasound is recognised as a developing alternative technique for muscle quantity and quality assessment. Ultrasound has benefits in that serial measurements can be taken with ease in a variety of environments including the outpatient department, inpatient wards, and in the community. It is safe, non-invasive, does not involve ionising radiation, and requires minimal training. However, preliminary research has suggested that muscle quantity and quality may be affected by hypervolaemia in post-operative patients [16, 49].

At present, acute sarcopenia is best identified as part of a comprehensive assessment. Anthropometry may lead to falsely elevated results in the presence of increased oedema. However, demonstration of reductions in calf circumference should prompt multidisciplinary assessment and management including nutrition, physical activity, and review of medical management, e.g., drugs. Where a dynamometer is not available, serial assessment of patients' abilities to complete chair stands can be used to demonstrate responsiveness of muscle strength, provided the patient is able to comply with instructions and sit out in a chair. Integration of the Hierarchical Assessment of Balance and Mobility (HABAM) into clinical practice in acute settings enables monitoring of function in the same way as vital signs [50]. Further research is necessary to assess the sensitivity to change of measures such as fatigue resistance in the acute setting, the time for force to decline by more than 50% of peak strength [51].

10.5   Proposed Interventions

Most effective prevention and intervention strategies are unknown [3]. However, it is conceivable that effective interventions will target any or all of the potential mechanisms described. This is likely to include a combination of physical activity (e.g., resistance exercise to combat negative effects of bedrest), nutritional (e.g., high protein supplementation in view of anabolic resistance), and pharmaceutical interventions (e.g., vitamin D, DHEA-s, novel agents). Neuromuscular electrical stimulation uses low-frequency, low-amplitude electrical current to activate motor neurones resulting in muscle contraction, and has been proposed as another potential treatment [3]. A recent systematic review of interventions to ameliorate negative changes in muscle quantity and function in hospitalised older adults provides an assimilation of evidence towards interventions for acute sarcopenia [52]. There is currently no definitive evidence for effective interventions; effect sizes for intervention types differed between trials, and there was high heterogeneity in terms of interventions that were trialled and outcome measures. However, many interventions have been trialled and shown to be safe and feasible. This is a rapidly growing research field, and knowledge that trials of complex interventions in complex populations are feasible should assist in driving further effectiveness trials, with potential for direct clinical implementation.

10.6 Recommendations for Future Research

Clinical characterisation studies [53] will assist to enhance understanding of the prevalence and outcomes of acute sarcopenia across multiple settings. Detailed evaluation will enable risk stratification towards targeted interventions. Research should strive to enhance knowledge of underlying mechanisms and expected intervention efficacy, whilst pragmatically trialling interventions for effectiveness. Increased understanding of mechanisms may also enable the identification of novel biomarkers for incorporation into clinical practice. Research that evaluates the long-term consequences of acute sarcopenia is strongly encouraged.

10.7 Conclusions

Acute sarcopenia is defined by the development of incident sarcopenia within six months and is normally proceeded by a stressor event. The longer term consequences of acute sarcopenia are unknown, but it is considered to increase the risk of developing chronic sarcopenia over time. Acute sarcopenia is considered to arise due to a combination of bedrest and inflammatory surge; these effects may be enhanced by underlying predisposition with age and frailty. Incorporation of serial measurements of muscle quantity and function in clinical practice will enable early identification of acute sarcopenia development. Further research is necessary to increase understanding of underlying mechanisms and enable targeted interventions.

References

1. Cruz-Jentoft AJ, Bahat G, Bauer J, Boirie Y, Bruyere O, Cederholm T, et al. Sarcopenia: revised European consensus on definition and diagnosis. Age Ageing. 2019;48(1):16–31.
2. Cruz-Jentoft AJ. Sarcopenia, the last organ insufficiency. Eur Geriatr Med. 2016;7(3):195–6.
3. Welch C, Hassan-Smith Z, Greig C, Lord J, Jackson T. Acute sarcopenia secondary to hospitalisation—an emerging condition affecting older adults. Aging Dis. 2018;9(1):151–64.
4. Cruz-Jentoft AJ, Sayer AA. Sarcopenia. Lancet. 2019;393(10191):2636–46.
5. Kortebein P, Ferrando A, Lombeida J, Wolfe R, Evans WJ. Effect of 10 days of bed rest on skeletal muscle in healthy older adults. JAMA. 2007;297(16):1772–4.
6. Tanner RE, Brunker LB, Agergaard J, Barrows KM, Briggs RA, Kwon OS, et al. Age-related differences in lean mass, protein synthesis and skeletal muscle markers of proteolysis after bed rest and exercise rehabilitation. J Physiol. 2015;593(18):4259–73.
7. Jones SW, Hill RJ, Krasney PA, O'Connor B, Peirce N, Greenhaff PL. Disuse atrophy and exercise rehabilitation in humans profoundly affects the expression of genes associated with the regulation of skeletal muscle mass. FASEB J. 2004;18(9):1025–7.

8. Hamburg NM, McMackin CJ, Huang AL, Shenouda SM, Widlansky ME, Schulz E, et al. Physical inactivity rapidly induces insulin resistance and microvascular dysfunction in healthy volunteers. Arterioscler Thromb Vasc Biol. 2007;27(12):2650–6.

9. Bergouignan A, Schoeller DA, Normand S, Gauquelin-Koch G, Laville M, Shriver T, et al. Effect of physical inactivity on the oxidation of saturated and monounsaturated dietary fatty acids: results of a randomized trial. PLoS Clin Trials. 2006;1(5):e27-e.

10. Crossland H, Skirrow S, Puthucheary ZA, Constantin-Teodosiu D, Greenhaff PL. The impact of immobilisation and inflammation on the regulation of muscle mass and insulin resistance: different routes to similar end-points. J Physiol. 2019;597(5):1259–70.

11. Welch C, Greig C, Masud T, Wilson D, Jackson T. COVID-19 and acute sarcopenia. Aging Dis. 2021;11(6):1345–51.

12. Smeets BJJ, Brinkman DJ, Horsten ECJ, Langius JAE, Rutten HJT, de Jonge WJ, et al. The effect of Myopenia on the inflammatory response early after colorectal surgery. Nutr Cancer. 2018;70(3):460–6.

13. Butcher SK, Killampalli V, Lascelles D, Wang K, Alpar EK, Lord JM. Raised cortisol:DHEAS ratios in the elderly after injury: potential impact upon neutrophil function and immunity. Aging Cell. 2005;4(6):319–24.

14. Paddon-Jones D, Sheffield-Moore M, Cree MG, Hewlings SJ, Aarsland A, Wolfe RR, et al. Atrophy and impaired muscle protein synthesis during prolonged inactivity and stress. J Clin Endocrinol Metabol. 2006;91(12):4836–41.

15. Bodine SC, Latres E, Baumhueter S, Lai VK-M, Nunez L, Clarke BA, et al. Identification of ubiquitin ligases required for skeletal muscle atrophy. Science. 2001;294(5547):1704–8.

16. Welch C, Greig CA, Hassan-Smith ZK, Pinkney TD, Lord JM, Jackson TA. A pilot observational study measuring acute sarcopenia in older colorectal surgery patients. BMC Res Notes. 2019;12(1):24.

17. Landi F, Calvani R, Tosato M, Martone AM, Ortolani E, Savera G, et al. Anorexia of aging: risk factors, consequences, and potential treatments. Nutrients. 2016;8(2):69.

18. Simmons SF, Schnelle JF. Individualized feeding assistance care for nursing home residents: staffing requirements to implement two interventions. J Gerontol A Biol Sci Med Sci. 2004;59(9):M966–73.

19. Jardine M, Miles A, Allen J. Dysphagia onset in older adults during unrelated hospital admission: quantitative videofluoroscopic measures. Geriatrics (Basel). 2018;3(4):66.

20. Lang CH, Frost RA, Nairn AC, MacLean DA, Vary TC. TNF-α impairs heart and skeletal muscle protein synthesis by altering translation initiation. Am J Physiol Endocrinol Metab. 2002;282(2):E336–E47.

21. Hassan-Smith ZK, Jenkinson C, Smith DJ, Hernandez I, Morgan SA, Crabtree NJ, et al. 25-hydroxyvitamin D3 and 1,25-dihydroxyvitamin D3 exert distinct effects on human skeletal muscle function and gene expression. PLoS One. 2017;12(2):e0170665.

22. Hirose Y, Onishi T, Miura S, Hatazawa Y, Kamei Y. Vitamin D attenuates FOXO1-target atrophy gene expression in C2C12 muscle cells. J Nutr Sci Vitaminol. 2018;64(3):229–32.

23. Reid D, Toole BJ, Knox S, Talwar D, Harten J, O'Reilly DS, et al. The relation between acute changes in the systemic inflammatory response and plasma 25-hydroxyvitamin D concentrations after elective knee arthroplasty. Am J Clin Nutr. 2011;93(5):1006–11.

24. van Deursen JM. The role of senescent cells in ageing. Nature. 2014;509(7501):439–46.

25. Coppé J-P, Patil CK, Rodier F, Sun Y, Muñoz DP, Goldstein J, et al. Senescence-associated secretory phenotypes reveal cell-nonautonomous functions of oncogenic RAS and the p53 tumor suppressor. PLoS Biol. 2008;6(12):e301.

26. De Larichaudy J, Zufferli A, Serra F, Isidori AM, Naro F, Dessalle K, et al. TNF-α- and tumor-induced skeletal muscle atrophy involves sphingolipid metabolism. Skelet Muscle. 2012;2(1):2.

27. Gomes MD, Lecker SH, Jagoe RT, Navon A, Goldberg AL. Atrogin-1, a muscle-specific F-box protein highly expressed during muscle atrophy. Proc Natl Acad Sci U S A. 2001;98(25):14440–5.

28. Junnila RK, List EO, Berryman DE, Murrey JW, Kopchick JJ. The GH/IGF-1 axis in ageing and longevity. Nat Rev Endocrinol. 2013;9(6):366–76.
29. Barclay RD, Burd NA, Tyler C, Tillin NA, Mackenzie RW. The role of the IGF-1 signaling cascade in muscle protein synthesis and anabolic resistance in aging skeletal muscle. Front Nutr. 2019;6:146.
30. Kawamura Y, Okazaki H, O'Brien PC, Dyck PJ. Lumbar Motoneurons of man: I. Number and diameter histogram of alpha and gamma axons of ventral root. J Neuropathol Exp Neurol. 1977;36(5):853–60.
31. Gonzalez-Freire M, de Cabo R, Studenski SA, Ferrucci L. The neuromuscular junction: aging at the crossroad between nerves and muscle. Front Aging Neurosci. 2014;6:208.
32. Health Aging Body Composition Study. Longitudinal study of muscle strength, quality, and adipose tissue infiltration. Am J Clin Nutr. 2009;90(6):1579–85.
33. Tuttle LJ, Sinacore DR, Mueller MJ. Intermuscular adipose tissue is muscle specific and associated with poor functional performance. J Aging Res. 2012;2012:172957.
34. Miljkovic I, Kuipers AL, Cvejkus R, Bunker CH, Patrick AL, Gordon CL, et al. Myosteatosis increases with aging and is associated with incident diabetes in African ancestry men. Obesity. 2016;24(2):476–82.
35. Kern PA, Ranganathan S, Li C, Wood L, Ranganathan G. Adipose tissue tumor necrosis factor and interleukin-6 expression in human obesity and insulin resistance. Am J Physiol Endocrinol Metab. 2001;280(5):E745–E51.
36. Clegg A, Young J, Iliffe S, Rikkert MO, Rockwood K. Frailty in elderly people. Lancet. 2013;381(9868):752–62.
37. Wilson D, Jackson T, Sapey E, Lord JM. Frailty and sarcopenia: the potential role of an aged immune system. Ageing Res Rev. 2017;36:1–10.
38. Pillon NJ, Bilan PJ, Fink LN, Klip A. Cross-talk between skeletal muscle and immune cells: muscle-derived mediators and metabolic implications. Am J Physiol Endocrinol Metab. 2013;304(5):E453–65.
39. Wilson D, Drew W, Jasper A, Crisford H, Nightingale P, Newby P, et al. Frailty is associated with neutrophil dysfunction which is correctable with phosphoinositol-3-kinase inhibitors. J Gerontol A Biol Sci Med Sci. 2020;75(12):2320–5.
40. Hawkins RB, Raymond SL, Stortz JA, Horiguchi H, Brakenridge SC, Gardner A, et al. Chronic critical illness and the persistent inflammation, immunosuppression, and catabolism syndrome. Front Immunol. 2018;9:1511.
41. Persico I, Cesari M, Morandi A, Haas J, Mazzola P, Zambon A, et al. Frailty and delirium in older adults: a systematic review and meta-analysis of the literature. J Am Geriatr Soc. 2018;66(10):2022–30.
42. Vasunilashorn SM, Ngo L, Inouye SK, Libermann TA, Jones RN, Alsop DC, et al. Cytokines and postoperative delirium in older patients undergoing major elective surgery. J Gerontol Ser A. 2015;70(10):1289–95.
43. Geense W, Zegers M, Dieperink P, Vermeulen H, van der Hoeven J, van den Boogaard M. Changes in frailty among ICU survivors and associated factors: results of a one-year prospective cohort study using the Dutch clinical frailty scale. J Crit Care. 2020;55:184–93.
44. Lang PO, Michel JP, Zekry D. Frailty syndrome: a transitional state in a dynamic process. Gerontology. 2009;55(5):539–49.
45. Wee TC, Tan YL. Should we be concerned about "acute sarcopenia" in the inpatient population? Is there a role for ultrasound evaluation? Am J Phys Med Rehabil. 2018;97(8):e74–e5.
46. Gordon S, Grimmer KA, Barras S. Assessment for incipient hospital-acquired deconditioning in acute hospital settings: a systematic literature review. J Rehabil Med. 2019;51(6):397–404.
47. Van Ancum JM, Scheerman K, Jonkman NH, Smeenk HE, Kruizinga RC, Meskers CGM, et al. Change in muscle strength and muscle mass in older hospitalized patients: a systematic review and meta-analysis. Exp Gerontol. 2017;92:34–41.
48. Nakanishi N, Tsutsumi R, Okayama Y, Takashima T, Ueno Y, Itagaki T, et al. Monitoring of muscle mass in critically ill patients: comparison of ultrasound and two bioelectrical impedance analysis devices. J Intensive Care. 2019;7(1):61.

49. Fischer A, Spiegl M, Altmann K, Winkler A, Salamon A, Themessl-Huber M, et al. Muscle mass, strength and functional outcomes in critically ill patients after cardiothoracic surgery: does neuromuscular electrical stimulation help? The Catastim 2 randomized controlled trial. Crit Care. 2016;20:30.
50. MacKnight C, Rockwood K. A hierarchical assessment of balance and mobility. Age Ageing. 1995;24(2):126–30.
51. Bautmans I, Njemini R, Lambert M, Demanet C, Mets T. Circulating acute phase mediators and skeletal muscle performance in hospitalized geriatric patients. J Gerontol Ser A. 2005;60(3):361–7.
52. Welch C, Majid Z, Greig C, Gladman J, Masud T, Jackson T. Interventions to ameliorate reductions in muscle quantity and function in hospitalised older adults: a systematic review towards acute sarcopenia treatment. Age Ageing. 2021;50(2):394–404.
53. Welch C, Greig CA, Masud T, Pinkney T, Jackson TA. Protocol for understanding acute sarcopenia: a cohort study to characterise changes in muscle quantity and physical function in older adults following hospitalisation. BMC Geriatr. 2020;20(1):239.

Sarcopenic Obesity

11

Shaun Sabico and Nasser M. Al-Daghri

11.1 Introduction

The term "sarcopenic obesity" was first coined in 1996 by Heber and colleagues, a type of body composition characterized by *"reduced lean mass with excess fat as a percentage of body weight"* [1]. As a separate entity and under normal physiologic conditions, sarcopenia is expected, given the age-related decline in muscle mass and strength. This is supported by a recent study by Santos and colleagues, where data from a large retrospective cohort of more than 400,000 anonymized participants showed that while the evolution of BMI varies widely overtime, there is a distinct pattern of progressive increase in total body fat with age, with a similar trajectory observed in lean body mass but plateauing in mid-40s, and followed by an opposing, uninterrupted decrease as the age progresses [2]. The universally accepted definition of sarcopenia, which is loss of muscle mass, strength, and physical performance, is in a way eclipsed by the heterogencity of diagnostic cut-offs used and other factors to clinically identify a patient with sarcopenia [3]. Hence, the prevalence is largely dependent on the cut-offs applied and may range from 6 to 12% in large-scale studies [4].

On the other hand, obesity or excessive fat accumulation is a by-product of unhealthy behaviors such as sedentary lifestyle and overeating, to name a few [5]. The global prevalence of adult obesity has increased to pandemic proportions since 1975 [6], with trends predicting an even higher prevalence reaching 18% in men and 21% in women by the year 2025 [7].

Sarcopenia and obesity have been observed to coexist particularly among the elderly, given the age-related alterations in body composition. Globally and as of 2019, there were an estimated 703 million individuals aged 65 years and above, and

S. Sabico (✉) · N. M. Al-Daghri
Chair for Biomarkers of Chronic Diseases, Biochemistry Department, College of Science, King Saud University, Riyadh, Saudi Arabia
e-mail: ssabico@ksu.edu.sa; ndaghri@ksu.edu.sa

© Springer Nature Switzerland AG 2021
N. Veronese et al. (eds.), *Sarcopenia*, Practical Issues in Geriatrics,
https://doi.org/10.1007/978-3-030-80038-3_11

this is expected to increase by as much as 1.5 billion in 2050 [8]. It makes sense therefore to anticipate that the incidence of sarcopenic obesity will also increase. In this chapter, we intend to shed light on what is already known in the emerging field of sarcopenic obesity, its implications, and current clinical approaches.

11.2 Pathogenesis

The pathogenesis of sarcopenic obesity has been comprehensively discussed in various literature and will not be further covered in this chapter [9–13]. In brief, non-modifiable risk factors affecting the muscle tissue (aging and age-related loss of anabolic signals that initiate decrease in muscle tissue mass), in combination with modifiable risk factors associated with obesity (physical inactivity and decreased protein intake that promote increased adiposity which triggers low-grade inflammation, insulin resistance, and hormonal changes) impair the complex cross talk between adipose and muscle tissue, leading to sarcopenic obesity. Figure 11.1 shows the simplified mechanisms leading to sarcopenic obesity.

11.3 Evolving Definition

Given the inconsistencies of preliminary available literature, early investigations on the combination of obesity with low muscle strength cautioned on the use of the terms sarcopenic obesity, and instead referred to it as obesity/muscle impairment geriatric syndrome, a type of obesity in the elderly that are at special risk for adverse outcomes [14]. Even at present, there is no consensus on the exact operational

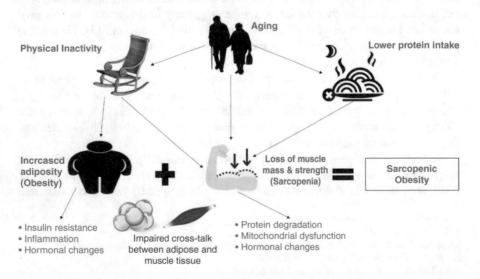

Fig. 11.1 Proposed etiology of sarcopenic obesity

diagnosis of sarcopenic obesity, making epidemiologic studies virtually incomparable. Existing definitions are based on the individual cut-offs used to diagnose sarcopenia and obesity, respectively, with both entities also having multiple cut-offs to choose from. Batsis and Villareal, in their recent comprehensive review, assembled some of the selected working definitions of sarcopenic obesity as seen in Table 11.1 [13]. Baumgartner was the first to use dual-energy X-ray absorptiometry (DXA) among the elderly obese to assess sarcopenia in combination with body fat percentage (%) [15], and also the first to identify sarcopenic obesity to be independently associated with incident disability [16]. The first study observed increasing prevalence of sarcopenic obesity from 2% among 60–69 years of age to about 10% in those >80 years [15], while the second study provided a working definition for sarcopenic obesity, which was the combination of an ALM index of <7.26 kg/m^2 and body fat mass of >28% in men; or <5.45 kg/m^2 and body fat mass of >40% in women [16, 17]. In another study, Newman and colleagues analyzed anthropometrics of more than 3000 men and women using the conventional definition of obesity (body mass index, BMI >30 kg/m^2) [17] and determined the prevalence of sarcopenia among obese participants using two definitions. Their results showed that none of the obese participants had sarcopenia using the conventional appendicular lean mass divided by height squared method (ALM/ht^2). However, when relative lean mass was adjusted for fat mass and height, and using the residuals' 20th percentile as a cut-off for sarcopenia, the prevalence was 11.5% in obese men and 21% in

Table 11.1 Selected definitions of sarcopenia with obesity

Author (year)	Sarcopenia definition	Measurement cut-off points	Obesity definition	Population
Baumgartner (2000) [15]	ALM/ht^2	DXA (men <7.26 kg/ m^2; women <5.45 kg/ m^2)	Body fat (men >27%; women >38%)	New Mexico aging process study
Newman et al. (2003) [17]	ALM/ht^2	DXA (men <7.23 kg/ m^2; women <5.67 kg/ m^2)	BMI (≥30 kg/ m^2)	New Mexico elder health survey
	ALM divided by height and fat mass	DXA (lowest 20th percentile of residuals (sex-specific))	BMI (≥30 kg/ m^2)	Health ABC study
Baumgartner et al. (2004) [16]	ALM/ht^2	DXA (men <7.26 kg/ m^2; women <5.45 kg/ m^2)	Body fat mass (men ≥28%; women ≥40%)	New Mexico elder health survey
Villareal et al. (2005), ASN–TOS [18]	ALM/ht^2	ALM (<5.45 kg/m^2, sex is not specified)	BMI (≥30 kg/ m^2)	Young healthy population
Bouchard et al. (2009) [19]	ALM/ht^2	DXA (men <8.51 kg/ m^2; women <6.29 kg/ m^2)	Body fat (men ≥28%; women ≥35%)	Nutrition as a determinant of successful aging study

Note: *ABC* ageing, body, and body composition, *ALM* appendicular lean mass, *DXA* dual-energy X-ray absorptiometry, *ht^2* height squared; The Obesity Society. Modified table taken from Batsis and Villareal [13]

women, highlighting the importance of fat mass in the evaluation of sarcopenia among the obese [18]. Lastly, Bouchard and colleagues' working definition of sarcopenic obesity was based on body fat percentage cut-off defined by the American College of Sports Medicine and ALM index based on previously obtained data of young adults aged 20–35 years (<6.29 kg/m^2 in women and <8.51 kg/m^2 in men) [19]. A summary of working definitions has been provided in Table 11.1.

Clearly, while the operational definitions provided in this chapter are in no way exhaustive, it is reasonable to assume that low muscle mass and strength maybe pathologically associated with increased adiposity in the elderly. For future investigations on sarcopenic obesity, researchers and clinicians are encouraged to use DXA as the modality of choice for body composition analysis, given its accessibility and superiority in providing the essential information, with excellent correlation compared to more expensive but gold standard methods such as the computed tomography (CT) scan and magnetic resonance imaging (MRI). Other body composition tools such as bioelectrical impedance and conventional anthropometric measures can also be used but should be interpreted with extreme caution, given its low precision and accuracy in distinguishing different components of body mass [20]. While the absence of a consensus definition for sarcopenic obesity is amplified by the abundance of thresholds and reference populations to name a few, the clinical implications of sarcopenic obesity as a single disease entity are much more established.

11.4   Complications of Sarcopenic Obesity

In previous chapters, the consequences of sarcopenia such as disability, fractures, hospitalization, and mortality, to name a few, have already been elaborately described. Majority, if not all, also apply to sarcopenic obesity. In addition, given that obesity alone is independently associated with reduced functional capacity and quality of life among the elderly, the combination of obesity-related cardiometabolic diseases such as type 2 diabetes (T2D) and atherosclerosis with sarcopenia accelerates functional decline and mortality among individuals with sarcopenic obesity [21–23]. In a recent study involving more than 2400 middle-aged and elderly Chinese, sarcopenia or obesity alone showed no higher risk for atrial fibrillation, but the coexistence of both was associated with more than fivefold risk (odds ratio, OR, 5.68 [95% confidence interval, CI, 1.3–24.1], p-value = 0.019) even after adjustment for multiple confounders [24].

Aside from the diseases mentioned, sarcopenic obesity has also been associated with depression and poor mental health. In a large-scale study involving 3862 community-dwelling elderly, those who were obese with lower grip strength twice as likely to have depressive symptoms (OR = 1.97 [95% CI, 1.22–3.17]) compared to their nonobese with stable grip strength counterparts [25]. Lastly, an emerging complication of sarcopenic obesity that remains under investigated is its coexistence with osteoporosis, or osteosarcopenic obesity [26]. The overlap of weakened bone health, impaired muscle mass, and strength with increased body fat has been observed, but causality is yet to be established. In a recent systematic review by Bauer and colleagues, collected evidence was insufficient to consider it as a distinct disease entity and whether the cluster of diseases mentioned cumulatively raises additional adverse outcomes aside from the ones already identified [27].

11.5 Management

Physical inactivity is arguably the single most important preventable and modifiable risk factor for sarcopenia, obesity, and sarcopenic obesity [28]. In a 2013 review involving 23 reports from seven countries, it was estimated that 65% of adults above 60 years were sedentary for almost 9 h per day [29]. Physical inactivity, which is an established risk factor for obesity, is also common in older adults due to progressive loss of physical fitness. Increased physical activity therefore is central to the management of sarcopenic obesity, in terms of increasing muscle strength and decreasing excess adiposity [28, 30, 31]. Aside from exercise, nutritional strategies are also warranted. In a comprehensive review done by Trouwbost and colleagues, they recommended that a combination of a diet ideal for moderate weight loss, combined with exercise and a high animal protein intake ($\geq$1.2 g/kg/day) spread throughout the day, has the greatest benefit in improving different components of sarcopenic obesity [32]. Other potential therapies are listed in Table 11.2 [13].

Table 11.2 Recommended therapies in sarcopenic obesity

Component	Goal	Proposed approach
Calorie restriction	Body fat loss and enhance physical function	500–1000 kcal per day
		~0.5 kg per week aiming for 8–10% weight loss at 6 months followed by weight loss maintenance
Aerobic exercises	Enhance cardiorespiratory fitness	2.5 h per week of moderate to vigorous aerobic exercise
Resistance exercises	Enhance muscle strength and mass; reduce muscle and bone loss during weight loss	60–75 min of resistance training three times weekly, separated by 1 day focusing on strength, balance, and flexibility
Protein supplementation	Lessen muscle mass and strength loss	1.0–1.2 g/kg of protein in divided doses (25–30 g daily)
		2.5–2.8 g leucine daily
Calcium supplementation	Prevent adverse disturbances in bone metabolism	1200 mg per day preferably through dietary measures
Vitamin D supplementation		1000 IU vitamin D per day, ideally maintaining blood levels $\geq$30 ng/mL

Note: IU international units. Modified table taken from Batsis and Villareal [13]

11.6 Conclusion

Sarcopenic obesity is an important clinical entity in geriatric medicine that may get worse overtime, given the increasing elderly population and the still uncontrolled pandemic of obesity. A unified consensus in its definition maybe the first step to determine a more accurate picture of the disease burden. While lifestyle interventions remain the hallmark strategies for managing sarcopenic obesity, further investigations are warranted to identify promising therapies that target harmonization of the muscle and adipose tissue cross talk among at risk populations, especially the elderly.

References

1. Heber D, Ingles S, Ashley JM, Maxwell MH, Lyons RF, Elashoff RM. Clinical detection of sarcopenic obesity by bioelectrical impedance analysis. Am J Clin Nutr. 1996;64(3 Suppl):472S–7S.
2. Santos MD, Buti M, López-Cano C, Sánchez E, Vidal A, Hernández M, Lafarga A, Gutiérrez-Carrasquilla L, Rius F, Bueno M, Lecube A. Dynamics of anthropometric indices in a large paired cohort with 10 years of follow-up: paving the way to sarcopenic obesity. Front Endocrinol (Lausanne). 2020;11:209.
3. Cruz-Jentoft AJ, Sayer AA. Sarcopenia. Lancet. 2019;393(10191):2636–46.
4. Shimokata H, Shimada H, Satake S, Endo N, Shibasaki K, Ogawa S, Arai H. Chapter 2. Epidemiology of sarcopenia. Geriatr Gerontol Int. 2018;18(Suppl 1):13–22.
5. Prospective Studies Collaboration, Whitlock G, Lewington S, Sherliker P, Clarke R, Emberson J, Halsey J, Qizilbash N, Collins R, Peto R. Body-mass index and cause-specific mortality in 900 000 adults: collaborative analyses of 57 prospective studies. Lancet. 2009;373(9669):1083–96.
6. Blüher M. Obesity: global epidemiology and pathogenesis. Nat Rev Endocrinol. 2019;15(5):288–98.
7. NCD Risk Factor Collaboration (NCD-RisC). Trends in adult body-mass index in 200 countries from 1975 To 2014: a pooled analysis of 1698 population-based measurement studies with 19·2 million participants. Lancet. 2016;387(10026):1377–96.
8. United Nations, Department of Economic and Social Affairs, Population Division. World Population Ageing 2019 (ST/ESA/SER.A/444). 2020. https://www.un.org/en/development/desa/population/publications/pdf/ageing/WorldPopulationAgeing2019-Report.pdf. Accessed 14 Sept 2020.
9. Koliaki C, Liatis S, Dalamaga M, Kokkinos A. Sarcopenic obesity: epidemiologic evidence, pathophysiology, and therapeutic perspectives. Curr Obes Rep. 2019;8(4):458–71.
10. Sieber CC. Malnutrition and sarcopenia. Aging Clin Exp Res. 2019;31(6):793–8.
11. Zamboni M, Rubele S, Rossi AP. Sarcopenia and obesity. Curr Opin Clin Nutr Metab Care. 2019;22(1):13–9.
12. Barazzoni R, Bischoff S, Boirie Y, Busetto L, Cederholm T, Dicker D, Toplak H, Van Gossum A, Yumuk V, Vettor R. Sarcopenic obesity: time to meet the challenge. Obes Facts. 2018;11(4):294–305.
13. Batsis JA, Villareal DT. Sarcopenic obesity in older adults: aetiology, epidemiology and treatment strategies. Nat Rev Endocrinol. 2018;14(9):513–37.
14. Stenholm S, Harris TB, Rantanen T, Visser M, Kritchevsky SB, Ferrucci L. Sarcopenic obesity: definition, cause and consequences. Curr Opin Clin Nutr Metab Care. 2008;11(6):693–700.
15. Baumgartner RN. Body composition in healthy aging. Ann N Y Acad Sci. 2000;904:437–48.

16. Baumgartner RN, Wayne SJ, Waters DL, Janssen I, Gallagher D, Morley JE. Sarcopenic obesity predicts instrumental activities of daily living disability in the elderly. Obes Res. 2004;12(12):1995–2004.
17. Newman AB, Kupelian V, Visser M, Simonsick E, Goodpaster B, Nevitt M, Kritchevsky SB, Tylavsky FA, Rubin SM, Harris TB, Health ABC Study Investigators. Sarcopenia: alternative definitions and associations with lower extremity function. J Am Geriatr Soc. 2003;51(11):1602–9.
18. Villareal DT, Apovian CM, Kushner RF, Klein S, American Society for Nutrition; NAASO, The Obesity Society. Obesity in older adults: technical review and position statement of the American Society for Nutrition and NAASO, the Obesity Society. Obes Res. 2005;13(11):1849–63.
19. Bouchard DR, Dionne IJ, Brochu M. Sarcopenic/obesity and physical capacity in older men and women: data from the nutrition as a determinant of successful aging (NuAge)-the Quebec longitudinal study. Obesity (Silver Spring). 2009;17(11):2082–8.
20. Ponti F, Santoro A, Mercatelli D, Gasperini C, Conte M, Martucci M, Sangiorgi L, Franceschi C, Bazzocchi A. Aging and imaging assessment of body composition: from fat to facts. Front Endocrinol (Lausanne). 2020;10:861.
21. Habib SS, Alkahtani S, Alhussain M, Aljuhani O. Sarcopenia coexisting with high adiposity exacerbates insulin resistance and dyslipidemia in Saudi adult men. Diabetes Metab Syndr Obes. 2020;13:3089–97.
22. Nakano R, Takebe N, Ono M, Hangai M, Nakagawa R, Yashiro S, Murai T, Nagasawa K, Takahashi Y, Satoh J, Ishigaki Y. Involvement of oxidative stress in atherosclerosis development in subjects with sarcopenic obesity. Obes Sci Pract. 2017;3(2):212–8.
23. Itani L, Kreidieh D, El Masri D, Tannir H, El Ghoch M. The impact of Sarcopenic obesity on health-related quality of life of treatment-seeking patients with obesity. Curr Diabetes Rev. 2020;16(6):635–40.
24. Xia MF, Chen LY, Wu L, Ma H, Li XM, Li Q, Aleteng Q, Hu Y, He WY, Gao J, Lin HD, Gao X. Sarcopenia, sarcopenic overweight/obesity and risk of cardiovascular disease and cardiac arrhythmia: a cross-sectional study. Clin Nutr. 2020;S0261-5614(20):30293–4.
25. Hamer M, Batty GD, Kivimaki M. Sarcopenic obesity and risk of new onset depressive symptoms in older adults: English longitudinal study of ageing. Int J Obes (Lond). 2015;39(12):1717–20.
26. Ilich JZ. Another impairment in older age: what does osteosarcopenic obesity syndrome mean for middle-aged and older women? J Am Med Dir Assoc. 2017;18(8):648–50.
27. Bauer JM, Cruz-Jentoft AJ, Fielding RA, Kanis JA, Reginster JY, Bruyère O, Cesari M, Chapurlat R, Al-Daghri N, Dennison E, Kaufman JM, Landi F, Laslop A, Locquet M, Maggi S, McCloskey E, Perna S, Rizzoli R, Rolland Y, Rondanelli M, Szulc P, Vellas B, Vlaskovska M, Cooper C. Is there enough evidence for Osteosarcopenic obesity as a distinct entity? A critical literature review. Calcif Tissue Int. 2019;105(2):109–24.
28. Ribeiro Santos V, Dias Correa B, De Souza Pereira CG, Alberto GL. Physical activity decreases the risk of sarcopenia and Sarcopenic obesity in older adults with the incidence of clinical factors: 24-month prospective study. Exp Aging Res. 2020;46(2):166–77.
29. Harvey JA, Chastin SF, Skelton DA. Prevalence of sedentary behavior in older adults: a systematic review. Int J Environ Res Public Health. 2013;10(12):6645–61.
30. Hsu KJ, Liao CD, Tsai MW, Chen CN. Effects of exercise and nutritional intervention on body composition, metabolic health, and physical performance in adults with Sarcopenic obesity: a meta-analysis. Nutrients. 2019;11(9):2163.
31. Langhammer B, Bergland A, Rydwik E. The importance of physical activity exercise among older people. Biomed Res Int. 2018;2018:7856823.
32. Trouwborst I, Verreijen A, Memelink R, Massanet P, Boirie Y, Weijs P, Tieland M. Exercise and nutrition strategies to counteract Sarcopenic obesity. Nutrients. 2018;10(5):605.

The Role of Physical Activity in Sarcopenia

12

Lee Smith and Shaea Alkahtani

12.1   An Overview of Physical Activity

Physical activity may be defined as any bodily movement caused by contraction of skeletal muscle that results in energy expenditure [1]. Physical activity can be categorised by its intensity measured in metabolic equivalents or METs. One MET is defined as the amount of oxygen consumed while sitting at rest and is equal to 3.5 mL O_2 per kg body weight per min [2]. Zero to 1.5 METs is classed as sedentary behaviour (activities such as TV viewing and computer use), 1.5 to 3 METs is categorised as light intensity physical activity (activities such as arts and crafts), 3 to 6 METS as moderate physical activity (activities such as walking and vacuuming) and 6+ METs as vigorous physical activity (activities such as riding a bike or running) [3], (Fig. 12.1).

There is a plethora of literature to show that regular and sustained participation in physical activity is beneficial for almost every facet of health, for example, with preventive benefits being observed in relation to cancer, cardiovascular disease, depression and anxiety. Moreover, physical activity has been found to be a useful tool in the treatment/reduction of severity in several noncommunicable diseases such as cardiovascular disease and depression. Physical activity improves physical and mental health via many mechanisms, such a discussion is beyond the scope of this chapter and we refer the interested reader to [4, 5]. It should be noted here that the greatest health benefits from physical activity are acquired at a moderate or

L. Smith (✉)
The Cambridge Centre for Sport and Exercise Sciences, Anglia Ruskin University, Cambridge, UK
e-mail: Lee.Smith@anglia.ac.uk

S. Alkahtani
Department of Exercise Physiology, College of Sport Sciences and Physical Activity, King Saud University, Riyadh, Saudi Arabia
e-mail: shalkahtani@ksu.edu.sa

© Springer Nature Switzerland AG 2021
N. Veronese et al. (eds.), *Sarcopenia*, Practical Issues in Geriatrics,
https://doi.org/10.1007/978-3-030-80038-3_12

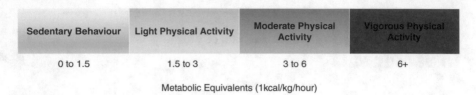

Sedentary Behaviour	Light Physical Activity	Moderate Physical Activity	Vigorous Physical Activity
0 to 1.5	1.5 to 3	3 to 6	6+

Metabolic Equivalents (1kcal/kg/hour)

Fig. 12.1 The Energy Expenditure Continuum

higher intensity. However, participation in light physical activity is beneficial to health if one is replacing sedentary time [3].

12.2 Physical Activity and Its Role in Preventing and Managing Sarcopenia

Importantly, regular participation in physical activity is an essential tool for older adults to utilise to aid in the prevention and/or management of several noncommunicable diseases. One such condition is sarcopenia. Sarcopenia is broadly defined here as "age-related muscle loss, affecting a combination of appendicular muscle mass, muscle strength, and/or physical performance measures" [6]. The prevalence of sarcopenia is high in older adults. For example, a recent meta-analysis suggested that sarcopenia prevalence in older adults is approximately 10% [7]. The reader is referred to Chap. 2 for a detailed discussion on the prevalence of sarcopenia and Chap. 3 on the health consequence of sarcopenia.

Owing to the high prevalence of sarcopenia and its associated detrimental impact on physical as well as mental health, it is essential that intervention strategies are implemented to aid in the prevention and management of sarcopenia, one potentially effective strategy is the promotion of physical activity. Indeed, there is a large body of literature to suggest that participation in physical activity is beneficial for the prevention of sarcopenia and for improvement in sarcopenia-related outcomes in those who are sarcopenic. For example, in one systematic review, ten studies were identified of which seven studies were randomized controlled trials, and three were cross-sectional or longitudinal. The results of eight studies indicated significant improvement in muscle mass, muscle strength, and physical performance through exercise (one domain of physical activity) intervention, as determined by long-term observation. Consequently, the review concluded that participation in physical activity is an effective protective strategy for sarcopenia in geriatric populations [8]. However, it is important to note that the review highlights there was no consistency in the measurement of sarcopenia. This is indeed a key limitation and one that limits the whole field of sarcopenia. Another systematic review identified 37 randomised controlled trials utilising exercise interventions in relation to sarcopenic outcomes. In 79% of studies, muscle mass increased with exercise and muscle strength increased in 82.8% of the studies. Finally, the majority of studies showed an increase of physical performance following exercise intervention. The review concluded that exercise has a positive impact on muscle mass and muscle function in subjects aged 60 years and older. The biggest effect of exercise intervention, of any type, was observed in relation to physical performance (gait speed, chair rising test, balance, etc.) [9]. Another systematic review summarised the available literature on the effects of exercise interventions on sarcopenia-related outcome measures in community-dwelling older people. A total of nine studies were identified including eight randomised controlled trials. The review reports that in exercise-only interventions a significant improvement in muscle mass in one study, muscle strength in two studies, and physical performance in two studies were observed. It should also be noted that the review found similar outcomes with combined physical activity and nutrition interventions [10].

Taken together the evidence presented in these systematic reviews unquestionably supports the promotion of physical activity in the prevention and management of sarcopenia. Participation in physical activity likely protects against onset sarcopenia and aids in the management of sarcopenia as it can lead to an increase in muscle mass and muscle strength [11]. Moreover, participation in physical activity can also improve the status of skeletal muscle [8]. For example, mitochondrial volume and enzyme activity increase after aerobic exercise demonstrate that muscle protein synthesis and muscle quality improve irrespective of age [12].

12.3   Aerobic Physical Activity and Sarcopenia

Participation in aerobic activity and particularly that of at least a moderate intensity has been found to preserve muscle function with age, as well as motor units, mitochondrial function, and proteostasis [13]. Consequently, aiding in the prevention of onset sarcopenia. In those who are sarcopenic and participate in aerobic exercise, beneficial outcomes have also been observed. Literature has shown that aerobic exercise may suppress the apoptotic pathway in skeletal muscle and helps maintain the expression of autophagy protein as well as increases the expressions of autophagy-related proteins in skeletal muscle [14]. Moreover, several studies have shown that aerobic exercise controls mRNA expression of myostatin. These molecular factors are associated with age-related sarcopenia, and thus it is likely that aerobic physical activity has a protective effect against sarcopenic-related outcomes. For example, one study examined potential age-specific adaptations in skeletal muscle size and myofiber contractile physiology in response to 12 weeks of cycle ergometer training. The study found that in both young males (20 ± 1 years) and older males (74 ± 3 years) improvements in muscle size and aerobic capacity were similar, while adaptations in myofiber contractile function showed a general improvement in older males only. Training-related increases in slow and fast myofibers peak power suggest that skeletal muscle of older males is responsive to aerobic exercise training and further support the use of aerobic exercise for improving skeletal muscle health in older individuals [15].

12.4 Resistance Exercise and Sarcopenia

In addition to aerobic activity having a beneficial influence in the prevention and management of sarcopenia, there is a growing body of literature to support the benefits of resistance exercise [16]. Resistance exercise stimulates muscle hypertrophy and increases muscle strength [17] by promoting muscle protein synthesis [18]. In a systematic review of 121 trials including over 6700 participants, it was concluded that "*progressive resistance training is an effective intervention for improving physical functioning in older people, including improving strength and the performance of some simple and complex activities*" [19]. Moreover, the majority of included trials involved high intensity training two to three times per week. Participation in these trials resulted in large positive effects on both muscle mass (hypertrophy) and strength. In one controlled trial, residents of Nursing Care Facilities (85.9 ± 7.5 years; $n = 42$) were required to participate in a resistance and balance exercise program twice a week for 6 months. A total of 35.7% of participants had sarcopenia at baseline, with prevalence increasing in the control group post-intervention (42.9%–52.4%). Following intervention, the exercise group experienced a significant increase in grip strength when compared to controls ($p = 0.02$), and a within-group decrease in body mass index and increase in grip strength ($p \leq 007$) [20]. These findings provide further evidence for the implementation of resistance exercise for the prevention and management of sarcopenia.

In adults, a decline in voluntary muscle contraction of 1–2% per year after the sixth decade occurs. Importantly, the effect of aging is more pronounced in concentric (muscle shortening) than eccentric (muscle lengthening) contraction, which may be linked to "the stiffer muscle structures and prolonged myosin cross-bridge cycles of aged muscles" [21]. Eccentric exercise requires less demand on cardiopulmonary system, and therefore for some individuals, it can be advantageous as it allows for an "easier" increase in workload and/or to perform exercise at a low metabolic effort. For example, 19 older and 19 young adults completed a program of eccentric and concentric leg squats, 5–7 days apart. Cardiovascular and pulmonary measures including heart rate, systolic blood pressure, cardiac index and expired ventilation were significantly lower during eccentric compared to concentric exercise in young and old participants [22]. Two sessions per week of conventional resistance training and eccentric ergometer training for 12 weeks were compared in older men and women. Maximal isometric leg extension strength, eccentric muscle coordination and loss of body and thigh fat were significantly improved with eccentric ergometer training, whereas both training increased thigh lean mass [23]. A greater preservation of muscle strength and force during eccentric compared to concentric contraction was observed in older adults, and residual force enhancement after lengthening contraction was greater in old than young muscle fibres. The decline in mobility with aging is partially due to change in muscle force–velocity relationship, and eccentric exercise can help to increase the velocity of contraction to improve muscle force–velocity [24]. However, senescence can affect inflammatory (TNF-α and IL-1β) and anti-inflammatory (interleukin-6 (IL-6) and TGF-β1) cytokines in response to exercise-induced injury [25], which could suggest performing eccentric resistance exercise at moderate intensity and impose a recovery period of 48–72 h for the trained muscle group. Ninety elderly obese women completed an acute eccentric resistance exercise session, and the responses of muscle damage-induced hormones (e.g. creatine kinase and IL-6) were monitored throughout 48 h post exercise. There were wide variations among participants who were classified as high and normal responders [26]. It was suggested that optimal resistance training is to implement eccentric and concentric contractile on the same force–velocity curve with different load even for a short period [27], but this model is not practically feasible in the long term.

12.5   Combined Aerobic and Resistance Exercise and Sarcopenia

It seems plausible that a combination of both aerobic and resistance exercise will yield the greatest benefits in the prevention and management of sarcopenia. As age increases, levels of physical activity decrease predisposing individuals to positive energy balance and increasing fat mass. With a decreased muscle mass due to sarcopenia symptoms, old individuals are expected to develop sarcopenic obesity promoting insulin resistance, metabolic syndrome, and inflammatory markers [28]. Whether sarcopenia and obesity act synergistically or not, sarcopenic obesity is a pathogenic multifactorial chronic condition increasing worldwide and causing a major public health problem [29]. Therefore, physical activity interventions should aim to increase energy expenditure to reduce fat mass via aerobic training and to increase muscle mass mainly via resistance exercise. In one study, 100 breast cancer survivors (53 ± 10.4 years) were randomly assigned to either an exercise condition, consisting of moderate-to-vigorous intensity aerobic and resistance exercise three times per week for 16 weeks, or control condition. It was found that the intervention effectively attenuated metabolic syndrome, sarcopenic obesity and relevant biomarkers in an ethnically diverse sample of sedentary, overweight or obese survivors of breast cancer [30]. The effectiveness of a 6-month obesity management program plus three types of training (aerobic, resistance or combined) was compared in 160 obese older adults. Maximal oxygen consumption significantly increased more in the combination and aerobic groups than in the resistance group, and strength significantly increased more in the combination and resistance groups than in the aerobic group. Body weight similarly decreased in all exercise groups, and lean mass decreased less in the combination and resistance groups than in the aerobic group [31]. Combined training can also exhibit a greater improvement in metabolic markers such as insulin resistance and chemerin protein than resistance exercise alone [32]. Interestingly, Shiotsu and Yanagita [33] examined the effect of the order of resistance and aerobic exercise in older adults and found that there was no different effect of exercise order on body composition and strength, but performing aerobic after resistance exercise reduced arterial stiffness to a greater extent than performing aerobic before resistance exercise and the control group. The same authors repeated the study at low- and moderate-intensity resistance exercise and found that all groups improved body composition, functional performance and muscle strength, whereas only moderate resistance intensity independent of aerobic and resistance exercise orders improved functional reach test which reflects dynamic balance capacity [34]. The increase in resistance exercise intensity could be a suggested strategy in age-related sarcopenia, which can increase protein synthesis, improve muscle strength and to some extent improve muscle hypertrophy, although there is lack of data of long-term interventions in older adults [35]. Moreover, decreased muscle mass and increased fat mass may be associated with decreased bone density, which synergistically can accelerate falls risk and fractures. A cross-sectional study found that osteoporosis increased among low appendicular skeletal muscle mass group, and further deficiency in gait speed and balance in sarcopenic obesity group [36]. Indeed, a recent review on physical activity and sarcopenia concluded that combined exercise training regimes (aerobic and resistance) have been shown to produce the most beneficial preventive and therapeutic effects for sarcopenia [18].

## 12.6	Neuromotor Exercise and Sarcopenia

Decreased postural stability and increased risks for falls are main challenges to address in relation to older adults. It should be noted that loss of muscle mass and strength and neuromuscular deficiency in the low extremities are the main causes of fall. Neuromotor fitness is important among older adults, and training of balance and coordination should be implemented in the exercise prescription for sarcopenia in older adults. Tai Chi is an ancient Chinese martial art embracing the mind, body and spirit and consisting of a series of slow and continuous movements of the human body, which is simple, easy to learn and does not need to require high metabolic demand [37]. It has been suggested that Tai Chi can benefit older people to prevent falls because of its positive effect on strength, balance, posture and concentration [38]. The effects of long-term Tai Chi exercise on muscle strength of lower extremities were tested in 205 older adults who practiced in Tai Chi compared with 205 matched controls who did not practice in Tai Chi. The strength of low extremities (e.g. iliopsoas, quadriceps femoris, tibialis anterior and hamstrings) in the Tai Chi group was significantly higher than that in the control group, and the strength of the muscles within the Tai Chi group was not different between age subgroups (60 and 69, 70 and 79, and 80 and 89 years) [39]. Another study found that people who practiced in Tai Chi had significantly higher knee extensor strength at all speeds tested than people who did not practice in Tai Chi, but no significant difference existed in knee flexors between the two groups. Moreover, eccentric strength of knee extensors was correlated to the foot centre of pressure, which demonstrates the importance of long-term Tai Chi training on postural muscles in the lower extremities [40]. However, it has been shown that a 16-week intervention of Tai Chi training is not a sufficient duration to enhance biomechanical characteristic changes of lower extremity muscles [41], which means long-term practice of Tai Chi may be required to elicit a positive effect on muscle and balance. Another intervention study with 12-week training also found a modest improvement or no changes in older men and women [42]. A systematic review showed evidence of Tai Chi combined with resistance training intervention, lasting 12 weeks to 12 months, on physical function and muscle strength of adults aged 50 years and older, but reported the limitations including sample size and study type in most available studies [43]. Another systematic review and meta-analysis showed a moderate to strong evidence of Tai Chi intervention starting from 12 weeks to maintain and improve lower limb proprioception in adults older than 55 years [44]. Finally, another review reported that there is limited evidence to support the role of Tai Chi on postural balance and fall prevention [38].

12.7   Sedentary Behaviour and Sarcopenia

There is currently a small but growing body of literature investigating the relationship between sedentary (0 to 1.5 METs) time and sarcopenia. Importantly, older adults spend the majority of their waking day in sedentary activities as opposed to being physically active [45]. In a recent study examining the cross-sectional association between sedentary behaviour and sarcopenia among 14,585 adults aged ≥ 65 years from low-middle income countries, it was found that compared to sedentary behaviour of 0–<4 h/day, ≥ 11 h/day was significantly associated with 2.14 (95%CI = 1.06–4.33) times higher odds for sarcopenia. Other studies have found similar findings, ([46, 47].

It may be that the association between sedentary behaviour and sarcopenia is the reverse of the association between light physical activity and sarcopenia. However, higher levels of sedentary behaviour have been shown to be associated with higher levels of liver adiposity and visceral/subcutaneous abdominal fat ratio [48]. Importantly, deep adipose tissue and visceral adiposity have been shown to be associated with an increase in pro-inflammatory cytokines and a decrease in anti-inflammatory markers, which can have a catabolic effect on muscle by promoting protein degradation [49]. Interestingly, sedentary behaviour per se has been shown to be associated with higher levels of chronic low-grade inflammation, and thus, potentially directly associated with a higher risk of sarcopenia [50].

12.8   Summary

To sum up, sarcopenia is predominantly a geriatric condition with a high global prevalence. The literature overwhelmingly suggests that physical activity per se is an important tool that can be utilised to aid in prevention and support the management of sarcopenia. To yield the greatest health benefits, a combination of aerobic and resistance exercise should be promoted. Additional, benefits in the prevention and management of sarcopenia may be observed from the parallel reduction in sedentary time. Future research taking a holistic approach where combined aerobic and resistance exercise interventions and sedentary behaviour reduction techniques are simultaneously employed are warranted, such an intervention may produce greater benefits than those observed to date.

References

1. Caspersen CJ, Powell KE, Christenson GM. Physical activity, exercise, and physical fitness: definitions and distinctions for health-related research. Public Health Rep. 1985;100(2):126–31.
2. Jette M, Sidney K, Blumchen G. Metabolic equivalents (METS) in exercise testing, exercise prescription, and evaluation of functional capacity. Clin Cardiol. 1990;13(8):555–65. https://doi.org/10.1002/clc.4960130809.
3. Smith L, Ekelund U, Hamer M. The potential yield of non-exercise physical activity energy expenditure in public health. Sports Med (Auckland, NZ). 2015;45(4):449–52. https://doi.org/10.1007/s40279-015-0310-2.
4. Sheikholeslami S, Ghanbarian A, Azizi F. The impact of physical activity on non-communicable diseases: findings from 20 years of the Tehran Lipid and Glucose Study. Int J Endocrinol Metab. 2018;16(4 Suppl):e84740-e. https://doi.org/10.5812/ijem.84740.
5. Health H. Exercise is an all-natural treatment to fight depression. Cambridge, MA: Harvard Health Publishing, Harvard University; 2013. https://www.health.harvard.edu/mind-and-mood/exercise-is-an-all-natural-treatment-to-fight-depression. Accessed 9 Mar 2020.
6. Woo J. Sarcopenia. Clin Geriatr Med. 2017;33(3):305–14. https://doi.org/10.1016/j.cger.2017.02.003.
7. Mayhew AJ, Amog K, Phillips S, Parise G, McNicholas PD, de Souza RJ, et al. The prevalence of sarcopenia in community-dwelling older adults, an exploration of differences between studies and within definitions: a systematic review and meta-analyses. Age Ageing. 2019;48(1):48–56. https://doi.org/10.1093/ageing/afy106.
8. Lee S-Y, Tung H-H, Liu C-Y, Chen L-K. Physical activity and sarcopenia in the geriatric population: a systematic review. J Am Med Dir Assoc. 2018;19(5):378–83. https://doi.org/10.1016/j.jamda.2018.02.003.
9. Beaudart C, Dawson A, Shaw SC, Harvey NC, Kanis JA, Binkley N, et al. Nutrition and physical activity in the prevention and treatment of sarcopenia: systematic review. Osteoporos Int. 2017;28(6):1817–33. https://doi.org/10.1007/s00198-017-3980-9.
10. Miyazaki R, Takeshima T, Kotani K. Exercise intervention for anti-sarcopenia in community-dwelling older people. J Clin Med Res. 2016;8(12):848–53. https://doi.org/10.14740/jocmr2767w.
11. Marzetti E, Calvani R, Tosato M, Cesari M, Di Bari M, Cherubini A, et al. Physical activity and exercise as countermeasures to physical frailty and sarcopenia. Aging Clin Exp Res. 2017;29(1):35–42. https://doi.org/10.1007/s40520-016-0705-4.
12. Short KR, Vittone JL, Bigelow ML, Proctor DN, Nair KS. Age and aerobic exercise training effects on whole body and muscle protein metabolism. Am J Physiol Endocrinol Metab. 2004;286(1):E92–101. https://doi.org/10.1152/ajpendo.00366.2003.
13. Laurin JL, Reid JJ, Lawrence MM, Miller BF. Long-term aerobic exercise preserves muscle mass and function with age. Curr Opin Physio. 2019;10:70–4. https://doi.org/10.1016/j.cophys.2019.04.019.
14. Lira VA, Okutsu M, Zhang M, Greene NP, Laker RC, Breen DS, et al. Autophagy is required for exercise training-induced skeletal muscle adaptation and improvement of physical performance. FASEB J. 2013;27(10):4184–93.
15. Harber MP, Konopka AR, Undem MK, Hinkley JM, Minchev K, Kaminsky LA, et al. Aerobic exercise training induces skeletal muscle hypertrophy and age-dependent adaptations in myofiber function in young and older men. J Appl Physiol (1985). 2012;113(9):1495–504. https://doi.org/10.1152/japplphysiol.00786.2012.

16. Law TD, Clark LA, Clark BC. Resistance exercise to prevent and manage sarcopenia and Dynapenia. Annu Rev Gerontol Geriatr. 2016;36(1):205–28. https://doi.org/10.1891/0198-8794.36.205.
17. Johnston AP, De Lisio M, Parise G. Resistance training, sarcopenia, and the mitochondrial theory of aging. Appl Physiol Nutr Metab. 2008;33(1):191–9. https://doi.org/10.1139/h07-141.
18. Yoo S-Z, No M-H, Heo J-W, Park D-H, Kang J-H, Kim SH, et al. Role of exercise in age-related sarcopenia. J Exerc Rehabil. 2018;14(4):551–8. https://doi.org/10.12965/jer.1836268.134.
19. Liu C-J, Latham N. Can progressive resistance strength training reduce physical disability in older adults? A meta-analysis study. Disabil Rehabil. 2011;33(2):87–97. https://doi.org/10.3109/09638288.2010.487145.
20. Hassan BH, Hewitt J, Keogh JWL, Bermeo S, Duque G, Henwood TR. Impact of resistance training on sarcopenia in nursing care facilities: a pilot study. Geriatr Nurs. 2016;37(2):116–21. https://doi.org/10.1016/j.gerinurse.2015.11.001.
21. Vandervoort AA. Aging of the human neuromuscular system. Muscle Nerve. 2002;25(1):17–25. https://doi.org/10.1002/mus.1215.
22. Vallejo AF, Schroeder ET, Zheng L, Jensky NE, Sattler FR. Cardiopulmonary responses to eccentric and concentric resistance exercise in older adults. Age Ageing. 2006;35(3):291–7. https://doi.org/10.1093/ageing/afj082.
23. Mueller M, Breil FA, Vogt M, Steiner R, Lippuner K, Popp A, et al. Different response to eccentric and concentric training in older men and women. Eur J Appl Physiol. 2009;107(2):145–53. https://doi.org/10.1007/s00421-009-1108-4.
24. Lim J-Y. Therapeutic potential of eccentric exercises for age-related muscle atrophy. Integr Med Res. 2016;5(3):176–81.
25. Hamada K, Vannier E, Sacheck JM, Witsell AL, Roubenoff R. Senescence of human skeletal muscle impairs the local inflammatory cytokine response to acute eccentric exercise. FASEB J. 2005;19(2):264–6. https://doi.org/10.1096/fj.03-1286fje.
26. Tajra V, Tibana RA, Vieira DCL, de Farias DL, Teixeira TG, Funghetto SS, et al. Identification of high responders for interleukin-6 and creatine kinase following acute eccentric resistance exercise in elderly obese women. J Sci Med Sport. 2014;17(6):662–6. https://doi.org/10.1016/j.jsams.2013.09.012.
27. Reeves ND, Maganaris CN, Longo S, Narici MV. Differential adaptations to eccentric versus conventional resistance training in older humans. Exp Physiol. 2009;94(7):825–33. https://doi.org/10.1113/expphysiol.2009.046599.
28. Roubenoff R. Sarcopenic obesity: the confluence of two epidemics. Obes Res. 2004;12(6):887–8. https://doi.org/10.1038/oby.2004.107.
29. Polyzos SA, Margioris AN. Sarcopenic obesity. Hormones. 2018;17(3):321–31. https://doi.org/10.1007/s42000-018-0049-x.
30. Dieli-Conwright CM, Courneya KS, Demark-Wahnefried W, Sami N, Lee K, Buchanan TA, et al. Effects of aerobic and resistance exercise on metabolic syndrome, sarcopenic obesity, and circulating biomarkers in overweight or obese survivors of breast cancer: a randomized controlled trial. J Clin Oncol. 2018;36(9):875–83. https://doi.org/10.1200/JCO.2017.75.7526.
31. Villareal DT, Aguirre L, Gurney AB, Waters DL, Sinacore DR, Colombo E, et al. Aerobic or resistance exercise, or both, in dieting obese older adults. N Engl J Med. 2017;376(20):1943–55.
32. Kim D-I, Lee DH, Hong S, Jo S-W, Won Y-S, Jeon JY. Six weeks of combined aerobic and resistance exercise using outdoor exercise machines improves fitness, insulin resistance, and chemerin in the Korean elderly: a pilot randomized controlled trial. Arch Gerontol Geriatr. 2018;75:59–64. https://doi.org/10.1016/j.archger.2017.11.006.
33. Shiotsu Y, Yanagita M. Intervention study on the exercise order of combined aerobic & resistance training in the elderly. J Sports Sci. 2017;5:322–31.
34. Shiotsu Y, Yanagita M. Comparisons of low-intensity versus moderate-intensity combined aerobic and resistance training on body composition, muscle strength, and functional performance in older women. Menopause. 2018;25(6):668–75. https://doi.org/10.1097/gme.0000000000001060.

35. Porter MM. The effects of strength training on sarcopenia. Can J Appl Physiol. 2001;26(1):123–41. https://doi.org/10.1139/h01-009.
36. Waters DL, Hale L, Grant AM, Herbison P, Goulding A. Osteoporosis and gait and balance disturbances in older sarcopenic obese new Zealanders. Osteoporos Int. 2010;21(2):351–7. https://doi.org/10.1007/s00198-009-0947-5.
37. Lam P. Tai Chi for Health Institute. Australia. 2018. https://taichiforhealthinstitute.org/what-is-tai-chi/. Accessed 8 Mar 2020.
38. Wu G. Evaluation of the effectiveness of tai chi for improving balance and preventing falls in the older population—a review. J Am Geriatr Soc. 2002;50(4):746–54. https://doi.org/10.1046/j.1532-5415.2002.50173.x.
39. Zhou M, Peng N, Dai Q, Li H-W, Shi R-G, Huang W. Effect of tai chi on muscle strength of the lower extremities in the elderly. Chin J Integr Med. 2016;22(11):861–6. https://doi.org/10.1007/s11655-015-2104-7.
40. Wu G, Zhao F, Zhou X, Wei L. Improvement of isokinetic knee extensor strength and reduction of postural sway in the elderly from long-term tai chi exercise. Arch Phys Med Rehabil. 2002;83(10):1364–9. https://doi.org/10.1053/apmr.2002.34596.
41. Li JX, Xu DQ, Hong Y. Changes in muscle strength, endurance, and reaction of the lower extremities with tai chi intervention. J Biomech. 2009;42(8):967–71. https://doi.org/10.1016/j.jbiomech.2009.03.001.
42. Woo J, Hong A, Lau E, Lynn H. A randomised controlled trial of tai chi and resistance exercise on bone health, muscle strength and balance in community-living elderly people. Age Ageing. 2007;36(3):262–8. https://doi.org/10.1093/ageing/afm005.
43. Qi M, Moyle W, Jones C, Weeks B. Tai chi combined with resistance training for adults aged 50 years and older: a systematic review. J Geriatr Phys Ther. 2020;43(1):32–41. https://doi.org/10.1519/jpt.0000000000000218.
44. Zou L, Han J, Li C, Yeung AS, Hui SS, Tsang WWN, et al. Effects of Tai Chi on lower limb proprioception in adults aged over 55: a systematic review and meta-analysis. Arch Phys Med Rehabil. 2019;100(6):1102–13. https://doi.org/10.1016/j.apmr.2018.07.425.
45. Leung PM, Ejupi A, van Schooten KS, Aziz O, Feldman F, Mackey DC, et al. Association between sedentary behaviour and physical, cognitive, and psychosocial status among older adults in assisted living. Biomed Res Int. 2017;2017:9160504. https://doi.org/10.1155/2017/9160504.
46. Aggio DA, Sartini C, Papacosta O, Lennon LT, Ash S, Whincup PH, et al. Cross-sectional associations of objectively measured physical activity and sedentary time with sarcopenia and sarcopenic obesity in older men. Prev Med. 2016;91:264–72. https://doi.org/10.1016/j.ypmed.2016.08.040.
47. Gianoudis J, Bailey CA, Daly RM. Associations between sedentary behaviour and body composition, muscle function and sarcopenia in community-dwelling older adults. Osteoporos Int. 2015;26(2):571–9. https://doi.org/10.1007/s00198-014-2895-y.
48. Smith L, Thomas EL, Bell JD, Hamer M. The association between objectively measured sitting and standing with body composition: a pilot study using MRI. BMJ Open. 2014;4(6):e005476. https://doi.org/10.1136/bmjopen-2014-005476.
49. Peake J, Gatta PD, Cameron-Smith D. Aging and its effects on inflammation in skeletal muscle at rest and following exercise-induced muscle injury. Am J Physiol Regul Integr Comp Physiol. 2010;298(6):R1485–R95. https://doi.org/10.1152/ajpregu.00467.2009.
50. Dalle S, Rossmeislova L, Koppo K. The role of inflammation in age-related sarcopenia. Front Physiol. 2017;8:1045. https://doi.org/10.3389/fphys.2017.01045.

Nutritional Approaches for Sarcopenia

13

Ailsa A. Welch and Richard P. G. Hayhoe

13.1 Introduction

Sarcopenia is associated with the conditions of frailty, falls, osteoporosis and risk of fracture, as well as with malnutrition [1–3]. In addition, there are metabolic consequences of loss of skeletal muscle mass during aging which include reduced energy expenditure, which affects obesity as well as glucose dysregulation, effects of glycaemic control and the onset of type-2 diabetes [1, 4]. The loss of, and changes to, skeletal muscle mass with aging also contribute to age-associated reduction in utilisation of dietary protein and fat [1].

In this chapter, the term 'sarcopenic factors' refers to the loss of skeletal muscle strength or function or loss or changes in skeletal muscle mass or combinations of these. The term 'fat free mass' (FFM) is used, since FFM is often measured and used as a proxy for skeletal muscle mass (SMM). Since FFM increases both with increased body weight and size, measurements of FFM in human studies are scaled for body size by height (skeletal muscle mass index—SMI), percentage of total body weight or Body Mass Index (BMI) (FFM/$_{BMI}$, FFM divided by BMI).

Nutrition is a modifiable lifestyle factor that can interact with the mechanisms of loss of skeletal muscle mass and function, as well as with the mechanisms of aging, and previous research has focused on a number of nutrients that are relevant for

A. A. Welch (✉)
Department of Epidemiology and Public Health, Faculty of Medicine and Health Sciences, Norwich Medical School, University of East Anglia, Norwich, UK
e-mail: a.welch@uea.ac.uk

R. P. G. Hayhoe
Department of Epidemiology and Public Health, Faculty of Medicine and Health Sciences, Norwich Medical School, University of East Anglia, Norwich, UK

Faculty of Health, Education, Medicine and Social Care, School of Allied Health, Anglia Ruskin University, Chelmsford, UK
e-mail: richard.hayhoe@aru.ac.uk

© Springer Nature Switzerland AG 2021
N. Veronese et al. (eds.), *Sarcopenia*, Practical Issues in Geriatrics,
https://doi.org/10.1007/978-3-030-80038-3_13

skeletal muscle physiology and metabolism. However, the major focus to date has been on protein intake. Lesser focus has been centred on the micronutrient vitamins and minerals, and on intake of fats and fatty acids. There have also been some recent studies examining the relevance of patterns of dietary intake. The relevance of dietary patterns may be due to the individual nutrients such as protein or the micronutrients which are associated with the optimal dietary patterns as well as to the synergistic effects of these nutrients and the foods within these dietary patterns.

This chapter covers the foods, nutrients and dietary patterns that have been linked to either prevention or treatment of sarcopenia and suggests areas for future research in relation to aspects of nutrition and prevention of sarcopenia.

13.2 Nitrogen Balance and Exogenous Antioxidants

Maintaining the balance between the continuous anabolism and catabolism of protein occurring in the body and thus ensuring *nitrogen balance* does not become negative are crucial for conserving skeletal muscle during aging [1, 5–8]. Thus, factors that interfere with this process such as inflammaging and insulin resistance have an adverse impact on nitrogen balance. There is also an increase in *anabolic resistance,* i.e. lower myofibrillar synthesis of protein, during aging.

A number of micronutrient vitamins or minerals are known to act as exogenous antioxidants or help counteract the increased circulating concentrations of inflammatory cytokines associated with aging, and thus may be beneficial to muscle health and prevention of sarcopenia. These include vitamins C, E, and D, the carotenoids and the minerals, magnesium, selenium and zinc, but there is also evidence for specific dietary patterns being relevant. Specific relationships between the mechanisms of aging with nutrients and patterns of dietary intake are described in the following sections.

13.2.1 Important Dietary Factors

13.2.1.1 Protein

Skeletal muscle is the main reserve of protein in the body, and protein is required to maintain this reserve of protein in the muscle through protein synthesis. It is thus logical that there has been extensive research into the relevance of protein intake to conservation and prevention of sarcopenia during aging [2, 3, 5, 6, 9]. As the relevance of protein to maintenance of sarcopenic factors and prevention of sarcopenia during aging has been studied extensively a summary of the importance of protein as well, as the most recent developments in this area of research are covered in this chapter. Readers may refer to the earlier work in the following publications [2, 3, 5, 6, 9].

A recent review of nutritional interventions to improve sarcopenic factors and sarcopenia found that the evidence was generally not of high quality and was insufficient to establish with any certainty the effects of supplementation with protein, essential amino acids or creatine, or ß-hydroxy-ß-methylbutyrate [10]. The authors determined that the level of evidence supporting most recommendations was low to moderate, but that the best evidence related to the amino acid leucine which has a significant effect on muscle mass in older people with sarcopenia. However, the review also recommended that increases in protein intake designed to increase muscle mass and strength should be accompanied by resistance exercise programmes [10]. By contrast, another systematic review found that protein does not augment the effects of resistance exercise on skeletal muscle mass and function in older people [11]. However, most recent research and clinical recommendations have noted that reducing the decline in sarcopenic factors during aging requires that the increase in intake of protein should accompanied by resistance exercise [9, 12–15]. This is because an increase in physical activity synergises with increased protein intake to affect regulation of protein synthesis.

Variability in Response to Interventions with Dietary Protein

The limited effectiveness of interventions with protein in older people and the variability in response to interventions with dietary protein may be due to a number of reasons including the anabolic resistance that occurs during aging [5, 15]. Recent research studied the effect of protein supplementation on muscle disuse in young men and found substantial declines in muscle mass and myofibrillar protein synthesis rates during inactivity [16]. The authors also found that the high intake of protein used in their intervention, 1.6 g/kg body weight per day, did not attenuate the decreases in quadriceps muscle volume that occurred during inactivity when compared with the control interventions with low, or no, protein intake; the control groups received either 0.5 g or 0.15 g/kg/day, respectively [9, 16]. Therefore, increased protein intake did not counteract the reduced myofibrillar protein synthesis rates that occurred during inactivity, even in young men. Other recent work has also demonstrated that the incorporation of amino acids such as leucine into skeletal muscle, during muscle protein synthesis, occurs only for a period of 2–3 h in a rested state. This is known as the *muscle full phenomenon* which means that muscle becomes unresponsive to higher doses of protein intake after a short period following protein consumption [13]. This phenomenon may also explain the limited effectiveness of increases in protein intake that are designed to overcome the anabolic resistance to protein synthesis in muscle during older age.

Other factors such as sex and race potentially also influence the effectiveness of protein intake in interventions to improve sarcopenic factors during aging. Recent research found that associations between protein intake and sarcopenic factors differed according to sex and race, in a longitudinal study [17].

Some of the variability in response to interventions with protein may also be due to the type of protein used since protein from animal sources such as meat or dairy foods is more biologically available than protein from vegetable sources such as pulses (beans and lentils) and vegetables [18]. Animal sources of protein have a profile of amino acids that is higher in indispensable amino acids, including the branch chain amino acids that stimulate the production of mTOR that is required to increase the synthesis of protein [7]. However, a recent population study, The

NU-AGE Study, found an interaction between plant and animal protein intakes on the risk of sarcopenia [19]. Though the risk of sarcopenia decreased with increased intakes of total protein, this decrease was greater when intakes of vegetable protein were also higher [19].

A number of the dietary interventions with protein-containing foods have found variability in sarcopenic outcomes which may be due to not only the protein composition of the foods that were administered but also to the associated nutrients in the foods. For instance, one intervention in an Australian population that was accompanied by resistance exercise training found positive effects of a red meat intervention on lean muscle mass in women when compared with a control group [20]. However, the increase in protein intake in the group provided with red meat was also accompanied by a significant increase in intake of zinc which may also have increased the effectiveness of the intervention. In a further study of similar design, which also included men, no significant effect of increased intake of meat was found. However, a similar increase in zinc intake occurred during the study that was also associated with the group with increased meat intake [21].

Finally, variation in the interaction between protein intake and the composition of the microbiome in the gut may occur. Thus, it has been hypothesised that the gut microbiome may modulate individual response to dietary protein and thus have effects on sarcopenia and sarcopenic factors [22, 23].

Intake of Dietary Amino Acids

To date, there is little data on intakes of amino acids in general populations of middle and older age who are at risk of sarcopenia. In recent unpublished research, we investigated the full range of amino acids in the diet and contributors to sarcopenia, skeletal muscle mass and function and found a number of differences in the associations between individual amino acids and sarcopenic factors in both younger and older women in the UK-Twin cohort.

Current Clinical Recommendations for Protein Intake

Current recommendations regarding protein intake during aging include increasing total protein intakes, between 1.0 g and 1.5 g protein per kg body weight per day, for individuals older than 65 years [5]. However, other reviews and dietary recommendations do not recommend intakes higher than 1.0 g protein/kg/day in older age groups [24]. It has also been suggested that ensuring protein intake balanced across meal occasions is important in older people, to ensure maximal utilisation of protein and muscle protein synthesis [5, 14].

In summary, adequate protein is undoubtably important for the maintenance of skeletal muscle function and structure during aging, but to date the evidence is mixed for the effectiveness of dietary interventions with protein to rectify or prevent sarcopenia. Accompanying increases in protein intake with sufficient micronutrient vitamins and minerals or as part of improvements in overall dietary intakes may be important in the prevention and treatment of sarcopenia, as described in the following sections.

13.2.1.2 The B Group Vitamins

The B vitamins are a diverse group of vitamins with important biological functions. Several of the B vitamins are highly relevant to muscle, acting as cofactors in processes involved in muscle synthesis and as neurotrophic agents that maintain neural integrity and function [25, 26]. In addition, deficiencies of a number of B vitamins result in neuromuscular problems (e.g. beri beri) and neurological symptoms (e.g. pellagra). So, maintenance of vitamin B status may be important for prevention of sarcopenia. However, very few studies have investigated relationships between dietary intake of B vitamins and circulating blood concentrations [25]. One study in the Netherlands found associations between dietary folate, vitamin B_6, and B_{12} intakes and physical function in older adults in the Netherlands [27]. Another study, in adults older than 65 years, found lower intakes of vitamin B_6 and folic acid in adults with sarcopenia compared with those without [28]. Two further studies found that lower intakes and concentrations of circulating vitamin B_{12} were associated with low SMI, sarcopenia or dynapenia [29, 30]. Lastly, in unpublished work from our group, using the Twins UK Study of adult women aged 18–79 years, significant positive associations were evident in multivariable models between dietary B vitamin intakes (niacin, folate, pantothenate, riboflavin, thiamine and B_6) and measures of fat-free mass. Similarly, positive trends were observed across niacin, folate, pantothenate, riboflavin and thiamine dietary intakes and leg explosive power (measured using a Nottingham Power Rig). Therefore, although more research is required, the current evidence suggests that dietary intake of B vitamins is important for both skeletal muscle mass and function.

13.2.1.3 Vitamin C

Vitamin C has several mechanistic functions relevant to skeletal muscle metabolism and physiology, which could prevent age-related loss of skeletal muscle. Vitamin C in muscle is involved in synthesis of carnitine, an important factor involved in energy production, and collagen, an essential structural component of muscle [31, 32]. It also has a strong capability to act as an electron donor. Reactive oxygen species (ROS) are produced during normal oxidative metabolism in muscle, but capable of cellular damage if uncontrolled [33]. Under normal physiological conditions, the presence of ROS is controlled by antioxidant and enzymatic defence systems including superoxide dismutase and glutathione peroxidase as well as antioxidants from the diet [33, 34]. Age-related increases in ROS due to mitochondrial dysfunction, modification to enzymatic defences and changes to muscle fibres may lead to cellular damage in muscle, as does the age-related increase in circulating concentrations of inflammatory cytokines [33, 35]. If in sufficient supply, the antioxidant capacity of vitamin C may therefore help to reduce oxidative damage to muscle, as well as reducing potentially damaging concentrations of inflammatory cytokines in the circulation [35]. In previous observational studies, positive associations between dietary vitamin C and measures of skeletal muscle function were found in the Italian InCHIANTI Study, and for women only in the UK [36–39]. One study examined both FFM and muscle function with intake as well as circulating vitamin C, finding positive associations between measures of physical function but not FFM [38]. A further study found intake of vitamin C was associated with FFM after 2.6 years of follow up [36]. More recent observational evidence in women of all ages found that higher intakes of vitamin C were associated with significantly higher indices of FFM and leg explosive power [40]. The differences between the highest intakes in quintile 5 versus those in quintile 1 ranged between 2.0% and 12.8% ($P < 0.01$–0.02) [40]. Further observational study evidence shows positive associations of both dietary and circulating vitamin C with measures of skeletal muscle mass in middle- and older-aged men and women [41]. Overall, the evidence thus points towards potential protective effects of vitamin C on measures of skeletal muscle mass and function.

13.2.1.4 Vitamin D

Vitamin D may be protective for development of sarcopenia through a number of direct or indirect mechanisms [7]. Receptors for vitamin D are found in skeletal muscle, but discussion is still ongoing as to the importance of this and the relevance to aging, such as whether levels or expression of these receptors decline during aging and whether they are important for the morphological changes that affect both skeletal muscle mass and function during aging [42]. Known roles of vitamin D are participation in myogenesis, cell proliferation, differentiation and regulation of cell signalling cascades, as well as signalling for potential genomic targets [43]. The functional effects of vitamin D in muscle may be through calcium and phosphate handling and signalling, particularly in relation to muscle strength and contraction [42]. Deficiency of vitamin D leads to muscle weakness which is one of the symptoms found in rickets in children, as well as in adults, where it is accompanied by muscle pain, in the condition of osteomalacia [42].

A recent systematic review summarised the evidence for supplementation of vitamin D in community-dwelling older adults aged 65 years and older in relation effects on muscle strength and function [44]. Studies included were those testing supplementation with vitamin D alone, or alongside calcium supplementation. Of the 15 studies included in the review, the majority found no improvement in muscle strength and mobility after administration of vitamin D with or without calcium supplements. In the meta-analyses performed, non-significant changes in hand-grip strength were found in the seven studies analysed and a small, but significant, increase in the timed-up and-go test of 0.3 s (95% CI = 0.1–0.5 s) in five studies. However, there was a high degree of heterogeneity between the studies. The overall conclusion was supplementation with vitamin D or with calcium did not result in improvements in skeletal muscle function [44]. A more recent intervention study with vitamin D in men aged 60 years and over, with low concentrations of circulating vitamin D, found no effect on lower extremity power, strength or lean mass over a period of 12 months of supplementation [45]. Further recent intervention studies, over shorter periods of 3–6 months, found either effects on appendicular skeletal muscle mass, but not grip strength [46], or improvements in skeletal muscle mass, but not strength.

There is also limited evidence that co-administration of vitamin D alongside the amino acid leucine is more likely to improve the efficacy of leucine supplementation on skeletal muscle mass [47]. It is clear from the existing evidence that vitamin D plays a role in maintenance of skeletal muscle mass strength or function, but in older populations the effects of supplementation on sarcopenic outcomes are mixed. Differences in the findings of intervention trials with vitamin D may be due to initial concentrations of circulating vitamin D, as well as to dosages used in the interventions, the age of the intervention groups and duration of the studies.

13.2.1.5 Vitamin E

Vitamin E, like vitamin C, has the potential to act as an antioxidant, preventing build-up of free radicals in cell membranes and in plasma lipoproteins. Vitamin E consists of two classes of molecules, tocopherols and tocotrienols, which are categorised according to the saturation of their phytyl tail groups. Observational data of individuals 65 years or over has shown a positive association between plasma alpha-tocopherol concentration and knee extension strength and physical performance, and between gamma-tocopherol and physical performance [48, 49]. In addition, low circulating vitamin E concentrations have been identified in frail individuals, compared to non-frail individuals, suggesting a lack of vitamin E may be linked to the transition from non-frail to frail [50]. Other cross-sectional analyses, of data from women aged 18–79 years in the Twins UK cohort, found that higher intake of vitamin E was associated with higher indices of skeletal muscle mass, but not function [40]. Further work in the EPIC-Norfolk study has found potentially protective associations in fat-free mass with higher intakes of dietary vitamin E or circulating concentrations of α-tocopherol [51].

The observational data are supported by mechanistic evidence from a number of animal studies, which demonstrate the role of vitamin E as an antioxidant and anti-inflammatory agent. This includes evidence that: in a rat model, vitamin E prevents increased nuclear translocation of NF-kB, increased expression of chemokines and the resultant leukocyte infiltration associated with H_2O_2-induced oxidative stress [52]; and in a mouse model, vitamin E reduces lipopolysaccharide (LPS)-induced inflammation by modulating the LPS-induced, and NF-kB mediated, upregulation of IL-6 gene and protein expression [53].

13.2.1.6 Carotenoids

The carotenoid family of phytochemical vitamins is found in yellow, orange and green leafy fruits and vegetables and includes β-carotene, β-cryptoxanthin, lycopene, lutein and zeaxthanin. These carotenoids function as exogenous antioxidants and anti-inflammatory agents thus interacting with the mechanisms of muscle aging.

Relatively few studies have investigated the relevance of total carotene, carotenoid intakes, or circulating concentrations, in relation to sarcopenia and sarcopenic factors. Two studies from a UK cohort found positive associations between higher intakes of carotene on grip strength or physical activity, with the latter finding of associations only in women [37, 39]. Several studies also found protective associations with higher circulating concentrations of β-carotene and indices of knee strength or function, or rate of decline in walking speed [49, 51–57].

Few studies have investigated associations with more detailed dietary intakes of the individual carotenoids and sarcopenic factors. In the UK Twin cohort, we found that higher intakes of total and individual carotenoids were significantly associated with indices of FFM and leg explosive power with differences across quintiles of between 1.0 and 7.5% [41]. The strongest associations for indices of FFM were found with α-carotene intake (Q5-Q1 0.24 kg/m 2 ± 0.1 P-trend = 0.03), a 1.6% difference across quintiles. Significant associations were also found with FFM% for ß-cryptoxthanin and with FFM% and FFM$_{BMI}$ for lutein and zeaxthanin, with inter-quintile differences ranging from 1.1 to 7.2% [40]. LEP was associated significantly with carotenoid intakes, with the exception of α-carotene, with differences in LEP ranging from 6.3 to 7.5% when comparing extreme quintiles of carotenoid intakes [40]. A previous study found that dietary carotenoid intake as total carotene, ß-cryptoxthanin, and combined lutein and zeaxanthin was positively associated with FFM, expressed as percentage body weight, in both men and women, with lycopene associated only in women [58]. The greatest association was found for combined lutein and zeaxanthin in women with an interquintile difference of 2.5%. A more recent longitudinal analysis from the Framingham cohort study also found protective effects with higher intakes of total carotenoids, lycopene and combined lutein and zeathanin with annualised change in grip strength or faster gait speed, over a period of follow up which ranged from 4.5 to 15.4 years [59]. However, replication of the analyses in the Cardiovascular Heart Study found no associations between total carotenoid intake and either grip strength or gait speed [59]. The research findings, though limited, indicate that future intervention studies with carotenoid containing foods are warranted.

13.2.1.7   Minerals: Magnesium

Skeletal muscle acts as a major store of magnesium where it is important for energy metabolism, protein synthesis and turnover, transmembrane transport and muscle contraction and relaxation [60, 61]. Magnesium is also integral to function of the mitochondria thus influencing muscle performance through energy metabolism (ATP generation).

A number of observational studies have shown dietary magnesium intake, serum magnesium or muscle magnesium concentrations are positively associated with measures of skeletal muscle mass [62, 63] and function [64]. Magnesium supplementation has also been shown to increase the muscle strength in young adults gained through exercise [65] and improve physical performance in older individuals [66]. Lower magnesium intake has also been associated with sarcopenia [28, 29]. However, the mechanisms by which magnesium may be acting in muscle are not fully understood. Cell culture and animal studies have demonstrated that magnesium depletion can cause structural damage to muscle cells due to oxidative stress and disrupted calcium homeostasis [67]. It has also been suggested that magnesium protects against inflammaging, a known risk factor for sarcopenia [7]. Indeed, circulating concentrations of inflammatory cytokines, including C-reactive protein (CRP), IL-6 and TNF-α, have been negatively associated with skeletal muscle measures of both mass and function in a number of studies [64, 68–70]. Systematic review evidence also indicates that dietary magnesium intake is inversely associated with serum CRP concentration [71]. Furthermore, it is relevant that age-related physiological decline in function of the gastrointestinal and renal systems may lead to an increased susceptibility of older individuals to develop low magnesium status [72].

13.2.1.8   Minerals and Trace Elements: Calcium, Iron, Potassium, Phosphorus, Selenium and Zinc

Although a number of minerals and trace elements, such as selenium, zinc, potassium, iron and phosphorus, play roles in muscle metabolism and function, comparatively little research has focused on this area [7, 73]. The minerals calcium, potassium, and sodium are necessary for healthy muscle and nerve activity. Calcium is the main regulatory signalling molecule for skeletal muscle fibres. Also, low iron blood serum concentrations may be associated with poor physical performance. Phosphorus can lead to muscle weakness, and selenium deficiency is associated with several muscular diseases that also include symptoms of weakness. Both selenium and zinc potentially play a role in protecting skeletal muscle from oxidative damage, and zinc is also integral to protein synthesis, and in animal studies, zinc deficiency has been shown to impaired protein synthesis in skeletal muscle [74].

One observational study in older people found that higher iron, phosphorus and zinc intakes were associated with conservation of lean mass over a period of 2.6 years, indicating a potential role for minerals in sarcopenic factors or prevention of sarcopenia [36]. A more recent systematic review identified only six studies investigating the role of minerals on prevention or treatment of sarcopenia in individuals, aged 65 years or over [73]. Evidence was provided mainly from observational studies, finding that serum selenium and calcium intakes were significantly associated with muscle mass, and selenium, iron, and zinc intakes were significantly and positively associated with physical performance in older adults [73]. Also, selenium, calcium and phosphorus intakes were associated with the prevalence of sarcopenia [74]. Although the majority of studies in this review reported on dietary intakes only, a study of community-dwelling older individuals that measured selenium in the serum of participants found that those in the lowest tertile of circulating selenium concentrations were at an increased risk of low skeletal muscle mass [75]. Also, an earlier study in men and women, which was not included in the review, found those individuals in the lowest quartile of circulating selenium concentration had lower measures of grip, knee and hip strength [76].

As comparatively little research has involved the relevance of minerals and trace elements to skeletal muscle health and sarcopenia, further research is needed to improve our knowledge and understanding in this area.

13.2.1.9   Fatty Acids

Dietary sources of fat exist as a combination of different classes of fatty acid. Thus, dietary fat intake may vary significantly between individuals with regard to both total consumption and the ratios of different fatty acids including saturated (SFA), monounsaturated (MUFA), polyunsaturated (PUFA) and trans (TFA) fatty acids [77, 78].

There are several aspects to the rationale for dietary fat being important to muscle health. During aerobic exercise, fatty acids provide energy by acting as a critical substrate for production of ATP [79]. Phospholipid fatty acids also act as key structural components of muscle cell membranes (sarcolemma), and incorporation of different types of fatty acids may influence cellular signalling and function [80]. Fatty acids may also affect inflammatory pathways, which could have consequences on muscle. Indeed, in general terms, it is though that higher SFA and total fat intakes are associated with higher risk of inflammation, while other fatty acids, including n-3 PUFA, are associated with anti-inflammatory properties and protein synthesis [81].

A number of observational studies have suggested a role for fatty acids and their dietary profiles and measures of skeletal muscle mass or sarcopenia. In an analysis of Twins UK data, positive associations were evident between the PUFA to SFA ratio and indices of FFM, and negative associations were evident with the proportion of energy from fat in the diet, and SFA, MUFA and TFA, individually as a percentage of total dietary energy [82]. There is also some suggestion that a higher omega-3: omega-6 ratio is desirable as omega-3 fatty acids may provide protective effects for muscle, while omega-6 has pro-inflammatory effects which result in adverse effects. However, a recent systematic review showed no significant effects of total PUFA or specific omega-3 or omega-6 fatty acids on indices of skeletal muscle mass [83]. In conclusion therefore, there is rationale for the importance of different profiles of fatty acid in the diet, with ratios of different fatty acids relevant to measures of muscle health and sarcopenic risk factors. However, further investigation is required before definitive conclusions can be made, and recommendations given to optimise fatty acid intakes for muscle health.

13.2.2 Dietary Patterns

Most previous research has studied associations between individual components of the diet and musculoskeletal health, but it is likely that the balance of dietary components is also important. Indeed, we consume nutrients in combinations in food, and thus there may be synergistic and cumulative effects of different dietary components including protein and micronutrients on health and disease which might not be seen by examining the effects of nutrients or foods individually.

The Mediterranean diet (MD) pattern is characterised by high intakes of fruits and vegetables, legumes, nuts, cereals and olive oil with low intakes of saturated fat, moderately high intakes of fish, low to moderate intakes of dairy products, low intake of meat and regular but moderate intake of alcohol [84]. This micronutrient rich diet is associated with a number of favourable health outcomes, including overall mortality and protective effects on cardiovascular disease, hypertension and cancer [85, 86]. Comparatively few studies have explored the relationship between the MD and sarcopenia or sarcopenic factors [87]. In terms of muscle health and relevance to sarcopenia, observational studies, including data from the Twins UK study of adult women, have demonstrated that higher adherence to the MD is associated with higher measures of fat-free mass, and leg explosive power [88]. Likewise in the EPIC-Norfolk cohort, higher adherence to a Mediterranean diet was associated with significantly higher indices of FFM [89].

Potential Renal Acid Load (PRAL) is a means to quantify acid-base load of the diet as well as the effect of diet on systemic acid-base balance. A more alkalinogenic load, low PRAL, is considered protective. Fruits and vegetables have a low PRAL and tend to promote systemic alkalinity due to the bicarbonate present, while hepatic oxidation of the sulphur-containing amino acids, cysteine and methionine found in meats, grains and cheeses generates hydrogen ions and thus has the opposite effect [90].

Metabolic acidosis may be detrimental to skeletal muscle by decreasing protein synthesis and increasing proteolysis and oxidation of amino acids, through actions of the ubiquitin proteasome pathway and insulin-like growth factor-1 signalling [91]. It has been associated with muscle wasting in patients with chronic renal failure [92], and in acidotic obese individuals undergoing very low calorie diets for weight loss [93, 94]. While this process is a useful adaptive response to acidosis resulting in release of amino acids in the blood as a substrate for synthesis of glutamine and in turn ammonia, which helps mop up excess hydrogen ions for excretion as ammonium ions and thus reduce the acidosis [95], it does nevertheless occur to the detriment of muscle. A number of population studies have therefore investigated PRAL in relation to muscle health in young and old individuals [96, 97]. For example, evidence from the Twins UK study in women [97] aged 18–79 years showed a positive association between a more alkaline diet and muscle mass indexes, and this association was also evident in the middle- to older aged men and women in the EPIC-Norfolk cohort [98].

13.3   Summary, Recommendations, and Guidelines

To date, published observational studies, both cross-sectional and longitudinal in design, have demonstrated significant relationships between specific dietary factors and dietary patterns with muscle measures of mass and function, and thus sarcopenic risk factors. They have also highlighted a number of differences in these relationships according to sex. The major evidence for micronutrients that may be relevant during muscle aging involves vitamin C and the mineral magnesium, with much less evidence available for the carotenoids, vitamin E, and other minerals and trace elements including iron, selenium, calcium and phosphorus. Many of these findings have not been translated into intervention study designs, but evidence from observational studies is nevertheless somewhat convincing. There is also a small but growing body of evidence to suggest that adherence to specific dietary patterns, including the Mediterranean diet, and diets with a more alkalinogenic, low PRAL, also has improved muscle measures and thus reduced sarcopenic risk factors. Within the observational studies for both micronutrients and dietary patterns, there are differences between extremes of population intakes of a magnitude that could be clinically relevant. These suggest that more optimal dietary intakes may have beneficial effects on sarcopenic factors during aging.

Until recently, the impact of nutrition on muscle health and sarcopenia has been largely underestimated. Indeed, efforts to promote or retain muscle mass and strength and thus reduce the risk of sarcopenia have mainly been focused on a combination of increased protein intake alongside resistance exercise. However, as summarised here, increasing evidence is emerging to show that overall diet quality and intake of a range of nutrients including vitamins and minerals, not only protein, may play an important role in muscle health in older people.

Dietary recommendations for older adults in relation to skeletal muscle health are limited. The current recommendations are summarised in Table 13.1. In making

Table 13.1 Current status of evidence for dietary nutrients and associations with sarcopenia and skeletal muscle health and a summary of dietary recommendations for older adults

Nutrient in diet	Overall strength of evidence	Recommendation daily intakes	Notes
Protein	+++	EFSA PRI 0.83 g/kg++ 0.80–1.0 g/kg +++ 1.0–1.2 g/kg ++	Divide intakes of protein across meal occasions during the day
Fat, fatty acids	+	+ Reduce total dietary fat as a percentage + Reduce dietary saturated fatty acids + Improve PUFA:SFA ratio ++ Improve n-3 PUFA intake	
Vitamin D	++	Meet recommendation of 15 µg/day	May require supplementation of 10 µg/day Ensure appropriate exposure to sun during summer months
Vitamin C	+	Meet recommendation of AR F: 80 mg/day, M: 90 mg/day	[a]Avoid supplementary doses of >500 mg/day due to potential prooxidant effects
Carotenoids	+	N/A	
Vitamin E	+	Meet diet recommendations	
B vitamins	+	Meet diet recommendations	
Magnesium	++	Meet recommendations of AI of F: 300 mg/day, M: 350 mg/day	Magnesium supplements can cause gastrointestinal upset. Interact with calcium supplementation
Minerals—Ca, Fe, P, K, Zn, Se	+	Meet diet recommendations	

Strength of evidence: +++ strong evidence ++ moderate evidence + emerging evidence. *N/A* not available, *AR* average requirement, *PRI* population reference intake, *AI* average intake
[a]Evidence for effectiveness of single doses of micronutrients is lacking. Supra-physiological doses should be avoided
Dietary recommenations taken from the EFSA Dietary Reference Values for nutrients Summary report European Food Safety Authority (EFSA) update 2019. https://doi.org/10.2903/sp.efsa.2017. e15121. https://www.efsa.europa.eu/en/supporting/pub/e15121

recommendations for intakes of specific nutrients for muscle health, it is important to consider that current dietary recommendations and clinical deficiency or sufficiency criteria have not been generated using muscle health outcomes. The current published recommended nutrient intakes or the body composition criteria utilised to derive dietary recommendations may therefore not be directly relevant to maintaining or improving muscle health. Indeed, it may be necessary to achieve higher intakes for optimal muscle health than might be predicted using other health outcomes, and further investigation will be required to determine this in the future. With this caveat, it is nevertheless reasonable to deduce from the current evidence that individuals should, in conjunction with an active lifestyle, aim to consume sufficient fruits and vegetables, and protein, and to limit their saturated fat intake, for muscle health in later life.

References

1. Welch AA, Hayhoe RPG, Cameron D. The relationships between sarcopenic skeletal muscle loss during ageing and macronutrient metabolism, obesity and onset of diabetes. Proc Nutr Soc. 2019:1–12.
2. Landi F, Camprubi-Robles M, Bear DE, Cederholm T, Malafarina V, Welch AA, et al. Muscle loss: the new malnutrition challenge in clinical practice. Clin Nutr. 2019;38(5):2113–20.
3. Deutz NEP, Ashurst I, Ballesteros MD, Bear DE, Cruz-Jentoft AJ, Genton L, et al. The under-appreciated role of low muscle mass in the management of malnutrition. J Am Med Dir Assoc. 2019;20(1):22–7.
4. Scott D, de Courten B, Ebeling PR. Sarcopenia: a potential cause and consequence of type 2 diabetes in Australia's ageing population? Med J Aust. 2017;207(2):89.
5. Wolfe RR, Miller SL, Miller KB. Optimal protein intake in the elderly. Clin Nutr. 2008;27(5):675–84.
6. Wolfe RR. The underappreciated role of muscle in health and disease. Am J Clin Nutr. 2006;84(3):475–82.
7. Welch AA. Nutritional influences on age-related skeletal muscle loss. Proc Nutr Soc. 2014;73(1):16–33.
8. Millward DJ. Limiting deconditioned muscle atrophy and strength loss with appropriate nutrition: can it be done? Am J Clin Nutr. 2020;112(3):499–500.
9. Deutz NE, Bauer JM, Barazzoni R, Biolo G, Boirie Y, Bosy-Westphal A, et al. Protein intake and exercise for optimal muscle function with aging: recommendations from the ESPEN expert group. Clin Nutr. 2014;33(6):929–36.
10. Gielen E, Beckwee D, Delaere A, De Breucker S, Vandewoude M, Bautmans I, et al. Nutritional interventions to improve muscle mass, muscle strength, and physical performance in older people: an umbrella review of systematic reviews and meta-analyses. Nutr Rev. 2021;79(2):121–47.
11. Thomas DK, Quinn MA, Saunders DH, Greig CA. Protein supplementation does not significantly augment the effects of resistance exercise training in older adults: a systematic review. J Am Med Dir Assoc. 2016;17(10):959 e1–9.
12. Cruz-Jentoft AJ, Dawson Hughes B, Scott D, Sanders KM, Rizzoli R. Nutritional strategies for maintaining muscle mass and strength from middle age to later life: a narrative review. Maturitas. 2020;132:57–64.
13. Deane CS, Ely IA, Wilkinson DJ, Smith K, Phillips BE, Atherton PJ. Dietary protein, exercise, ageing and physical inactivity: interactive influences on skeletal muscle proteostasis. Proc Nutr Soc. 2020:1–12.

14. Theodorakopoulos C, Jones J, Bannerman E, Greig CA. Effectiveness of nutritional and exercise interventions to improve body composition and muscle strength or function in sarcopenic obese older adults: a systematic review. Nutr Res. 2017;43:3–15.

15. Nowson C, O'Connell S. Protein requirements and recommendations for older people: a review. Nutrients. 2015;7(8):6874–99.

16. Kilroe SP, Fulford J, Jackman S, Holwerda A, Gijsen A, van Loon L, et al. Dietary protein intake does not modulate daily myofibrillar protein synthesis rates or loss of muscle mass and function during short-term immobilization in young men: a randomized controlled trial. Am J Clin Nutr. 2020;113(3):548–61.

17. Elstgeest LEM, Schaap LA, Heymans MW, Hengeveld LM, Naumann E, Houston DK, et al. Sex-and race-specific associations of protein intake with change in muscle mass and physical function in older adults: the health, aging, and body composition (health ABC) study. Am J Clin Nutr. 2020;112(1):84–95.

18. Aubertin-Leheudre M, Adlercreutz H. Relationship between animal protein intake and muscle mass index in healthy women. Br J Nutr. 2009;102(12):1803–10.

19. Montiel-Rojas D, Nilsson A, Santoro A, Bazzocchi A, de Groot L, Feskens EJM, et al. Fighting sarcopenia in ageing european adults: the importance of the amount and source of dietary proteins. Nutrients. 2020;12(12):3601.

20. Daly RM, O'Connell SL, Mundell NL, Grimes CA, Dunstan DW, Nowson CA. Protein-enriched diet, with the use of lean red meat, combined with progressive resistance training enhances lean tissue mass and muscle strength and reduces circulating IL-6 concentrations in elderly women: a cluster randomized controlled trial. Am J Clin Nutr. 2014;99(4):899–910.

21. Formica MB, Gianoudis J, Nowson CA, O'Connell SL, Milte C, Ellis KA, et al. Effect of lean red meat combined with a multicomponent exercise program on muscle and cognitive function in older adults: a 6-month randomized controlled trial. Am J Clin Nutr. 2020;112(1):113–28.

22. Bowyer RCE, Jackson MA, Pallister T, Skinner J, Spector TD, Welch AA, et al. Use of dietary indices to control for diet in human gut microbiota studies. Microbiome. 2018;6(1):77.

23. Ni Lochlainn M, Bowyer RCE, Steves CJ. Dietary protein and muscle in aging people: the potential role of the gut microbiome. Nutrients. 2018;10(7):929.

24. Committee on Medical Aspects of Food Policy. Panel on Dietary Reference V, Great Britain. Dept. of H. Dietary reference values for food energy and nutrients for the United Kingdom: Report of the Panel on Dietary Reference Values of the Committee on Medical Aspects of Food Policy. London: HMSO; 1991.

25. Aytekin N, Mileva KN, Cunliffe AD. Selected B vitamins and their possible link to the aetiology of age-related sarcopenia: relevance of UK dietary recommendations. Nutr Res Rev. 2018;31(2):204–24.

26. Hwang SY, Sung B, Kim ND. Roles of folate in skeletal muscle cell development and functions. Arch Pharm Res. 2019;42(4):319–25.

27. Behrouzi P, Grootswagers P, Keizer PLC, Smeets E, Feskens EJM, de Groot L, et al. Dietary intakes of vegetable protein, folate, and vitamins B-6 and B-12 are partially correlated with physical functioning of Dutch older adults using copula graphical models. J Nutr. 2020;150(3):634–43.

28. Ter Borg S, de Groot LC, Mijnarends DM, de Vries JH, Verlaan S, Meijboom S, et al. Differences in nutrient intake and biochemical nutrient status between Sarcopenic and Nonsarcopenic older adults-results from the Maastricht sarcopenia study. J Am Med Dir Assoc. 2016;17(5):393–401.

29. Verlaan S, Aspray TJ, Bauer JM, Cederholm T, Hemsworth J, Hill TR, et al. Nutritional status, body composition, and quality of life in community-dwelling sarcopenic and non-sarcopenic older adults: a case-control study. Clin Nutr. 2017;36(1):267–74.

30. Ates Bulut E, Soysal P, Aydin AE, Dokuzlar O, Kocyigit SE, Isik AT. Vitamin B12 deficiency might be related to sarcopenia in older adults. Exp Gerontol. 2017;95:136–40.

31. Rebouche CJ. Ascorbic acid and carnitine biosynthesis. Am J Clin Nutr. 1991;54(6 Suppl):1147S–52S.

32. Franceschi RT. The role of ascorbic acid in mesenchymal differentiation. Nutr Rev. 1992;50(3):65–70.
33. Gomes MJ, Martinez PF, Pagan LU, Damatto RL, Cezar MDM, Lima ARR, et al. Skeletal muscle aging: influence of oxidative stress and physical exercise. Oncotarget. 2017;8(12):20428–40.
34. Bowen TS, Schuler G, Adams V. Skeletal muscle wasting in cachexia and sarcopenia: molecular pathophysiology and impact of exercise training. J Cachexia Sarcopenia Muscle. 2015;6(3):197–207.
35. Cerullo F, Gambassi G, Cesari M. Rationale for antioxidant supplementation in sarcopenia. J Aging Res. 2012;2012:316943.
36. Scott D, Blizzard L, Fell J, Giles G, Jones G. Associations between dietary nutrient intake and muscle mass and strength in community-dwelling older adults: the Tasmanian older adult cohort study. J Am Geriatr Soc. 2010;58(11):2129–34.
37. Martin H, Aihie Sayer A, Jameson K, Syddall H, Dennison EM, Cooper C, et al. Does diet influence physical performance in community-dwelling older people? Findings from the Hertfordshire cohort study. Age Ageing. 2011;40(2):181–6.
38. Saito K, Yokoyama T, Yoshida H, Kim H, Shimada H, Yoshida Y, et al. A significant relationship between plasma vitamin C concentration and physical performance among Japanese elderly women. J Gerontol A Biol Sci Med Sci. 2012;67(3):295–301.
39. Robinson SM, Jameson KA, Batelaan SF, Martin HJ, Syddall HE, Dennison EM, et al. Diet and its relationship with grip strength in community-dwelling older men and women: the Hertfordshire cohort study. J Am Geriatr Soc. 2008;56(1):84–90.
40. Welch AA, Jennings A, Kelaiditi E, Skinner J, Steves CJ. Cross-sectional associations between dietary antioxidant vitamins C, E and carotenoid intakes and Sarcopenic indices in women aged 18–79 years. Calcif Tissue Int. 2020;106(4):331–42.
41. Lewis LN, Hayhoe RPG, Mulligan AA, Luben RN, Khaw KT, Welch AA. Lower dietary and circulating vitamin C in middle- and older-aged men and women are associated with lower estimated skeletal muscle mass. J Nutr. 2020;150(10):2789–98.
42. Girgis CM. Vitamin D and skeletal muscle: emerging roles in development, anabolism and repair. Calcif Tissue Int. 2020;106(1):47–57.
43. Montenegro KR, Cruzat V, Carlessi R, Newsholme P. Mechanisms of vitamin D action in skeletal muscle. Nutr Res Rev. 2019;32(2):192–204.
44. Rosendahl-Riise H, Spielau U, Ranhoff AH, Gudbrandsen OA, Dierkes J. Vitamin D supplementation and its influence on muscle strength and mobility in community-dwelling older persons: a systematic review and meta-analysis. J Hum Nutr Diet. 2017;30(1):3–15.
45. Shea MK, Fielding RA, Dawson-Hughes B. The effect of vitamin D supplementation on lower-extremity power and function in older adults: a randomized controlled trial. Am J Clin Nutr. 2019;109(2):369–79.
46. Suebthawinkul C, Panyakhamlerd K, Yotnuengnit P, Suwan A, Chaiyasit N, Taechakraichana N. The effect of vitamin D2 supplementation on muscle strength in early postmenopausal women: a randomized, double-blind, placebo-controlled trial. Climacteric. 2018;21(5):491–7.
47. El Hajj C, Fares S, Chardigny JM, Boirie Y, Walrand S. Vitamin D supplementation and muscle strength in pre-sarcopenic elderly Lebanese people: a randomized controlled trial. Arch Osteoporos. 2018;14(1):4.
48. Martinez-Arnau FM, Fonfria-Vivas R, Cauli O. Beneficial effects of leucine supplementation on criteria for sarcopenia: a systematic review. Nutrients. 2019;11(10):2504.
49. Cesari M, Pahor M, Bartali B, Cherubini A, Penninx BW, Williams GR, et al. Antioxidants and physical performance in elderly persons: the Invecchiare in chianti (InCHIANTI) study. Am J Clin Nutr. 2004;79(2):289–94.
50. Ble A, Cherubini A, Volpato S, Bartali B, Walston JD, Windham BG, et al. Lower plasma vitamin E levels are associated with the frailty syndrome: the InCHIANTI study. J Gerontol A Biol Sci Med Sci. 2006;61(3):278–83.
51. Mulligan AA, Hayhoe R, Luben R, Welch A. Positive associations of dietary intake and plasma concentrations of vitamin E with skeletal muscle mass, heel bone ultrasound attenuation and fracture risk in the EPIC-Norfolk cohort. Antioxidants (Basel). 2021. Accessed 17 Jan 2021.

52. Aoi W, Naito Y, Takanami Y, Kawai Y, Sakuma K, Ichikawa H, et al. Oxidative stress and delayed-onset muscle damage after exercise. Free Radic Biol Med. 2004;37(4):480–7.
53. Huey KA, Fiscus G, Richwine AF, Johnson RW, Meador BM. In vivo vitamin E administration attenuates interleukin-6 and interleukin-1beta responses to an acute inflammatory insult in mouse skeletal and cardiac muscle. Exp Physiol. 2008;93(12):1263–72.
54. Lauretani F, Semba RD, Bandinelli S, Dayhoff-Brannigan M, Giacomini V, Corsi AM, et al. Low plasma carotenoids and skeletal muscle strength decline over 6 years. J Gerontol A Biol Sci Med Sci. 2008;63(4):376–83.
55. Semba RD, Blaum C, Guralnik JM, Moncrief DT, Ricks MO, Fried LP. Carotenoid and vitamin E status are associated with indicators of sarcopenia among older women living in the community. Aging Clin Exp Res. 2003;15(6):482–7.
56. Semba RD, Varadhan R, Bartali B, Ferrucci L, Ricks MO, Blaum C, et al. Low serum carotenoids and development of severe walking disability among older women living in the community: the women's health and aging study I. Age Ageing. 2007;36(1):62–7.
57. Alipanah N, Varadhan R, Sun K, Ferrucci L, Fried LP, Semba RD. Low serum carotenoids are associated with a decline in walking speed in older women. J Nutr Health Aging. 2009;13(3):170–5.
58. Hayhoe RPG, Lentjes MAH, Luben RN, Khaw KT, Welch AA. Dietary carotenoid intake of individuals in the EPIC-Norfolk cohort is positively associated with percentage fat-free mass. Proc Nutr Soc. 2016;75(75):E216.
59. Sahni S, Dufour AB, Fielding RA, Newman AB, Kiel DP, Hannan MT, et al. Total carotenoid intake is associated with reduced loss of grip strength and gait speed over time in adults: the Framingham offspring study. Am J Clin Nutr. 2020;113(2):437–45.
60. Jahnen-Dechent W, Ketteler M. Magnesium basics. Clin Kidney J. 2012;5(Suppl 1):i3–i14.
61. de Baaij JH, Hoenderop JG, Bindels RJ. Magnesium in man: implications for health and disease. Physiol Rev. 2015;95(1):1–46.
62. Hayhoe RPG, Lentjes MAH, Mulligan AA, Luben RN, Khaw KT, Welch AA. Cross-sectional associations of dietary and circulating magnesium with skeletal muscle mass in the EPIC-Norfolk cohort. Clin Nutr. 2019;38(1):317–23.
63. Welch AA, Skinner J, Hickson M. Dietary magnesium may be protective for aging of bone and skeletal muscle in middle and younger older age men and women: cross-sectional findings from the UK Biobank Cohort. Nutrients. 2017;9(11):1189.
64. Welch AA, Kelaiditi E, Jennings A, Steves CJ, Spector TD, MacGregor A. Dietary magnesium is positively associated with skeletal muscle power and indices of muscle mass and may attenuate the association between circulating C-reactive protein and muscle mass in women. J Bone Miner Res. 2016;31(2):317–25.
65. Brilla LR, Haley TF. Effect of magnesium supplementation on strength training in humans. J Am Coll Nutr. 1992;11(3):326–9.
66. Veronese N, Berton L, Carraro S, Bolzetta F, De Rui M, Perissinotto E, et al. Effect of oral magnesium supplementation on physical performance in healthy elderly women involved in a weekly exercise program: a randomized controlled trial. Am J Clin Nutr. 2014;100(3):974–81.
67. Rock E, Astier C, Lab C, Vignon X, Gueux E, Motta C, et al. Dietary magnesium deficiency in rats enhances free radical production in skeletal muscle. J Nutr. 1995;125(5):1205–10.
68. Aleman H, Esparza J, Ramirez FA, Astiazaran H, Payette H. Longitudinal evidence on the association between interleukin-6 and C-reactive protein with the loss of total appendicular skeletal muscle in free-living older men and women. Age Ageing. 2011;40(4):469–75.
69. Schaap LA, Pluijm SM, Deeg DJ, Harris TB, Kritchevsky SB, Newman AB, et al. Higher inflammatory marker levels in older persons: associations with 5-year change in muscle mass and muscle strength. J Gerontol A Biol Sci Med Sci. 2009;64(11):1183–9.
70. Cesari M, Penninx BW, Pahor M, Lauretani F, Corsi AM, Rhys Williams G, et al. Inflammatory markers and physical performance in older persons: the InCHIANTI study. J Gerontol A Biol Sci Med Sci. 2004;59(3):242–8.
71. Dibaba DT, Xun P, He K. Dietary magnesium intake is inversely associated with serum C-reactive protein levels: meta-analysis and systematic review. Eur J Clin Nutr. 2014;68(4):510–6.

72. Veronese N, Zanforlini BM, Manzato E, Sergi G. Magnesium and healthy aging. Magnes Res. 2015;28(3):112–5.
73. van Dronkelaar C, van Velzen A, Abdelrazek M, van der Steen A, Weijs PJM, Tieland M. Minerals and sarcopenia; the role of calcium, Iron, magnesium, phosphorus, potassium, selenium, sodium, and zinc on muscle mass, muscle strength, and physical performance in older adults: a systematic review. J Am Med Dir Assoc. 2018;19(1):6–11 e3.
74. Giugliano R, Millward DJ. The effects of severe zinc deficiency on protein turnover in muscle and thymus. Br J Nutr. 1987;57(1):139–55.
75. Chen YL, Yang KC, Chang HH, Lee LT, Lu CW, Huang KC. Low serum selenium level is associated with low muscle mass in the community-dwelling elderly. J Am Med Dir Assoc. 2014;15(11):807–11.
76. Lauretani F, Semba RD, Bandinelli S, Ray AL, Guralnik JM, Ferrucci L. Association of low plasma selenium concentrations with poor muscle strength in older community-dwelling adults: the InCHIANTI study. Am J Clin Nutr. 2007;86(2):347–52.
77. Welch AA, Hayhoe RG. The relationship between dietary fat and sarcopenia, skeletal muscle loss, osteoporosis and risk of fractures in aging. In: Weaver CM, Bischoff-Ferrari H, Daly RM, Wong M-S, editors. Nutritional influences on bone health: 10th International Symposium. Cham: Springer; 2019. p. 211–27.
78. Welch A, Hayhoe R. The relationship between dietary fat and sarcopenia, skeletal muscle loss, osteoporosis and risk of fractures in aging. In: Weaver CM, Bischoff-Ferrari H, Daly RM, Wong M-S, editors. Nutritional influences on bone health. Cham: Springer; 2019. p. 211–25.
79. Melzer K. Carbohydrate and fat utilization during rest and physical activity. E-SPEN. 2011;6(2):e45–52.
80. Gerling CJ, Mukai K, Chabowski A, Heigenhauser GJF, Holloway GP, Spriet LL, et al. Incorporation of Omega-3 fatty acids into human skeletal muscle Sarcolemmal and mitochondrial membranes following 12 weeks of fish oil supplementation. Front Physiol. 2019;10:348.
81. Galli C, Calder PC. Effects of fat and fatty acid intake on inflammatory and immune responses: a critical review. Ann Nutr Metab. 2009;55(1–3):123–39.
82. Welch AA, Macgregor AJ, Minihane AM, Skinner J, Valdes AA, Spector TD, et al. Dietary fat and fatty acid profile are associated with indices of skeletal muscle mass in women aged 18–79 years. J Nutr. 2014;144(3):327–34.
83. Abdelhamid A, Hooper L, Sivakaran R, Hayhoe RPG, Welch A, Group P. The relationship between Omega-3, Omega-6 and Total polyunsaturated Fat and musculoskeletal health and functional status in adults: a systematic review and meta-analysis of RCTs. Calcif Tissue Int. 2019;105(4):353–72.
84. Milaneschi Y, Bandinelli S, Corsi AM, Lauretani F, Paolisso G, Dominguez LJ, et al. Mediterranean diet and mobility decline in older persons. Exp Gerontol. 2011;46(4):303–8.
85. Gotsis E, Anagnostis P, Mariolis A, Vlachou A, Katsiki N, Karagiannis A. Health benefits of the Mediterranean diet: an update of research over the last 5 years. Angiology. 2015;66(4):304–18.
86. Ostan R, Lanzarini C, Pini E, Scurti M, Vianello D, Bertarelli C, et al. Inflammaging and cancer: a challenge for the Mediterranean diet. Nutrients. 2015;7(4):2589–621.
87. Craig JV, Bunn DK, Hayhoe RP, Appleyard WO, Lenaghan EA, Welch AA. Relationship between the Mediterranean dietary pattern and musculoskeletal health in children, adolescents, and adults: systematic review and evidence map. Nutr Rev. 2017;75(10):830–57.
88. Kelaiditi E, Jennings A, Steves CJ, Skinner J, Cassidy A, MacGregor AJ, et al. Measurements of skeletal muscle mass and power are positively related to a Mediterranean dietary pattern in women. Osteoporos Int. 2016;27(11):3251–60.
89. Jennings A, Mulligan AA, Khaw KT, Luben RN, Welch AA. A Mediterranean diet is positively associated with bone and muscle health in a non-Mediterranean region in 25,450 men and women from EPIC-Norfolk. Nutrients. 2020;12(4):1154.
90. Remer T, Manz F. Potential renal acid load of foods and its influence on urine pH. J Am Diet Assoc. 1995;95(7):791–7.
91. Workeneh BT, Mitch WE. Review of muscle wasting associated with chronic kidney disease. Am J Clin Nutr. 2010;91(4):1128S–32S.

92. Garibotto G, Russo R, Sofia A, Sala MR, Sabatino C, Moscatelli P, et al. Muscle protein turnover in chronic renal failure patients with metabolic acidosis or normal acid-base balance. Miner Electrolyte Metab. 1996;22(1–3):58–61.
93. Vazquez JA, Adibi SA. Protein sparing during treatment of obesity: ketogenic versus nonketogenic very low calorie diet. Metabolism. 1992;41(4):406–14.
94. Bell JD, Margen S, Calloway DH. Ketosis, weight loss, uric acid, and nitrogen balance in obese women fed single nutrients at low caloric levels. Metabolism. 1969;18(3):193–208.
95. Dawson-Hughes B, Harris SS, Ceglia L. Alkaline diets favor lean tissue mass in older adults. Am J Clin Nutr. 2008;87(3):662–5.
96. Faure AM, Fischer K, Dawson-Hughes B, Egli A, Bischoff-Ferrari HA. Gender-specific association between dietary acid load and total lean body mass and its dependency on protein intake in seniors. Osteoporos Int. 2017;28(12):3451–62.
97. Welch AA, MacGregor AJ, Skinner J, Spector TD, Moayyeri A, Cassidy A. A higher alkaline dietary load is associated with greater indexes of skeletal muscle mass in women. Osteoporos Int. 2013;24(6):1899–908.
98. Hayhoe RPG, Abdelhamid A, Luben RN, Khaw KT, Welch AA. Dietary acid-base load and its association with risk of osteoporotic fractures and low estimated skeletal muscle mass. Eur J Clin Nutr. 2020;74(Suppl 1):33–42.

The Future of Drugs in Sarcopenia

14

Maria Beatrice Zazzara, Rose S. Penfold,
and Graziano Onder

14.1 Introduction

Sarcopenia is the age-related decline in muscle mass and strength and is associated with increased risk of adverse health outcomes including falls, morbidity, loss of independence, disability and mortality [1, 2].

The cause of sarcopenia is multifactorial, including alteration in the composition of muscle fibres, neurological factors related to the loss of motor neurons occurring with ageing, endocrine alterations resulting from the decrease of hormone levels and nutritional and lifestyle changes related to the adoption of sedentary habits [3, 4].

Starting from the fifth decade of life, muscle mass declines approximately 0.8% per year [5]. From the sixth decade of life, gradual loss in skeletal muscle mass and strength is estimated to be around 2% per year [6]. Other studies report a reduction in lean muscle mass by 3–8% per decade starting at age 30 [7, 8].

Lifestyle interventions (i.e. physical activity and nutrition) have proven to have significant impact in improving this condition [2, 9]. However, many of those with sarcopenia are unable to exercise or unable to maintain a healthy nutritional status.

M. B. Zazzara (✉)
Department of Gerontology, Fondazione Policlinico Gemelli IRCCS, Rome, Italy

R. S. Penfold
Department of Twin Research and Genetic Epidemiology, King's College London, St Thomas' Hospital, London, UK
e-mail: rose.penfold@kcl.ac.uk

G. Onder
Department of Cardiovascular, Endocrine-metabolic Diseases and Aging, Istituto Superiore di Sanità, Rome, Italy
e-mail: graziano.onder@iss.it

© Springer Nature Switzerland AG 2021
N. Veronese et al. (eds.), *Sarcopenia*, Practical Issues in Geriatrics,
https://doi.org/10.1007/978-3-030-80038-3_14

Despite important efforts to find effective drugs to address this condition, to date there are no official US Food and Drug Administration (FDA) or European Medicines Agency (EMA) approved drugs for the treatment of sarcopenia [10].

In this chapter, we review the implications of drugs developed with the aim of preventing, slowing progression, reversing sarcopenia, and increasing muscular outcomes in older adults.

14.2 Myostatin/Activin Pathway Antagonism

14.2.1 Myostatin Inhibitors

Myostatin, also known as growth differentiation factor-8 (GDF8), is a member of the transforming growth factor-β (TGF-β) family expressed in skeletal muscle. It inhibits myogenesis and activates protein degradation by interacting with several pathways of muscle cell growth and differentiation [11–14]. With ageing, the expression of myostatin within the muscle increases, leading to progressive muscle athrophy [12].

Myostatin forms tetrameric complexes through the binding of the receptor complex activin type 2B (ACVR2B) and activin-like kinase 4 (ALK4) which allows the phosphorylation of the serine and threonine residues of type 1 receptors through the kinase activity of type 2 receptors, with consequent activation of the transcription factors SMAD2 and SMAD3 that eventually downregulates genes involved in myogenic differentiation such as MyoD, myogenin, myf5 [8, 12] and MRF4/Myf6 [15].

Also, ageing itself is associated with an alteration in the differentiating capacity of satellite cells and with a reduced number of differentiating cells. The blockage of the myostatin pathway could therefore overcome this age-related modification and increase the rate of satellite cell differentiation into myo-tubes.

Furthermore myostatin, through the suppression of the Akt/mTOR axis, is involved in the direct activation of transcriptional factor FOXO which is connected to the expression of muscle-1 ring-finger protein-1 (MuRF-1) and other transcriptional factors in the ubiquitin-proteasome and autophagy pathways [8, 16].

The role of myostatin was primarily evaluated when mutations of the myostatin gene were found to be associated with muscle hypertrophy in children [17, 18]. Theoretically, agents targeting the myostatin pathway may be useful in increasing muscle mass and have been studied in order to find a molecular target that could play a significant role in age-related sarcopenia.

In murine ageing models, antibody directed against myostatin significantly improved muscle mass, fibre size and function [11, 19]. In middle-aged mice, antagonizing myostatin enhanced muscle tissue regeneration [20]. Recombinant human antibody, follistatin (a myostatin binding protein) or myostatin-antagonists such as trichostatin-A, also offers potential for treatment of sarcopenia [21].

There have been no in-human trials testing the efficacy of myostatin inhibitors for sarcopenia. Nevertheless, the first trial of myostatin inhibitors concerned muscular dystrophy patients and assessed efficacy of stamulumab (MYO-029), a recombinant human antibody. Stamulumab neutralizes the activity of myostatin protein by preventing myostatin from binding to ACVR2B [22]. MYO-29 has been tested in phase 2 trials for muscular dystrophy, and preliminary results have shown a good safety and tolerability profile [22]. However, it has been reported that muscle tissue may be more susceptible to muscle and tendon injuries in mice with myostatin deficiency [17].

In the last 10 years, two phase 2 randomized control trials have investigated the safety and efficacy of landogrozumab (LY-2495655), a humanized monoclonal antibody which neutralizes activity of the myostatin protein. The first study, in 400 adults aged ≥50 years who had undergone elective total hip surgery for osteoarthritis, found that subcutaneous injections of landogrozumab demonstrated a dose-dependent increase in appendicular lean body mass and decrease in fat mass in the intervention versus placebo group [23].

The second evaluated whether LY-2495655 increased appendicular lean body mass and physical performance in older fallers with low muscle strength. Participants aged 75 years or older were randomized to receive a subcutaneous injection of 315 mg of landogrozumab or placebo. A significant increase in lean mass and a trend of improvement of functional measures was found in the intervention as compared to placebo group [24]. Other phase 2 clinical trials of LY-2495655 in patients with sarcopenia are currently under review [10].

Another phase 2 trial determined the efficacy of trevogrumab (REGN1033), another myostatin antibody. The trial evaluated whether REGN1033 could be safe and effective in increasing muscle mass and function in patients affected by sarcopenia. Definitive results and evaluations have not been published yet [10, 25].

Development of a fusion protein of activin receptor type 2B and IgG1-Fc, ramatercept (ACE-031), for the treatment of muscular dystrophy, was discontinued due to safety concerns including minor nosebleeds, gum bleeding and small dilated blood vessels within the skin [13, 26].

Recently, a newer form of ACE-031 called ACE-083 has been designed for facioscapulohumeral muscular dystrophy (FSHD) and Charcot-Marie-Tooth (CMT) disease based on a modified form of human follistatin [13].

ACE-083 is a recombinant fusion protein consisting of a modified form of human follistatin linked to the human immunoglobulin G2 Fc domain [27].

Inhibition of the myostatin pathway with follistatin may have potential therapeutic benefits on skeletal muscle. Follistatin inhibits muscle growth signalling by binding activins A and B and myostatin, inducing muscle hypertrophy through satellite cell proliferation [27–29].

The results of a phase 1 clinical trial assessing safety and efficacy of a local injection of ACE-083 to the rectus femoris or tibialis anterior muscles in healthy postmenopausal women reported an increase in muscle volume directly related to an increase in the dose. However, no significant changes in muscle strength were noticed [30]. Phase 2 clinical trials are ongoing in patients with FSHD and CMT [10, 31].

14.2.2 Activin Inhibitors

Other potential targets are activin receptors.

As mentioned, myostatin acts as a negative regulator of muscle mass via the activin receptor type 2B (ACVR2B). ACVR2B binds numerous ligands, including the activins (activin A, B, C and E), GDF11, bone morphogenetic protein 9 (BMP9) and BMP10, suggesting the presence of additional negative regulators of muscle hypertrophy and more intricated mechanism in the development of sarcopenia [32].

Monoclonal antibodies have been produced with the aim of blocking this signalling pathway.

Bimagrumab (BYM-338) is a human monoclonal antibody that binds activin receptors ACVR2A and ACVR2B and prevents the binding of its ligands that usually act as inhibitors of muscle growth and protein anabolism.

By blocking these ligands, BYM-338 promotes differentiation of myoblasts and prevents the inhibition of differentiation induced by myostatin or activin A.

BYM-338 has been evaluated as a therapy for sporadic inclusion body myositis, an inflammatory myopathy that is characterized by progressive pathological muscle weakness and atrophy. BYM-338 also inhibits myostatin- or activin A-induced atrophy, thus sparing the myosin heavy chain from degradation.

Bimagrumab significantly increased skeletal muscle mass in mice, beyond the sole inhibition of myostatin [33].

The effect of a 24-week treatment with 30 mg/kg intravenous BYM-338 was evaluated in a randomized control study of community-dwelling adults aged 65 and older with sarcopenia and mobility limitations. It was safe and well tolerated by older adults [34]. After the first of two doses, patients showed an increase in outcomes including thigh muscle volume, lean body mass, appendicular lean mass and reductions in body fat mass as compared to the placebo group. Patients also showed improvements in mobility and physical function, as assessed by 6-min walk distance and gait speed.

The same authors evaluated the clinical potential of BYM-338 in the recovery of skeletal muscle volume from disuse atrophy in healthy young males in a double-blind, placebo-controlled trial. A full-length cast was placed on all participants on one of the lower extremities for 2 weeks. After cast removal, subjects were randomized to receive a single intravenous dose of either bimagrumab 30 mg/kg or placebo. Participants who received bimagrumab demonstrated a more rapid recovery of tight muscle volume [33, 35].

Principal studies addressing the myostatin/activin pathway antagonism are summarized in Table 14.1.

Table 14.1 Summary of the studies evaluating the myostatin/activin pathway antagonism

Study	Drug	Study design	Population	Interventions	Outcomes	Results
Wagner (2008) [22]	StamuLImab (MYO-029)	Phase 1 and 2 randomized, double-blind, placebo-controlled trial	Subjects aged ≥18 years with muscular dystrophy [Becker's muscular dystrophy (BMD), facioscapulohumeral dystrophy (FSHD), limb-girdle muscular dystrophy (LGMD)] N = 116 total participants (36 with BMD, 42 with FSHD and 38 with LGMD) Cohort 1: N = 27, mean age 37.2 (9.5), females 7 (25.9%) Cohort 2: N = 27, mean age 37.1 (13.6), females 5 (18.5%) Cohort 3: N = 27, mean age 40.2 (11.5), females 7 (25.9%) Cohort 4: N = 6, mean age 44.3 (10.2), females 1 (16.7%) Placebo cohort: N = 29, mean age 39.3 (13.3), females 8 (27.6%)	Cohort 1: 1 mg/kg Cohort 2: 3 mg/kg Cohort 3: 10 mg/kg Cohort 4: 30 mg/kg Placebo cohort • Way of administration: Intravenously every 2 weeks for 6 months (total of 13 doses) • Follow-up: 3 months after last administration	Primary outcome: 1. Safety and tolerability of MYO-029 Exploratory outcomes: 1. Biological activity assessed with muscle testing (MMT), quantitative muscle testing (QMT), timed function tests (TFTs), pulmonary function tests and subject reported outcomes 2. Muscle histology: An open muscle biopsy to evaluate presence of fibre necrosis, inflammation and muscle regeneration 3. Myostatin levels: Both free and total myostatin serum and in muscle biopsy samples though a validated enzyme-linked immunosorbent assay (ELISA) at baseline and 2 weeks after interventions	• MYO-029 demonstrated a good safety and tolerability except for cutaneous hypersensitivity at the 10 and 30 mg/kg doses in four subjects • No improvements in exploratory end points of muscle strength or function; in a limited number of subjects, there was a trend toward increased muscle size using dual-energy radiographic absorptiometry (DEXA) • In the 26 available muscle, biopsy MYO-029 had no observable adverse effect on muscle pathology • No observable changes in total and free myostatin serum levels or measurable free myostatin levels in serum at either week 6 or 36 compared with baseline in any group

(continued)

Table 14.1 (continued)

Study	Drug	Study design	Population	Interventions	Outcomes	Results
Woodhouse (2016) [23]	Landogrozumab (LY2495655)	Phase 2, randomized, parallel, double-blind, 12-week clinical trial	Subjects aged ≥50 years scheduled for elective total hip arthroplasty for osteoarthritis within 10 ± 6 days after randomization in 44 sites across 11 countries $N = 400$ total participants Group 1: $N = 104$, mean age 68.7 (8.1), females 70 (67.3%) Group 2: $N = 98$, mean age 67.9 (8.1), females 51 (52.0%) Group 3: $N = 100$, mean age 68.7 (8.0), females 54 (54.0%) Placebo group: $N = 98$, mean age 69.4 (8.9), females 59 (60.2%)	Group 1: 35 mg Group 2: 105 mg Group 3: 315 mg Placebo group • Way of administration: subcutaneous injections at weeks 0 (randomization date), 4, 8, and 12 • Follow-up: until week 24	Primary outcome: 1. Probability that LY2495655 increases appendicular lean mass (operated limb excluded) by at least 2.5% more than placebo at week 12, using dual-energy X-ray absorptiometry Exploratory outcomes: 1. Muscle strength 2. Performance-based and self-reported measures of physical function 3. Whole body composition over time	• Changes in lean mass did not meet the superiority threshold at week 12 in the treatment groups as compared to placebo • Significant progressive increases in appendicular lean mass were documented in group 1 and 2 as compared to placebo group at weeks 8 and 16 • In group 3, whole body fat mass significantly decreased as compared to placebo at weeks 8 and 16 • No meaningful differences were detected between groups in other exploratory outcomes • Injection site reactions occurred more often in the treatment groups as compared to placebo

| Becker (2015) [24] | Landogrozumab (LY2495655) | Proof-of-concept, randomized, placebo-controlled, double-blind, parallel, multicentre, phase 2 study | Subjects ≥75 years who had fallen in the past year from 21 investigator sites across Argentina, Australia, France, Germany, Sweden and the USA, with low performance on hand-grip strength and chair rise tests

N = 201 total participants
Intervention group: N = 102, mean age 82 (75–96), females 75 (74%)
Placebo group: N = 99, mean age 83 (75–99), females 65 (66%) | Intervention group: 315 mg
Placebo group
• Way of administration: subcutaneous injections at weeks 0 (randomization visit), 4, 8, 12, 16, and 20
• Follow-up: 16 weeks observation after the last visit | Primary outcome:
1. Change in appendicular lean body mass from baseline to 24 weeks
Secondary outcome:
2. Physical performance assessed with four-step stair climbing time, usual gait speed and time to rise five times from a chair without arms, or with arms for participants unable to do it without arms
Exploratory outcomes:
1. 12-step stair climbing test
2. 6-min walking distance
3. Fast gait speed
4. Hand-grip strength
5. Isometric leg extension strength | • At 24 weeks, there was a significant difference in an LBM between intervention and placebo group ($p < 0.0001$). This difference was not significant at week 12 ($p = 0.083$) but was maintained until week 36 ($p = 0.005$). Patients in the intervention group also had a greater increase in total lean mass ($p = 0.0007$) and a larger reduction in total fat mass ($p < 0.0001$) as compared to placebo
• Stair climbing time (four-step and 12-step tests), chair rise with arms and fast gait speed improved significantly from baseline to week 24 with
• No effect was detected for other performance-based measures |

(continued)

Table 14.1 (continued)

Study	Drug	Study design	Population	Interventions	Outcomes	Results
ClinicalTrials. gov identifier (NCT number: NCT01963598) [25]	Trevogrumab (REGN1033)	Randomized, double-blind, placebo-controlled, multicentre 3 months phase 2 study	Men and women aged ≥75 years (all women participating in the study must be postmenopausal) Subjects with sarcopenia *N* = 253 total participants	3 Experimental groups 1 placebo group • Way of administration: 3-month subcutaneous treatment	Primary outcomes: 1. Percent change in total lean body mass measured by DEXA from baseline (day 1) to week 12 (day 85) 2. Safety Secondary outcomes: 1. Adverse events from baseline (day 1) to the end of the study (day 141) 2. Changes from baseline in appendicular lean mass by DEXA; in maximal leg press strength (1-repetition max); in maximal chest press strength (1-repetition max); in 4-meter gait speed; in short physical performance battery (SPPB); in distance walked in the 6MWT (6-min walk test); in hand-grip strength by handheld dynamometer; in unloaded and loaded stair climb power 3. Change from baseline in regional and total fat mass by DEXA	• Ongoing

| Campbell (2016) [26] | Ramatercept (ACE-031) | Randomized, double-blind, placebo-controlled, multiple-ascending-dose, phase 2 clinical trial | Male subjects enrolled at 4 Canadian study site with age ≥4 years with confirmed Duchenne muscular dystrophy (DMD) with the ability to ambulate 10 m in <12 s, undergoing corticosteroid therapy for at least 1 year before enrolment were and clinical evidence of weakness of the neck flexors N = 24 Cohort 1: N = 9, mean age 9.3 (3.7) Cohort 2: N = 9, mean age 9.8 (2.5) Placebo cohort: N = 6, mean age 10.5 (3.6) | Cohort 1: 0.5 mg/kg every 4 weeks (4 doses total) Cohort 2: 1 mg/kg every 2 weeks (7 doses total) Placebo cohort • Way of administration: subcutaneously • Follow-up: Clinical evaluation continued until day 169 (57 days), 84 days after the last dose | Primary outcome: 1. Safety and tolerability (adverse drugs events) of repeated doses and multiple dose levels of ACE-031 Secondary outcomes: 1. Determine the maximum tolerated dose level of ACE-031 in terms of safety 2. Determine and characterize pharmacokinetic and pharmacodynamic effects on lean mass, fat mass, BMD and 6MWT | • ACE-031 was not associated with serious or severe adverse events • The study was stopped after the second dosing regimen due to potential safety concerns of epistaxis and telangiectasias. Epistaxis and telangiectasias were reported with greater frequency with increasing ACE-031 dose levels. Telangiectasias appeared after the seventh dose of study drug and faded or resolved approximately 1 month after drug discontinuation in most cases. No thrombocytopenia was noted to account for bleeding-related AEs • A non-significant increase in the 6-min walk test (6MWT) distance in the intervention groups compared with a decline in the placebo group was demonstrated |

(continued)

Table 14.1 (continued)

Study	Drug	Study design	Population	Interventions	Outcomes	Results
Glasser (2018) [30]	ACE-083 (modified form of human follistatin linked to the human immunoglobulin G2 Fc domain)	Phase 1, randomized, double-blind, placebo-controlled trial	Subjects were healthy postmenopausal women aged 45–75 years with a body mass index (BMI) range of 18.5–32 kg/m N = 58 total participants Cohorts 1–5: Intervention group: Total N = 30, median age 56.0 (45–70) Placebo group: total N = 10, median age 57.5 (55–73) Cohorts 6–7: Intervention group: Total N = 12, median age 55.5 (49–62) Placebo group: Total N = 6, median age 57.5 (45–65)	7 cohorts Cohorts 1–3: 50, 100 or 200 mg per muscle Cohorts 4 and 5: 100 or 200 mg per muscle Cohorts 6 and 7: 100 or 150 mg per muscle Placebo cohorts • Way of administration: ACE-083 or placebo was administered unilaterally in the right side only with electromyography guidance used to administer each dose as 2 or 4 equal volume injections (0.5–1.0 mL per injection), depending on the dose, using a 26-gauge Myoject needle Cohorts 1–3: ACE-083 was injected into the rectus femoris (RF) as a single dose Cohorts 4 and 5: ACE-083 was injected into the rectus femoris (RF) as 2 doses on days 1 and 22 Cohorts 6 and 7: ACE-083 was injected into the tibialis anterior (TA) as 2 doses on days 1 and 22 • Follow-up: 12 weeks after their final dose	Outcomes: 1. Safety assessed with evaluation of adverse events (AE), injection site reactions, clinical laboratory tests, electrocardiograms, vital signs, antidrug antibody (ADA) and physical examinations 2. Pharmacokinetics 3. Pharmacodynamics: assessed with MRI of the thigh (RF cohorts) and lower leg (TA cohorts) to measure muscle volume and intramuscular fat	• No serious AE dose-limiting toxicities, or discontinuations resulting from AEs occurred • AEs involving the injection site accounted for most AEs reported for both intervention and placebo groups. Injection site pain was the most common AE • Pharmacokinetics results were available for cohorts 6 and 7. Serum ACE-083 levels were detectable only during the first day after dosing • A significant increase in RF and TA muscle was demonstrated with effects in the contralateral noninjected muscle similar to placebo-injected muscles. Maximum volume increases were 14.5% (4.5%) and 8.9% (4.7%), respectively • No significant changes in mean muscle strength were observed

| Rooks (2017) [34] | Bimagrumab (BYM-338) | A phase 2, randomized, double-blind, placebo controlled, parallel-arm, proof-of-concept study | Subjects were community-living men and women aged ≥65 years with a 4 m gait speed between 0.4 and 1.0 m/s and an appendicular skeletal muscle index (ASMI; skeletal muscle in kg/height in m^2) of 7.25 kg/m^2 or less for men and 5.67 kg/m^2 or less for women using DEXA N = 44 total participants Intervention group: N = 19, mean age 71.6 (6.3), females 6 (32%) Placebo group: N = 21, mean age 72.4 (4.6), females 13 (62%) | Intervention group: 30 mg/kg Placebo group • Way of administration: intravenous infusion of bimagrumab 30 mg/kg on day 1 and day 57 • Follow-up: 24 weeks | Primary outcome: 1. Thigh muscle volume (TMV) assessed using magnetic resonance imaging (MRI) at the midthigh level Secondary outcomes: 1. Changes in total lean body mass (LBM) assessed with DEXA 2. Changes in grip strength from baseline between the intervention and placebo groups 3. Changes in gait speed from baseline between the intervention and placebo groups 4. Changes in 6-min walk distance (6MWD) from baseline between the intervention and placebo groups | • TMV increased significantly by week 2 in the intervention group versus placebo (5.15(2.19%) vs. 0.34(2.59%), $P < 0.001$) • Increase was sustained throughout the treatment period and remained above baseline at the end of study in the intervention group versus placebo (week 24: 4.80(5.81%) vs. 1.01(4.43%), $P = 0.002$) • DEXA analysis showed a greater increase in LBM and appendicular lean mass (ALM) and a greater decrease in fat mass in the intervention group as compared to placebo. A significant increase in ALM (kg ALM/m^2 of height) at week 8 of 5.7% vs. 0.5%, $P < 0.001$ from baseline in the intervention group • Significant improve in gait speed (mean 0.15 m/s, $P = 0.009$) and 6 MWD (mean 82 m, $P = 0.022$) was observed in patients with slower walking speed at baseline in the intervention group as compared to placebo • Non-significant improvement was noted in the grip strength of the dominant hand at weeks 8, 12 and 16 in the intervention group |

(continued)

Table 14.1 (continued)

Study	Drug	Study design	Population	Interventions	Outcomes	Results
Rooks (2017) [35]	Bimagrumab (BYM-338)	3:2 randomized, double-blind, placebo-controlled trial	Subjects were healthy young men aged 18–40 years with a BMI of 18 to 32 kg/m² A full-length cast was placed in one of the lower extremities for 2 weeks to induce disuse atrophy. Randomization occurred after cast removal *N* = 24 total participants Intervention group: *N* = 15, mean age 23.5 (4.9) Placebo group: *N* = 9, mean age 25.1 (8.2)	Intervention group: 30 mg/kg Placebo group • Way of administration: a single intravenous infusion of bimagrumab 30 mg/kg • Follow-up: 12 weeks	Primary outcome: 1. Thigh muscle volume (TVM), inter-muscular adipose tissue (IMAT) and subcutaneous adipose tissue (SCAT) were obtained using MRI scanner and Q-body coil Secondary outcome: 1. Changes in the maximum strength of a single limb knee extension from pre-cast levels were assessed in both legs 2. Safety: Determined based on physical examination, assessment of vital signs, electrocardiogram, blood tests, urinalysis and identification of AEs	• After cast removal, in the interventions group TMV recovered to within −0.8% ± 0.6% of the baseline value in 2 weeks, +1.3% ± 0.6% at week 4 and + 5.1% ± 0.9% at week 12 from baseline in the treatment group as compared to placebo • Changes in TMV were accompanied by treatment specific effects on IMAT and SCAT volumes • No change in maximum force production was noted in the non-casted limb, and no significant difference was observed in response to treatment • No serious severe AE was reported. The most commonly reported AEs were dermatitis acneiform, transient muscle spasms and pain in extremity

At time of writing, no other conclusive data have been reported from human studies [11]. Other monoclonal antibodies have been evaluated in primate and murine models suggesting that the blockage of the activin signalling pathway, in particular the blockage of activin A, may more prominently regulate muscle mass in primates than myostatin [32]. Although there are currently no clear drug candidates to directly inhibit sarcopenia, the inhibition of myostatin/ACVR2 signalling may improve muscle mass in patients with muscle wasting syndromes and could represent a potential therapeutic target for sarcopenia.

14.3 Hormones

The reduction of circulating hormones which occurs with ageing is believed to contribute to changes in muscle mass and function in older individuals [36]. Hormonal supplementation has therefore been studied as a potential therapeutic option for sarcopenia [37].

14.3.1 Androgen Supplementation

14.3.1.1 Testosterone

Testosterone is a steroid hormone secreted by the ovarian thecal cells in women and by the Lcydig cells in men.

Higher testosterone levels are associated with higher muscle mass and increased muscle protein anabolism [36].

Several randomized controlled studies support the relationship between decline in testosterone levels with age and loss of muscle mass and strength, suggesting a direct effect of testosterone on muscle mass and strength [38–42].

Testosterone induces muscle fibre hypertrophy and regulates muscle protein synthesis and breakdown. It also appears to increase the number of satellite cells in both animals and human studies [43, 44]. By modulating the differentiation of mesenchymal pluripotent cells, it promotes cellular commitment to the myogenic lineage and inhibits differentiation into the adipogenic lineage through an androgen receptor-mediated pathway. Testosterone administration is associated with an increase in the cross-sectional areas of both type I and II muscle fibers [45, 46].

As well as anabolic effects, testosterone is also purported to exert effects via its action on motor neurons. Motor neurons have androgen receptors [47]. With ageing, muscular junctions and fibres suffer from instability or denervation due to loss of motor neurones, reduction in axonal size and demyelination at the level of the peripheral nerve with consequent reduction in conduction speed. This process affects particularly larger motor neurons and its accompanied by a compensational remodelling of the motor units which increase in size which initially helps maintaining muscle function to some extent [4, 48], eventually leading to strength loss and fatigue [4].

Testosterone may enhance peripheral motor nerve regeneration following injury by stimulating the production of neuritin-a protein that is involved in the re-establishment of neuronal connectivity following traumatic damage to the nervous system [49].

Results from studies assessing testosterone replacement therapy in men are heterogenous, with differences among age of participants, level of plasma testosterone before the treatment and route of administration. Such studies heterogeneity makes it difficult to draw firm conclusions regarding the effect of testosterone replacing treatment on disability and physical performance. A meta-analysis performed in 2006, including data from 11 randomized-clinical trials, suggests that testosterone treatment produces a moderate increase in muscle strength compared to placebo [50]. A significant positive effect of testosterone supplementation on muscle mass in older participants was demonstrated by a 2018 umbrella review of systematic reviews and meta-analyses. However, sarcopenic status of participants was not systemically assessed, and effects on muscle strength and physical performance were minimal when compared to the effect on muscle mass, especially among men with low serum levels of testosterone ($<200-300$ ng/dL) [51].

In frail older men, administration of 50 mg per day of transdermal testosterone hydro-alcoholic gel for 6 months led to a significant increase in lean body mass and an increase in knee extensor strength [52]. Moreover, the combination with nutritional supplements or physical exercise enhanced the effects of transdermal supplementation of testosterone improved on muscle mass and function [53–56]. Similarly, a prospective study demonstrated an increase in upper body strength during resistance exercise alone following testosterone treatment of older patients with low to normal serum testosterone [57, 58].

Furthermore, testosterone replacement therapy can have possible side effects that need to be balanced against the potential benefits of treatment. Testosterone is associated with adverse effects including peripheral oedema, gynecomastia, polycythaemia and sleep apnoea [17]. Perhaps more importantly, there is a correlation between serum testosterone levels and prostate cancer. In the Baltimore Longitudinal Study on Ageing involving 781 subjects, likelihood of developing high-risk prostate cancer in men 65 years or older doubled for every 0.1 unit increase in free testosterone level [59]. Furthermore, testosterone was associated with increased risk of cardiovascular events [60]. In the Testosterone Trials (TTrials), testosterone supplementation increased the non-calcified plaque volume of coronary artery assessed with computed tomographic angiography [61]. However, the TTrials found no significant differences in number of cardiovascular or prostate adverse events with testosterone supplementation versus placebo [61].

Given current uncertainties, it may be recommended to treat only older men with repeatedly low serum testosterone levels and symptoms and signs consistent with androgen deficiency.

14.3.1.2 Selective Androgen Receptor Modulators

Selective androgen receptor modulators (SARMs) are synthetic androgen modulators and potential alternatives to testosterone. By improving tissue selectivity,

SARMs have a similar anabolic effect as testosterone on muscle tissue, without many of the undesirable side effects associated with traditional androgen therapies. They may also offer therapeutic options for androgen use in women.

One study demonstrated that 3 months treatment with a SARM called ostarine (MK-2866) induced a dose-dependent increase in muscle mass and stair-climbing power in healthy older adults [62, 63].

Another randomized control study, of 170 women aged ≥65 years with sarcopenia and moderate physical dysfunction, showed how 6 months of treatment with a SARM (MK-0773), in combination with vitamin D and protein supplementation, significantly increased lean body mass versus placebo, although no improvement was observed in muscle strength or physical performances [64].

Although early evidence is promising, future of SARMs for the treatment of sarcopenia depends on necessary further studies demonstrating safety and efficacy.

14.3.1.3   Dehydroepiandrosterone

Dehydroepiandrosterone (DHEA) is a hormone precursor that is converted to testosterone/oestrogen hormones at specific target tissues [65].

Animal models have demonstrated that skeletal muscle contains specific enzymes able of converting circulating DHEA to testosterone and dehydrotestosterone, the androgen that acts at a steroid receptors' level. Moreover, DHEA supplementation increases insulin growth-factor 1 (IGF-1) levels that stimulates the proliferation and migration of myogenic or muscle precursor cells [66].

Therefore, DHEA supplementation could potentially help enhance muscle mass and strength in both males and females and could be of particular importance in older subjects, where almost all of the total androgens are derived from these adrenal precursor steroids [67].

Unfortunately, there are few studies evaluating the impact of DHEA supplementation in older adults, and the effects on muscle mass and function are inconsistent.

In the inChianti study, authors found that circulating DHEA was independently correlated with muscle strength and calf muscle area in men aged 60–79 years [68].

However, a systematic review of eight studies investigating the effect of DHEA supplementation on body composition and physical performance in older adults found inconclusive results concerning muscle strength and physical function in older adults [67]. Other studies demonstrated that supplementation of DHEA increased the bone density but had no effects on muscle size, strength or function in aged men and women [65].

Improvement in strength and function may require a combination of DHEA and exercise. In a randomized trial of 99 older frail women (mean age 76.6), DHEA supplementation in combination with exercise improved lower extremity strength and function [54]. Similarly, another study showed improvement in strength in a group of healthy older adults from a combination of DHEA supplementation and high-resistance training [69].

Other researches have suggested that, in ageing adults, the effect of DHEA supplementation should be evaluated over a longer period of time, so that supplementation with DHEA would result in increased levels of circulating androgen levels as compared to young and healthy adults [65]. However, a study investigating the effects of 6 months of DHEA supplementation in women with adrenal failure found no effects on muscle and fat mass or bone tissue, with high frequency of documented side effects [70].

Overall, studies demonstrating safety and efficacy of androgens supplementation as a pharmacological treatment of sarcopenia are controversial. To this date probably only SERMs, thanks to reduced adverse effects due to higher tissue selectivity, may represent an important potential therapy for sarcopenia, but further studies are required to be able to recommend them as a standard therapy for sarcopenia.

14.3.2 Oestrogens and Phytoestrogens

Oestrogen levels in women are associated with muscle mass and strengths. Hormone changes after menopause, in association with a more sedentary lifestyle, contribute to both bone loss and loss of muscle mass and strength [71]. The role of oestrogens on body composition is uncertain, with studies suggesting they could increase lean body mass and decrease fat mass and other studies showing no effects [71].

Oestrogen is converted to testosterone mainly by the action of the aromatase, which converts testosterone to oestradiol and androstenedione to oestrone. As above, this has a known anabolic effect on muscle protein synthesis.

Moreover, it seems to have a suppressing effect on inflammatory cytokines that have catabolic effects on skeletal muscle [72].

In postmenopausal women, oestrogen therapy results in a higher myogenic regulatory factor gene expression, a greater myogenic response to physical exercise and a lower muscle damage after maximal eccentric exercise [73]. Oestrogen replacement treatment has been reported to also improve insulin response during physical activity, possibly activating the anabolic pathway related to insulin secretion [74].

Evidence demonstrating the association between hormonal replacement treatment and muscle mass and muscle strength is controversial.

Some trials showed a significant positive effect of oestrogens on muscle strength [75–77]; while other randomized controlled trials did not find any significant effect on muscle mass [78] or strength [79–81]. Despite significant differences in duration of observation periods and mean age of participants in these trials, overall treatment with oestrogens demonstrated no significant effects in older women as compared to younger ones.

These findings, given also the well-documented side effects associated with these drugs (such as breast cancer, endometrial cancer, ovarian cancer, venous thromboembolic risk and stroke), are inconclusive, and further research is needed before recommending oestrogens as treatment for sarcopenia.

In line with oestrogens supplementation, another potential approach to prevent or treat sarcopenia might be represented by phytoestrogens supplementation. Phytoestrogens or isoflavones are produced almost exclusively by the members of the leguminosae family. They have a high affinity for the oestrogen receptor-α, which is found in muscle, thus having a possible beneficial effect on muscle mass.

Isoflavone supplements are mainly found in soy products. Isoflavones have lipid-lowering effect, favour vasodilatation as well as arterial compliance and regulate fasting glucose and insulin levels, overall contributing to reducing chronic inflammation [82].

An animal study demonstrated that chronic high soy protein diet was effective to reduce the activation of pathway involved in muscle protein degradation [83].

In humans, results are contrasting. In obese-sarcopenic postmenopausal women, soy isoflavone supplementation was associated with a significant increase in fat-free mass [84, 85]. However, a study reported that, in postmenopausal women, 16 weeks supplementation of soy protein in combination with resistance training did not significantly impact on muscle mass as compared to physical exercise alone [86]. Similar results were found in a more recent study which showed that adding soy protein to milk resulted in a greater increase in muscle strength but not in muscle gain after 16 weeks of resistance training in healthy postmenopausal women [87]. To this date, supplementation of phytoestrogens as a treatment for sarcopenia remains inconclusive.

14.3.3 Tibolone

Tibolone is a synthetic steroid with weak estrogenic, progestogenic and androgenic activity. Tibolone can have an impact on muscle anabolism acting by binding androgen receptors in muscle fibres and increasing serum-free testosterone, growth hormone and insulin growth-factor 1 (IGF-1) levels [88]. Tibolone demonstrated also a positive effect on muscle strength, increasing the plasma levels of nitric oxide that mediates satellite cell activation, and positively impacting on chronic inflammation [72, 89].

Some studies have documented a significant positive effect of tibolone on muscle strength [90] and muscle mass [91]. In particular, tibolone seems to increase fat-free mass and total body water content and reduce fat mass. Positive effects of tibolone were also shown when used in combination with oestrogens. In contrast, Hanggi et al. demonstrated that tibolone treatment had no impact on muscle mass [91]. Finally, it is worth mentioning that only a few of the clinical studies on oestrogens and on tibolone described included older women [80]. Once again, similarly to androgens supplementation, the available evidence is yet too controversial and insufficient to be able to systemically recommend oestrogens, phytoestrogens or tibolone as a standard treatment for sarcopenia.

14.3.4 Growth Hormone

Levels of growth hormone (GH) are usually lower in older subjects and this is one of the reasons why there is increasing interest surrounding the effect of GH in preventing age-related muscle mass loss and its potential in treatment of sarcopenia.

The effects of GH on muscle are principally mediated via insulin growth factor 1 (IGF-1), produced by the liver and the skeletal muscle in response to GH. IGF-1 stimulates the Akt/mTOR pathway which promotes muscle anabolism and protein synthesis in response to exercise [92], resulting in the proliferation of muscle satellite cells and the increase of synthesis of contractile proteins. In addition, IGF-1 suppresses proteolysis, promotes the delivery of amino acids and glucose to myocytes and stimulates myoblast proliferation and differentiation. Systemic IGF-1 administration enhances the rate of muscle functional recovery after injury and improves endurance and contractile muscle function, and low IGF-1 levels have been associated with poorer physical performance and strength [93].

Moreover, IGF-1 expression modulates systemic inflammation by decreasing plasma levels of pro-inflammatory cytokines, such as tumour necrosis factor alpha (TNF-α) and interleukin-1 beta (IL-1β).

The impact on sarcopenia could be mediated by muscle expression of IGF-1 accelerating the regenerative process of injured muscle, regulating the inflammatory response and limiting the development of fibrosis [94].

Furthermore, given that a low-grade chronic inflammation has been linked to the etiopathogenesis of sarcopenia [1], GH supplementation, downregulating systemic inflammation, could have an impact in preventing onset of sarcopenia.

Studies addressing GH supplementation in non-GH-deficient older adults found differing results, with most documenting inefficacy of GH treatment on muscle mass and strength.

A meta-analysis on the effects of GH administration on aerobic exercise capacity and muscle strength in GH-deficient adults, analyzing 15 randomized, double-blind, placebo-controlled trials, reported that GH replacement in GH-deficient adults was associated with a significant positive effect on aerobic exercise capacity and muscle mass [95]. However, 1 year later, another meta-analysis, restricted to eight high-quality studies involving 231 patients in nine cohorts, does not support a beneficial effect of GH replacement on strength in GH deficiency adults [96].

In 2002, Brill et al. demonstrated that 1 month supplementation of GH in combination with testosterone ameliorated balance and physical function but had no effect on muscle strength [97].

In another previous study, among healthy subjects aged 69 years and older, 6 months GH treatment increased muscle mass and decreased fat mass, without improving physical performance [98]. Blackman et al. found that supplementation with GH marginally increased muscle strength in men treated with GH and testosterone, but found no significant effect on muscle strength among healthy older women [99]. Another study documented that, in a group of older men, a combined supplementation of GH with testosterone for 4 months significantly increased muscle mass and muscle strength, while it decreased the fat mass [100].

Some other studies reported an increase of muscle mass and strength in healthy older persons after GH supplementation [17, 65].

Inefficacy of recombinant human GH was also reported in combination with an exercise program in older men [101] and moderately obese postmenopausal women [102].

Also in 2002, Lange et al. conducted a randomized clinical trial examining the effects of GH alone, exercise alone and GH combined with exercise. This study showed that GH alone had no effect on muscle mass, strength and power as compared to the other two intervention groups [103].

Furthermore, most GH supplementation trials have reported a high occurrence of adverse reactions, such as orthostatic hypotension, diabetes, fluid retention, soft tissue oedema, carpal tunnel syndrome, arthralgias and gynecomastia.

Numerous causes may explain the ineffectiveness of GH supplementation to improve muscle mass and strength, such as the failure of exogenous GH administration to mimic the pulsatile pattern of natural GH secretion or the induction of GH-related insulin resistance [17].

Once again, based on the current evidence, GH treatment should not be considered as a safe strategy to improve body composition and functionality in older individuals.

14.3.5 Ghrelin and Melanocortin

Ghrelin is a peptide hormone secreted by the stomach in response to fasting that stimulates the release of GH through an activation of the GH secretagogue-receptor (GHS-R1a) present in the hypothalamus. Ghrelin concentrations have been reported to be strongly correlated with the amount of skeletal muscle mass—presumably through stimulation of appetite, or is it direct effect [104]. However, very few clinical studies have been conducted in older subjects.

Promising results have been reported in a sample of 25 subjects with chronic obstructive pulmonary disease and reduced mobility, where subcutaneous injections of a synthetic ghrelin analogue tended to increase the lean mass and physical performance [11]. In another study of healthy older adults without sarcopenia, 2 years of an oral ghrelin mimetic agent increased the GH and IGF-1 blood levels and muscle mass, without significant changes in strength or physical function [105]. Given the important role of malnutrition in development of sarcopenia, further studies on the impact of ghrelin supplementation are recommended.

The effect of ghrelin is partially related to the melanocortin receptor antagonism that modulates food intake [11]. The melanocortin-4 receptor (MC4R) is a G-protein receptor that is expressed in the hypothalamus [11, 38] which is thought to be related to the pathogenesis of cachexia. In murine models, stimulation of the MC4R modulated food-seeking behaviour, increased basal metabolic rate and decreased lean body mass [11]. Blockage of central melanocortin signalling increased both lean body mass and fat mass in a rat model of cardiac cachexia [106].

In humans, mutations of the MC4R are associated with obesity [107]. Inhibition of the melanocortin system either through antagonism or by an antibody against the MC4R has shown encouraging results in animal models of cachexia [11]. This possible therapeutic target is yet to be properly evaluated in humans.

14.3.6 Pathways of Sarcopenia and Possible Future Target Treatment

Molecular mechanisms behind the development of sarcopenia are not completely defined and represent an intense area of research, given their potential as target therapy [4, 8, 108].

A complex interaction of genetic and molecular pathways has been implicated in the development of the age-related muscle loss and the onset of sarcopenia [8]. Sarcopenia could in same ways represent one of the epiphenomena of the complex mechanisms which represent the hallmarks of ageing.

Age-related intracellular changes in the DNA damages repairing system of muscle cells, cellular senescence hallmark such as the reduction of telomers length and alteration in the mitochondrial function of the muscle cells, are among the mechanisms that have been evaluated. However, these alterations might hardly constitute easily usable pharmaceutical targets.

Moreover, alterations in the proteolytic system, antioxidative system and systemic inflammation have also been acknowledged to explain the intricated mechanism leading to sarcopenia [8, 109] and could potentially be targeted pharmaceutically.

In particular, the proteolytic processes involving the ubiquitin-proteasome system plays a key role in controlling size of muscle fibres [110] and could represent a potential target therapy which has not been yet evaluated for pharmacological purposes.

In fact, preliminary studies have indicated that atrogin-1 and muscle-1 ring-finger protein-1 (MuRF-1), two ubiquitin ligases, are upregulated in situations of muscle atrophy. Their expression has also been observed in autophagy-related muscle degeneration processes. Atrogin-1 and MuRF-1 activations seem to be modulated by the FOXO family of transcriptional factors, which integrates signals generated by nutrient deprivation and stress circumstances, stimulating the degradation systems of ubiquitin-proteasome and autophagy pathways and favouring the degradation of muscle proteins [4, 110]. In addition, MuRF-1 may also be associated with mechanisms that cause neuromuscular junction alterations [4, 14, 111], another mechanism that is thought to lead to muscle degeneration and concur to the development of sarcopenia.

Moreover, oxidative stress and systemic inflammation seems to play a key role in the onset of sarcopenia, and their exogenous modulation may have potential as another possible target for new potential treatments.

The ageing process is associated with an unbalanced production of free radicals which are not counteracted by antioxidant and repairing systems. Free radicals are a product of reactive oxygen (ROS), which are produced especially by the mitochondria, and nitrogen species (RNS), which are a product of nitric oxide synthase (NOS) in which arginine, one of the essential amino acids, is a fundamental substrate [4, 8].

Because of high metabolic rate, myocytes are particularly susceptible to oxidative damage and, especially in older persons, are particularly predisposed to accumulate oxidatively damaged molecules. Also, skeletal muscle accounts for a large share of total oxygen consumption, increasing the risk of collateral mitochondria-derived production of ROS, such as hydrogen peroxide that can cause progressive cellular damage, determining enzymatic dysfunction and affecting the proteolytic system, facilitating an imbalance between protein synthesis and breakdown. Increased susceptibility to oxidative stress alters both structure and function of the muscular cells and affecting metabolism and muscle contraction, ultimately contributing to the appearance of sarcopenia and delay of muscle regeneration in the elderly [4, 8, 112]. Oral antioxidant supplementation has been suggested as a potential treatment to reduce muscle wasting, but so far, results from different studies have been inconsistent and poorly relevant in a clinical environment [113]. Potential of this pathway could relay in downregulating the synthesis of RNS, thanks to molecules inhibiting the inducible form of NOS (iNOS) [114]. Those inhibitors have demonstrated a significant efficiency to prevent symptoms of muscle wasting [114], albeit further studies are needed.

Furthermore, ageing is knowingly associated with a low-grade chronic inflammation due to increased circulating pro-inflammatory cytokines—among which the tumour necrosis factor-α (TNF-α) and interleukin-6 (IL-6)—and presence of dysfunctional immune systems determining the condition of immune-senescence and inflammaging [115–118].

Inflammation in the long term can progressively lead to muscle deterioration [118], affecting skeletal muscle regeneration capacity and inducing a reduction in the number of satellite cells and in the neurohormonal response [4, 118].

Increased serum levels of TNF-α and IL-6 can be considered as a marker of the impact of inflammation on the development of sarcopenia and are associated with the release of other inflammatory markers such as C-reactive protein (CRP), one of the acute-phase reactive proteins produced by the liver [4, 118]. TNF-α activates local vascular endothelial cells via the release of NO, increasing vascular permeability and allowing the passage of pro-inflammatory cells that contribute to systemic inflammation. High plasma levels of TNF-α and IL-6 have been respectively correlated to lower muscle mass and strength [119], fatigue and disability associated with muscle destruction and are related with a decrease in physical performance and a greater degree of disability [4, 120].

Pro-inflammatory cytokines could be potential pharmacological targets in sarcopenia treatment, although results of treatment in the TNF-α signalling pathways have not been promising.

14.4   Conclusion

To this date, there are no licensed drugs for the treatment of sarcopenia. However, the impact of sarcopenia is detrimental to healthy ageing, increasing the risk of adverse outcomes and reducing quality of life.

Developing treatments for sarcopenia is vital. Despite new discoveries and the development of new drugs, non-pharmacological options should also be considered for prevention and treatment of changes in muscle mass, strength and function associated with ageing [4]. Positive effects on muscle have been reported with nutritional supplements and exercise training which are strongly recommended in the prevention of sarcopenia and reduction of negative outcomes by slowing the process of age-related muscle wasting [121–123].

In order to be able to revert sarcopenia, possible future hybrid therapies combining myostatin/activin inhibitors, hormonal therapy—SERM in particular—in combination with physical exercise and nutritional therapy could represent a novel approach in the treatment of sarcopenia [13]; however, further studies are needed in order to derive conclusive guidance and standard treatment approaches and before these therapy will be incorporated into mainstream clinical practise.

References

1. Landi F, Calvani R, Cesari M, et al. Sarcopenia: an overview on current definitions, diagnosis and treatment. Curr Protein Pept Sci. 2017;19(7):633–8. https://doi.org/10.217 4/1389203718666170607113459.
2. Marzetti E, Calvani R, Tosato M, et al. Sarcopenia: an overview. Aging Clin Exp Res. 2017;29(1):11–7. https://doi.org/10.1007/s40520-016-0704-5.
3. Cruz-Jentoft AJ, Bahat G, Bauer J, et al. Sarcopenia: revised European consensus on definition and diagnosis. Age Ageing. 2019;48(1):16–31. https://doi.org/10.1093/ageing/afy169.
4. Pascual-Fernández J, Fernández-Montero A, Córdova-Martínez A, Pastor D, Martínez-Rodríguez A, Roche E. Sarcopenia: molecular pathways and potential targets for intervention. Int J Mol Sci. 2020;21(22):1–16. https://doi.org/10.3390/ijms21228844.
5. Phillip SM. Physiologic and molecular bases of muscle hypertrophy and atrophy: impact of resistance exercise on human skeletal muscle (protein and exercise dose effects). Appl Physiol Nutr Metab. 2009;34(3):403–10. https://doi.org/10.1139/H09-042.
6. Hughes VA, Frontera WR, Roubenoff R, Evans WJ, Fiatarone Singh MA. Longitudinal changes in body composition in older men and women: role of body weight change and physical activity. Am J Clin Nutr. 2002;76(2):473–81. https://doi.org/10.1093/ajcn/76.2.473.
7. Paddon-Jones D, Rasmussen BB. Dietary protein recommendations and the prevention of sarcopenia. Curr Opin Clin Nutr Metab Care. 2009;12(1):86–90. https://doi.org/10.1097/MCO.0b013e32831cef8b.
8. Wiedmer P, Jung T, Castro JP, et al. Sarcopenia – molecular mechanisms and open questions. Ageing Res Rev. 2021;65:101200. https://doi.org/10.1016/j.arr.2020.101200.
9. Cruz-Jentoft AJ, Landi F, Schneider SM, et al. Prevalence of and interventions for sarcopenia in ageing adults: a systematic review. Report of the International Sarcopenia Initiative (EWGSOP and IWGS). Age Ageing. 2014;43(6):748–59. https://doi.org/10.1093/ageing/afu115.
10. Kwak JY, Kwon KS. Pharmacological interventions for treatment of sarcopenia: current status of drug development for sarcopenia. Ann Geriatr Med Res. 2019;23(3):98–104. https://doi.org/10.4235/agmr.19.0028.
11. Kung T, Springer J, Doehner W, Anker SD, Von Haehling S. Novel treatment approaches to cachexia and sarcopenia: highlights from the 5th Cachexia conference. In: Expert opinion on investigational drugs; 2010. https://doi.org/10.1517/13543781003724690.
12. Elkina Y, von Haehling S, Anker SD, Springer J. The role of myostatin in muscle wasting: an overview. J Cachexia Sarcopenia Muscle. 2011;2(3):143–51. https://doi.org/10.1007/s13539-011-0035-5.
13. Saitoh M, Ishida J, Ebner N, Anker SD, Von Haehling S. Myostatin inhibitors as pharmacological treatment for muscle wasting and muscular dystrophy. JCSM Clin Rep. 2017;2:1–10. https://doi.org/10.17987/jcsm-cr.v2i1.37.
14. Delfino GB, Peviani SM, Durigan JLQ, et al. Quadriceps muscle atrophy after anterior cruciate ligament transection involves increased mRNA levels of atrogin-1, muscle ring finger 1, and myostatin. Am J Phys Med Rehabil. 2013;92(5):411–9. https://doi.org/10.1097/PHM.0b013e3182643f82.
15. Domingues-Faria C, Vasson MP, Goncalves-Mendes N, Boirie Y, Walrand S. Skeletal muscle regeneration and impact of aging and nutrition. Ageing Res Rev. 2016;26:22–36. https://doi.org/10.1016/j.arr.2015.12.004.

16. Hoppeler H. Molecular networks in skeletal muscle plasticity. J Exp Biol. 2016;219(Pt 2):205–13. https://doi.org/10.1242/jeb.128207.
17. Burton LA, Sumukadas D. Optimal management of sarcopenia. Clin Interv Aging. 2010;5:217–28. https://doi.org/10.2147/cia.s11473.
18. Schuelke M, Wagner KR, Stolz LE, et al. Myostatin mutation associated with gross muscle hypertrophy in a child. N Engl J Med. 2004;350(26):2682–8. https://doi.org/10.1056/nejmoa040933.
19. Murphy KT, Koopman R, Naim T, et al. Antibody-directed myostatin inhibition in 21-mo-old mice reveals novel roles for myostatin signaling in skeletal muscle structure and function. FASEB J. 2010;24:4433–42. https://doi.org/10.1096/fj.10-159608.
20. Siriett V, Salerno MS, Berry C, et al. Antagonism of myostatin enhances muscle regeneration during sarcopenia. Mol Ther. 2007;15(8):1463–70. https://doi.org/10.1038/sj.mt.6300182.
21. Solomon AM, Bouloux PMG. Modifying muscle mass—the endocrine perspective. J Endocrinol. 2006;191:349–60. https://doi.org/10.1677/joe.1.06837.
22. Wagner KR, Fleckenstein JL, Amato AA, et al. A phase I/II trial of MYO-029 in adult subjects with muscular dystrophy. Ann Neurol. 2008;63:561–71. https://doi.org/10.1002/ana.21338.
23. Woodhouse L, Gandhi R, Warden SJ, et al. A phase 2 randomized study investigating the efficacy and safety of myostatin antibody LY2495655 versus placebo in patients undergoing elective total hip arthroplasty. J Frailty Aging. 2016;5:62–70. https://doi.org/10.14283/jfa.2016.81.
24. Becker C, Lord SR, Studenski SA, et al. Myostatin antibody (LY2495655) in older weak fallers: a proof-of-concept, randomised, phase 2 trial. Lancet Diabetes Endocrinol. 2015;3:948–57. https://doi.org/10.1016/S2213-8587(15)00298-3.
25. ClinicalTrials.gov [Internet]. Bethesda (MD): National Library of Medicine (US). 2000 Feb 29. Identifier NCT01963598, Study of the safety and efficacy of REGN1033 (SAR391786) in patients with sarcopenia; October 16, 2013 October 16. https://clinicaltrials.gov/ct2/show/NCT01963598. Accessed 11 Jan 2021.
26. Campbell C, McMillan HJ, Mah JK, et al. Myostatin inhibitor ACE-031 treatment of ambulatory boys with Duchenne muscular dystrophy: results of a randomized, placebo-controlled clinical trial. Muscle Nerve. 2017;55:458–64. https://doi.org/10.1002/mus.25268.
27. Rodino-Klapac LR, Haidet AM, Kota J, Handy C, Kaspar BK, Mendell JR. Inhibition of myostatin with emphasis on follistatin as a therapy for muscle disease. Muscle Nerve. 2009;39:283–96. https://doi.org/10.1002/mus.21244.
28. Pearsall R, Widrick J, Cotton E, et al. ACE-083 increases muscle hypertrophy and strength in C57BL/6 mice. Neuromuscul Disord. 2015;25:S218. https://doi.org/10.1016/j.nmd.2015.06.123.
29. Lee SJ, Huynh TV, Lee YS, et al. Role of satellite cells versus myofibers in muscle hypertrophy induced by inhibition of the myostatin/activin signaling pathway. Proc Natl Acad Sci U S A. 2012;109:E2353–60. https://doi.org/10.1073/pnas.1206410109.
30. Glasser CE, Gartner MR, Wilson D, Miller B, Sherman ML, Attie KM. Locally acting ACE-083 increases muscle volume in healthy volunteers. Muscle Nerve. 2018;57:921–6. https://doi.org/10.1002/mus.26113.
31. Pearsall RS, Davies MV, Cannell M, et al. Follistatin-based ligand trap ACE-083 induces localized hypertrophy of skeletal muscle with functional improvement in models of neuromuscular disease. Sci Rep. 2019;9:11392. https://doi.org/10.1038/s41598-019-47818-w.
32. Latres E, Mastaitis J, Fury W, et al. Activin A more prominently regulates muscle mass in primates than does GDF8. Nat Commun. 2017;8:15153. https://doi.org/10.1038/ncomms15153.
33. Lach-Trifilieff E, Minetti GC, Sheppard K, et al. An antibody blocking Activin type II receptors induces strong skeletal muscle hypertrophy and protects from atrophy. Mol Cell Biol. 2014;34:606–18. https://doi.org/10.1128/mcb.01307-13.
34. Rooks D, Praestgaard J, Hariry S, et al. Treatment of sarcopenia with Bimagrumab: results from a phase II, randomized, controlled, proof-of-concept study. J Am Geriatr Soc. 2017;65:1988–95. https://doi.org/10.1111/jgs.14927.

35. Rooks DS, Laurent D, Praestgaard J, Rasmussen S, Bartlett M, Tankó LB. Effect of bimagrumab on thigh muscle volume and composition in men with casting-induced atrophy. J Cachexia Sarcopenia Muscle. 2017;8:727–34. https://doi.org/10.1002/jcsm.12205.
36. Tenover JS. Effects of testosterone supplementation in the aging male. J Clin Endocrinol Metab. 1992;75:1092–8. https://doi.org/10.1210/jcem.75.4.1400877.
37. Dennison EM, Sayer AA, Cooper C. Epidemiology of sarcopenia and insight into possible therapeutic targets. Nat Rev Rheumatol. 2017;13:340–7. https://doi.org/10.1038/nrrheum.2017.60.
38. Rolland Y, Onder G, Morley JE, Gillette-Guyonet S, Abellan van Kan G, Vellas B. Current and future pharmacologic treatment of sarcopenia. Clin Geriatr Med. 2011;27:423–47. https://doi.org/10.1016/j.cger.2011.03.008.
39. Onder G, Della Vedova C, Landi F. Validated treatments and therapeutics prospectives regarding pharmacological products for sarcopenia. J Nutr Health Aging. 2009;13:746–56. https://doi.org/10.1007/s12603-009-0209-4.
40. Visvanathan R, Chapman I. Preventing sarcopaenia in older people. Maturitas. 2010;66:383–8. https://doi.org/10.1016/j.maturitas.2010.03.020.
41. Emmelot-Vonk MH, Verhaar HJJ, Nakhai Pour HR, et al. Effect of testosterone supplementation on functional mobility, cognition, and other parameters in older men: a randomized controlled trial. JAMA. 2008;299:39–52. https://doi.org/10.1001/jama.2007.51.
42. Ferrando AA, Sheffield-Moore M, Paddon-Jones D, Wolfe RR, Urban RJ. Differential anabolic effects of testosterone and amino acid feeding in older men. J Clin Endocrinol Metab. 2003;88:358–62. https://doi.org/10.1210/jc.2002-021041.
43. Serra C, Tangherlini F, Rudy S, et al. Testosterone improves the regeneration of old and young mouse skeletal muscle. J Gerontol Ser A Biol Sci Med Sci. 2013;88:358–62. https://doi.org/10.1093/gerona/gls083.
44. Sinha-Hikim I, Roth SM, Lee MI, Bhasin S. Testosterone-induced muscle hypertrophy is associated with an increase in satellite cell number in healthy, young men. Am J Physiol Endocrinol Metab. 2003;285:E197–205. https://doi.org/10.1152/ajpendo.00370.2002.
45. Verdijk LB, Snijders T, Beelen M, et al. Characteristics of muscle fiber type are predictive of skeletal muscle mass and strength in elderly men. J Am Geriatr Soc. 2010;58:2069–75. https://doi.org/10.1111/j.1532-5415.2010.03150.x.
46. Sinha-Hikim I, Artaza J, Woodhouse L, et al. Testosterone-induced increase in muscle size in healthy young men is associated with muscle fiber hypertrophy. Am J Physiol Endocrinol Metab. 2002;283:E154–64. https://doi.org/10.1152/ajpendo.00502.2001.
47. Palazzolo I, Gliozzi A, Rusmini P, et al. The role of the polyglutamine tract in androgen receptor. J Steroid Biochem Mol Biol. 2008;108:245–53. https://doi.org/10.1016/j.jsbmb.2007.09.016.
48. Aagaard P, Suetta C, Caserotti P, Magnusson SP, Kjær M. Role of the nervous system in sarcopenia and muscle atrophy with aging: strength training as a countermeasure. Scand J Med Sci Sports. 2010;20:49–64. https://doi.org/10.1111/j.1600-0838.2009.01084.x.
49. Fargo KN, Alexander TD, Tanzer L, Poletti A, Jones KJ. Androgen regulates neuritin mRNA levels in an in vivo model of steroid-enhanced peripheral nerve regeneration. J Neurotrauma. 2008;25:561–6. https://doi.org/10.1089/neu.2007.0466.
50. Ottenbacher KJ, Ottenbacher ME, Ottenbacher AJ, Acha AA, Ostir GV. Androgen treatment and muscle strength in elderly men: a meta-analysis. J Am Geriatr Soc. 2006;54:1666–73. https://doi.org/10.1111/j.1532-5415.2006.00938.x.
51. De Spiegeleer A, Beckwée D, Bautmans I, et al. Pharmacological interventions to improve muscle mass, muscle strength and physical performance in older people: an umbrella review of systematic reviews and meta-analyses. Drugs Aging. 2018;35:719–34. https://doi.org/10.1007/s40266-018-0566-y.
52. Srinivas-Shankar U, Roberts SA, Connolly MJ, et al. Effects of testosterone on muscle strength, physical function, body composition, and quality of life in intermediate-frail and frail elderly men: a randomized, double-blind, placebo-controlled study. J Clin Endocrinol Metab. 2010;95:639–50. https://doi.org/10.1210/jc.2009-1251.

53. Chapman IM, Visvanathan R, Hammond AJ, et al. Effect of testosterone and a nutritional supplement, alone and in combination, on hospital admissions in undernourished older men and women. Am J Clin Nutr. 2009;89:880–9. https://doi.org/10.3945/ajcn.2008.26538.
54. Kenny AM, Boxer RS, Kleppinger A, Brindisi J, Feinn R, Burleson JA. Dehydroepiandrosterone combined with exercise improves muscle strength and physical function in frail older women. J Am Geriatr Soc. 2010;58:1707–14. https://doi.org/10.1111/j.1532-5415.2010.03019.x.
55. Dos Santos MR, Sayegh ALC, Bacurau AVN, et al. Effect of exercise training and testosterone replacement on skeletal muscle wasting in patients with heart failure with testosterone deficiency. Mayo Clin Proc. 2016;91:575–86. https://doi.org/10.1016/j.mayocp.2016.02.014.
56. Skinner JW, Otzel DM, Bowser A, et al. Muscular responses to testosterone replacement vary by administration route: a systematic review and meta-analysis. J Cachexia Sarcopenia Muscle. 2018;9:465–81. https://doi.org/10.1002/jcsm.12291.
57. Hildreth KL, Barry DW, Moreau KL, et al. Effects of testosterone and progressive resistance exercise in healthy, highly functioning older men with low-normal testosterone levels. J Clin Endocrinol Metab. 2013;98:1891–900. https://doi.org/10.1210/jc.2012-3695.
58. Endo Y, Nourmahnad A, Sinha I. Optimizing skeletal muscle anabolic response to resistance training in aging. Front Physiol. 2020;11:874. https://doi.org/10.3389/fphys.2020.00874.
59. Pierorazio PM, Ferrucci L, Kettermann A, Longo DL, Metter EJ, Carter HB. Serum testosterone is associated with aggressive prostate cancer in older men: results from the Baltimore longitudinal study of aging. BJU Int. 2010;105:824–9. https://doi.org/10.1111/j.1464-410X.2009.08853.x.
60. Basaria S, Coviello AD, Travison TG, et al. Adverse events associated with testosterone administration. N Engl J Med. 2010;363:109–22. https://doi.org/10.1056/NEJMoa1000485.
61. Snyder PJ, Bhasin S, Cunningham GR, et al. Lessons from the testosterone trials. Endocr Rev. 2018;39:369–86. https://doi.org/10.1210/er.2017-00234.
62. Morley J. Developing novel therapeutic approaches to frailty. Curr Pharm Des. 2009;15:3384–95. https://doi.org/10.2174/138161209789105045.
63. Dalton JT, Barnette KG, Bohl CE, et al. The selective androgen receptor modulator GTx-024 (enobosarm) improves lean body mass and physical function in healthy elderly men and post-menopausal women: results of a double-blind, placebo-controlled phase II trial. J Cachexia Sarcopenia Muscle. 2011;2:153–61. https://doi.org/10.1007/s13539-011-0034-6.
64. Papanicolaou DA, Ather SN, Zhu H, et al. A phase IIA randomized, placebo-controlled clinical trial to study the efficacy and safety of the selective androgen receptor modulator (SARM), MK-0773 in female participants with sarcopenia. J Nutr Health Aging. 2013;17:533–43. https://doi.org/10.1007/s12603-013-0335-x.
65. Jones TE, Stephenson KW, King JG, Knight KR, Marshall TL, Scott WB. Sarcopenia—mechanisms and treatments. J Geriatr Phys Ther. 2009;32:83–9. https://doi.org/10.1519/00139143-200932020-00008.
66. Sato K, Iemitsu M, Aizawa K, Ajisaka R. Testosterone and DHEA activate the glucose metabolism-related signaling pathway in skeletal muscle. Am J Physiol Endocrinol Metab. 2008;294:E961–8. https://doi.org/10.1152/ajpendo.00678.2007.
67. Baker WL, Karan S, Kenny AM. Effect of dehydroepiandrosterone on muscle strength and physical function in older adults: a systematic review. J Am Geriatr Soc. 2011;59:997–1002. https://doi.org/10.1111/j.1532-5415.2011.03410.x.
68. Valenti G, Denti L, Maggio M, et al. Effect of DHEAS on skeletal muscle over the life span: the InCHIANTI study. J Gerontol Ser A Biol Sci Med Sci. 2004;59:466–72. https://doi.org/10.1093/gerona/59.5.m466.
69. Villareal DT, Holloszy JO. DHEA enhances effects of weight training on muscle mass and strength in elderly women and men. Am J Physiol Endocrinol Metab. 2006;291:E1003–8. https://doi.org/10.1152/ajpendo.00100.2006.
70. Christiansen JJ, Bruun JM, Christiansen JS, Jørgensen JO, Gravholt CH. Long-term DHEA substitution in female adrenocortical failure, body composition, muscle function, and bone metabolism: a randomized trial. Eur J Endocrinol. 2011;165:293–300. https://doi.org/10.1530/EJE-11-0289.

71. Messier V, Rabasa-Lhoret R, Barbat-Artigas S, Elisha B, Karelis AD, Aubertin-Leheudre M. Menopause and sarcopenia: a potential role for sex hormones. Maturitas. 2011;68:331–6. https://doi.org/10.1016/j.maturitas.2011.01.014.
72. Wilson D, Jackson T, Sapey E, Lord JM. Frailty and sarcopenia: the potential role of an aged immune system. Ageing Res Rev. 2017;36:1–10. https://doi.org/10.1016/j.arr.2017.01.006.
73. Dieli-Conwright CM, Spektor TM, Rice JC, Schroeder ET. Hormone therapy attenuates exercise-induced skeletal muscle damage in postmenopausal women. J Appl Physiol. 2009;107:853–8. https://doi.org/10.1152/japplphysiol.00404.2009.
74. Huffman KM, Slentz CA, Johnson JL, et al. Impact of hormone replacement therapy on exercise training-induced improvements in insulin action in sedentary overweight adults. Metabolism. 2008;57:888–95. https://doi.org/10.1016/j.metabol.2008.01.034.
75. Sipila S, Taaffe DR, Cheng S, Puolakka J, Toivanen J, Suominen H. Effects of hormone replacement therapy and high-impact physical exercise on skeletal muscle in post-menopausal women: a randomized placebo-controlled study. Clin Sci. 2001;101:147–57. https://doi.org/10.1042/CS20000271.
76. Heikkinen J, Kyllönen E, Kurttila-Matero E, et al. HRT and exercise: Effects on bone density, muscle strength and lipid metabolism. A placebo controlled 2-year prospective trial on two estrogen-progestin regimens in healthy postmenopausal women. Maturitas. 1997;26:139–49. https://doi.org/10.1016/S0378-5122(96)01098-5.
77. Skelton DA, Phillips SK, Bruce SA, Naylor CH, Woledge RC. Hormone replacement therapy increases isometric muscle strength of adductor pollicis in post-menopausal women. Clin Sci. 1999;96:357–64. https://doi.org/10.1042/cs0960357.
78. Bea JW, Zhao Q, Cauley JA, et al. Effect of hormone therapy on lean body mass, falls, and fractures: 6-year results from the Women's health initiative hormone trials. Menopause. 2011;18:44–52. https://doi.org/10.1097/gme.0b013e3181e3aab1.
79. Ribom EL, Piehl-Aulin K, Ljunghall S, Ljunggren Ö, Naessén T. Six months of hormone replacement therapy does not influence muscle strength in postmenopausal women. Maturitas. 2002;42:225–31. https://doi.org/10.1016/S0378-5122(02)00079-8.
80. Ribom EL, Svensson P, Van Os S, Larsson M, Naessen T. Low-dose tibolone (1.25 mg/d) does not affect muscle strength in older women. Menopause. 2011;18:194–7. https://doi.org/10.1097/gme.0b013e3181e9d833.
81. Armstrong AL, Oborne J, Coupland CAC, Macpherson MB, Bassey EJ, Wallace WA. Effects of hormone replacement therapy on muscle performance and balance in post menopausal women. Clin Sci. 1996;91:685–90. https://doi.org/10.1042/cs0910685.
82. Candow DG, Chilibeck PD, Abeysekara S, Zello GA. Short-term heavy resistance training eliminates age-related deficits in muscle mass and strength in healthy older males. J Strength Cond Res. 2011;25:326–33. https://doi.org/10.1519/JSC.0b013e3181bf43c8.
83. Nikawa T, Ikemoto M, Sakai T, et al. Effects of a soy protein diet on exercise-induced muscle protein catabolism in rats. Nutrition. 2002;18:490–5. https://doi.org/10.1016/S0899-9007(02)00744-X.
84. Aubertin-Leheudre M, Lord C, Khalil A, Dionne IJ. Six months of isoflavone supplement increases fat-free mass in obese-sarcopenic postmenopausal women: a randomized double-blind controlled trial. Eur J Clin Nutr. 2007;61:1442–4. https://doi.org/10.1038/sj.ejcn.1602695.
85. Moeller LE, Peterson CT, Hanson KB, et al. Isoflavone-rich soy protein prevents loss of hip lean mass but does not prevent the shift in regional fat distribution in perimenopausal women. Menopause. 2003;10:322–31. https://doi.org/10.1097/01.GME.0000054763.94658.FD.
86. Candow DG, Vogt E, Johannsmeyer S, Forbes SC, Farthing JP. Strategic creatine supplementation and resistance training in healthy older adults. Appl Physiol Nutr Metab. 2015;40:689–94. https://doi.org/10.1139/apnm-2014-0498.
87. Orsatti FL, Maestá N, de Oliveira EP, et al. Adding soy protein to milk enhances the effect of resistance training on muscle strength in postmenopausal women. J Diet Suppl. 2018;15:140–52. https://doi.org/10.1080/19390211.2017.1330794.

88. Porcile A, Gallardo E, Duarte P, et al. Differential effects on serum IGF-1 of tibolone (5 mg/day) vs combined continuous estrogen/progestagen in post menopausal women. Rev Med Chil. 2003;131:1151–6.
89. Cicinelli E, Ignarro LJ, Galantino P, Pinto V, Barba B, Schonauer S. Effects of tibolone on plasma levels of nitric oxide in postmenopausal women. Fertil Steril. 2002;78:464–8. https://doi.org/10.1016/S0015-0282(02)03295-8.
90. Meeuwsen IBAE, Samson MM, Duursma SA, Verhaar HJJ. Muscle strength and tibolone: a randomised, double-blind, placebo-controlled trial. BJOG. 2002;109:77–84. https://doi.org/10.1111/j.1471-0528.2002.01213.x.
91. Boyanov MA, Shinkov AD. Effects of tibolone on body composition in postmenopausal women: a 1-year follow up study. Maturitas. 2005;51:363–9. https://doi.org/10.1016/j.maturitas.2004.09.003.
92. Bolster DR, Kubica N, Crozier SJ, et al. Immediate response of mammalian target of rapamycin (mTOR)-mediated signalling following acute resistance exercise in rat skeletal muscle. J Physiol. 2003;553:213–20. https://doi.org/10.1113/jphysiol.2003.047019.
93. Bian A, Ma Y, Zhou X, et al. Association between sarcopenia and levels of growth hormone and insulin-like growth factor-1 in the elderly. BMC Musculoskelet Disord. 2020;21:214. https://doi.org/10.1186/s12891-020-03236-y.
94. Carpenter V, Matthews K, Devlin G, et al. Mechano-growth factor reduces loss of cardiac function in acute myocardial infarction. Heart Lung Circ. 2008;17:33–9. https://doi.org/10.1016/j.hlc.2007.04.013.
95. Rubeck KZ, Bertelsen S, Vestergaard P, Jørgensen JOL. Impact of GH substitution on exercise capacity and muscle strength in GH-deficient adults: a meta-analysis of blinded, placebo-controlled trials. Clin Endocrinol (Oxf). 2009;71:860–6. https://doi.org/10.1111/j.1365-2265.2009.03592.x.
96. Matthew Widdowson W, Gibney J. The effect of growth hormone (GH) replacement on muscle strength in patients with GH-deficiency: a meta-analysis. Clin Endocrinol (Oxf). 2010;72:787–92. https://doi.org/10.1111/j.1365-2265.2009.03716.x.
97. Brill KT, Weltman AL, Gentili A, et al. Single and combined effects of growth hormone and testosterone administration on measures of body composition, physical performance, mood, sexual function, bone turnover, and muscle gene expression in healthy older men. J Clin Endocrinol Metab. 2002;87:5649–57. https://doi.org/10.1210/jc.2002-020098.
98. Papadakis MA, Grady D, Black D, et al. Growth hormone replacement in healthy older men improves body composition but not functional ability. Ann Intern Med. 1996;124:708–16. https://doi.org/10.7326/0003-4819-124-8-199604150-00002.
99. Blackman MR, Sorkin JD, Münzer T, et al. Growth hormone and sex steroid administration in healthy aged women and men: a randomized controlled trial. JAMA. 2002;288:2282–92. https://doi.org/10.1001/jama.288.18.2282.
100. Sattler FR, Castaneda-Sceppa C, Binder EF, et al. Testosterone and growth hormone improve body composition and muscle performance in older men. J Clin Endocrinol Metab. 2009;94:1991–2001. https://doi.org/10.1210/jc.2008-2338.
101. Taaffe DR, Pruitt L, Reim J, et al. Effect of recombinant human growth hormone on the muscle strength response to resistance exercise in elderly men. J Clin Endocrinol Metab. 1994;79:1361–6. https://doi.org/10.1210/jcem.79.5.7525633.
102. Thompson JL, Butterfield GE, Gylfadottir UK, et al. Effects of human growth hormone, insulin like growth factor 1, and diet and exercise on body composition of obese postmenopausal women 1. J Clin Endocrinol Metab. 1998;83:1477–84. https://doi.org/10.1210/jcem.83.5.4826.
103. Lange KHW, Andersen JL, Beyer N, et al. GH administration changes myosin heavy chain isoforms in skeletal muscle but does not augment muscle strength or hypertrophy, either alone or combined with resistance exercise training in healthy elderly men. J Clin Endocrinol Metab. 2002;87:513–23. https://doi.org/10.1210/jcem.87.2.8206.

104. Tai K, Visvanathan R, Hammond AJ, Wishart JM, Horowitz M, Chapman IM. Fasting ghrelin is related to skeletal muscle mass in healthy adults. Eur J Nutr. 2009;48:176–83. https://doi.org/10.1007/s00394-009-0779-2.

105. Nass R, Pezzoli SS, Oliveri MC, et al. Effects of an oral ghrelin mimetic on body composition and clinical outcomes in healthy older adults: a randomized trial. Ann Intern Med. 2008;149:601–11. https://doi.org/10.7326/0003-4819-149-9-200811040-00003.

106. Scarlett JM, Bowe DD, Zhu X, Batra AK, Grant WF, Marks DL. Genetic and pharmacologic blockade of central melanocortin signaling attenuates cardiac cachexia in rodent models of heart failure. J Endocrinol. 2010;206:121–30. https://doi.org/10.1677/JOE-09-0397.

107. Farooqi IS, Keogh JM, Yeo GSH, Lank EJ, Cheetham T, O'Rahilly S. Clinical Spectrum of obesity and mutations in the Melanocortin 4 receptor gene. N Engl J Med. 2003;348:1085–95. https://doi.org/10.1056/nejmoa022050.

108. Ng TP, Lu Y, Choo RWM, et al. Dysregulated homeostatic pathways in sarcopenia among frail older adults. Aging Cell. 2018;17:e12842. https://doi.org/10.1111/acel.12842.

109. Welle S. Cellular and molecular basis of age-related sarcopenia. Can J Appl Physiol. 2002;27:19–41. https://doi.org/10.1139/h02-002.

110. Sandri M, Sandri C, Gilbert A, et al. Foxo transcription factors induce the atrophy-related ubiquitin ligase atrogin-1 and cause skeletal muscle atrophy. Cell. 2004;117:399–412. https://doi.org/10.1016/S0092-8674(04)00400-3.

111. Gumucio JP, Mendias CL. Atrogin-1, MuRF-1, and sarcopenia. Endocrine. 2013;43:12–21. https://doi.org/10.1007/s12020-012-9751-7.

112. Fulle S, Protasi F, Di Tano G, et al. The contribution of reactive oxygen species to sarcopenia and muscle ageing. Exp Gerontol. 2004;39:17–24. https://doi.org/10.1016/j.exger.2003.09.012.

113. Cerullo F, Gambassi G, Cesari M. Rationale for antioxidant supplementation in sarcopenia. J Aging Res. 2012;2012:316943. https://doi.org/10.1155/2012/316943.

114. Hall DT, Ma JF, Marco S, Di Gallouzi IE. Inducible nitric oxide synthase (iNOS) in muscle wasting syndrome, sarcopenia, and cachexia. Aging (Albany NY). 2011;3:702–15. https://doi.org/10.18632/aging.100358.

115. Franceschi C, Campisi J. Chronic inflammation (Inflammaging) and its potential contribution to age-associated diseases. J Gerontol Ser A Biol Sci Med Sci. 2014;69:S4–9. https://doi.org/10.1093/gerona/glu057.

116. Hazeldine J, Lord JM, Hampson P. Immunesenescence and inflammaging: a contributory factor in the poor outcome of the geriatric trauma patient. Ageing Res Rev. 2015;24:349–57. https://doi.org/10.1016/j.arr.2015.10.003.

117. Hazeldine J, Lord JM. Innate immunesenescence: underlying mechanisms and clinical relevance. Biogerontology. 2015;16:187–201. https://doi.org/10.1007/s10522-014-9514-3.

118. Schaap LA, Pluijm SMF, Deeg DJH, et al. Higher inflammatory marker levels in older persons: associations with 5-year change in muscle mass and muscle strength. J Gerontol Ser A Biol Sci Med Sci. 2009;64:1183–9. https://doi.org/10.1093/gerona/glp097.

119. Visser M, Pahor M, Taaffe DR, et al. Relationship of interleukin-6 and tumor necrosis factor-α with muscle mass and muscle strength in elderly men and women: the health ABC study. J Gerontol Ser A Biol Sci Med Sci. 2002;57:M326–32. https://doi.org/10.1093/gerona/57.5.M326.

120. Schaap LA, Pluijm SMF, Deeg DJH, Visser M. Inflammatory markers and loss of muscle mass (sarcopenia) and strength. Am J Med. 2006;119:526.e9–526.e17. https://doi.org/10.1016/j.amjmed.2005.10.049.

121. Argilés JM, Busquets S, López-Soriano FJ, Costelli P, Penna F. Are there any benefits of exercise training in cancer cachexia? J Cachexia Sarcopenia Muscle. 2012;3:73–6. https://doi.org/10.1007/s13539-012-0067-5.

122. Coats AJS. Research on cachexia, sarcopenia and skeletal muscle in cardiology. J Cachexia Sarcopenia Muscle. 2012;3:219–23. https://doi.org/10.1007/s13539-012-0090-6.

123. Gould DW, Lahart I, Carmichael AR, Koutedakis Y, Metsios GS. Cancer cachexia prevention via physical exercise: molecular mechanisms. J Cachexia Sarcopenia Muscle. 2013;4:111–24. https://doi.org/10.1007/s13539-012-0096-0.

Sarcopenia and Covid-19: A New Entity?

15

Shaun Sabico and Nicola Veronese

15.1 Introduction

Since the Severe Acute Respiratory Syndrome Coronavirus-2's (SARS-CoV-2) discovery in late 2019 [1], our knowledge about the virus and the coronavirus disease-2019 (COVID-19) in general have exponentially evolved which, over time, translated to modest but substantial control in the pandemic's irreversible damages and progression. At the time of writing this chapter, COVID-19 has so far claimed more than three million human lives globally [2], with casualties concentrated disproportionately in older people and those with preexisting conditions [3]. Nevertheless, as more and more vulnerable people get access to several emergency-use COVID-19 vaccines, the promise of herd immunity is now within reach. Currently, the global medical community has started to shift its focus on the long-term effects of this disease, independent from its respiratory sequelae. In particular, given that the older population is arguably the most vulnerable group in the current pandemic, active management and identification of secondary consequences are crucial and warrant special attention in decreasing risk of unnecessary and highly preventable complications, either from COVID-19 itself or from the drastic measures to prevent COVID-19 that predisposes to anticipated acute disorders.

During the first wave of COVID-19, border lockdowns, quarantines, and social restrictions became the new normal. This prolonged period of confinement has significantly altered the diet and physical activity habits of the general population, resulting in acute and unfavorable metabolic changes [4]. Among the roster of

S. Sabico
Chair for Biomarkers of Chronic Diseases, Biochemistry Department, College of Science, King Saud University, Riyadh, Saudi Arabia
e-mail: ssabico@ksu.edu.sa

N. Veronese (✉)
Geriatrics Section, Department of Internal Medicine, University of Palermo, Palermo, Italy
e-mail: nicola.veronese@unipa.it

© Springer Nature Switzerland AG 2021
N. Veronese et al. (eds.), *Sarcopenia*, Practical Issues in Geriatrics,
https://doi.org/10.1007/978-3-030-80038-3_15

potential metabolic disorders is acute sarcopenic obesity, which is secondary to reduced physical activity and over nutrition, increasing both muscle loss and fat mass [5]. In COVID-19 patients, weight loss and decreased muscle mass and strength are common, in part because of anorexia and elevated inflammatory cytokines, leading to increased risk for cachexia and secondary sarcopenia [6]. Furthermore, it is known that among the critically ill, bed-ridden patients, rapid decreases in muscle mass and bone mineral density (BMD) are anticipated. In a recent study, Kilroe and colleagues demonstrated that muscle volume loss by as much as 1.7% as a consequence of just 2 days (short term) of leg immobilization, which rapidly deteriorates to 5.5% muscle volume loss after 1 week [7]. Finally, in terms of mental health, the pandemic restrictions have been a major factor in triggering several eating disorders across all populations [8]. COVID-19 in its mild forms is associated with weight loss, most likely from acute chemosensory alterations, but severe manifestations have been associated with anorexia and malnutrition [9].

In the present chapter, we highlight the limited yet expanding literature on the musculoskeletal and nutritional challenges encountered particularly in older adults in the ongoing pandemic, the associated risk of secondary sarcopenia among those with severe COVID-19, as well as the still evolving management options among patients with sarcopenia in the era of COVID-19. The chapter is by no means comprehensive, but nonetheless offers insights on the coexistence of sarcopenia and COVID-19, as well as the necessity to address the long lasting and probably lifelong rehabilitation of these patients.

15.2   Nutritional Problems in COVID-19

Preliminary retrospective studies of in-patients with confirmed SARS-CoV-2 have uncovered several risk factors associated with COVID-19 which included old age, male, ethnicity, and preexisting chronic conditions such as obesity, hypertension, diabetes, and cardiovascular diseases [10–12]. Individuals with these lifestyle-related diseases suffered inadvertently more during the imposed lockdowns, because of the sudden lack of access to proper care, negative changes in dietary habits, physical activity, and over-all mental health [13]. As the focus was geared towards the protection of the elderly and the immunocompromised, strategies to cope with pandemic-related stress, including proper nutrition and in-door exercises, were advised by major health institutions. As stated in a recent review by Wang and colleagues [14], hypothetically, the interaction between sarcopenia and COVID-19 could be bidirectional and may form a vicious circle, yet the therapies for sarcopenia can potentially break this cycle and benefit the treatment of both conditions (Fig. 15.1) [15].

Other major nutritional issues relative to sarcopenia during the pandemic are highlighted below, which include micronutrient deficiencies and access to nutritional care.

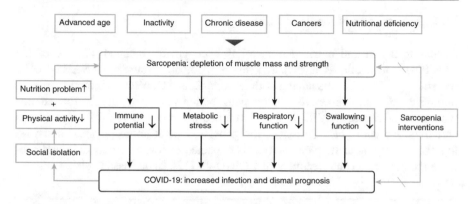

Fig. 15.1 A vicious circle of interactions between sarcopenia and COVID-19. Interventions targeting sarcopenia are anticipated to benefit the treatment of both conditions [15]

Table 15.1 Micronutrients associated with COVID-19

Micronutrient	Action	Ref.
Ascorbic acid or vitamin C	Decreases interleukin-6 which is elevated in severe COVID-19	[22]
Zinc	Inhibits enzymatic activity and replication of SARS-CoV-2 RNA polymerase and to some extent, ACE2 activity	[23]
Selenium	Demonstrates antiviral effect by regulating CD4+ T cell response; deficiency exacerbates progression of viral infections	[24]
Omega-3 fatty acids	As an anti-inflammatory, inhibits the production of mediators such as IL-1β, IL-6, tumor necrosis factor alpha (TNF-α) and may prevent cytokine storm	[25]
Magnesium	Decreases inflammation, oxidative stress, and bronchial smooth muscle relaxation	[26]

15.2.1 Micronutrient Deficiencies

A major part of the preventive management (other than hygiene and isolation measures) included boosting the immune system by correcting micronutrient deficiencies prevalent in the general and the aging population. Vitamin D deficiency, for instance, has been associated with increased mortality among COVID-19 patients [16–18], but evidence as to whether supplementation translates to better outcomes are still limited and not clinically meaningful [19]. Nevertheless, it is known the angiotensin converting enzyme 2 (ACE2) receptors, the point of entry for SARS-CoV-2, is downregulated in COVID-19, with evidence that vitamin D upregulates ACE2, which can bind to SARS-CoV-2 and prevent it from binding to ACE2 receptor [20]. Table 15.1 shows some of the other micronutrients of special interest during the pandemic that are used either as adjuvant or as prophylactic therapy against SARS-CoV-2 infection. The micronutrients have been studied, at varying levels, for their associations with physical performance, muscle mass and function especially in older individuals [21].

15.2.2 Access to Nutritional Care

Access to health and nutritional care has been greatly reduced because of the COVID-19 pandemic as in-person visits are potential sources of SARS-CoV-2 transmission [27]. Patients having both sarcopenia and COVID-19 infection require intensive care and aggressive management, which is also applicable for patients who survived severe COVID-19 and developed acute sarcopenia following illness and intensive care [14]. Currently, the provision of at-home physical activities together with protein supplementation is expected to reverse sarcopenia and promote the prevention and treatment of COVID-19 [15], as discussed below.

15.3   Muscle Mass Loss and Sarcopenia in COVID-19

15.3.1 Acute Sarcopenia in COVID-19

Muscle loss in COVID-19 is mainly acute, also because this condition is known from about 1 year; therefore, we do not know the long-term consequences on muscle mass.

The crucial occurrence in the train of events leading to sarcopenia in COVID-19 is practically due to two main factors, i.e., low physical activity and bedrest [6]. During the COVID-19 pandemic, the bedrest and low physical activity could be associated either with the acute disease or with the universal imposition of lockdown measures and social distancing. It is widely known that immobilization translates into significant changes of muscle cross-sectional area, volume, and mass, promoting the metabolic dysfunction and leading to impaired functionality and finally to disability [4, 28]. In one seminal paper, 10-day forced immobility of healthy older persons would translate to a significant decrease in lower limb lean body mass corresponding to a decrease of isokinetic force, stair-climbing force, and VO2 max [29, 30]. It is estimated that this loss roughly corresponds to the physiological loss of 10 years in healthy young people.

However, these data predate COVID-19 era. It is possible that due to the impact of SARS-CoV-2 infection on energy-producing capabilities, the abovementioned decreases could be even larger. Likewise, longer hospitalization times might translate to larger proportional damage to muscle, as the process may be rather exponential than linear. The immobilization during COVID-19 hospitalization differs markedly from the immobilization due to other conditions, e.g., hip fracture. The experience in COVID-19 suggests that the patient may experience profound weakness, spend hours on high-flow oxygen therapy or in the prone position, and stay in the intensive care unit which was associated per se in only 1 week with an important decrease in muscle mass and strength [31]. They may also develop the post-intensive care syndrome (PICS) which apart from muscular weakness encompasses fatigue, impaired thinking, difficulty swallowing, anxiety, depression, and sleep disturbances [32, 33].

Physical inactivity is also related to a relevant metabolic derangement [4]. The studies of step reduction, both in younger and older healthy adults, demonstrated decrease in insulin sensitivity and finally to higher insulin resistance [34, 35]. In this sense, unfortunately, the COVID-19 pandemic significantly changed patterns of physical activity. The Effects of home Confinement on multiple Lifestyle Behaviours during the COVID-19 outbreak (ECLB-COVID19) was a large multinational web-based questionnaire study that examined an impact of the lockdown measures associated with the first wave of COVID-19 in more than 1000 participants, with a consistent part of older persons [36]. In this study, the physical activity decreased, by approximately one-third, from the baseline vigorous, moderate, weak, and all physical activity estimates. Similarly, the sitting time increased from 5 to 8 h per day [36]. Another study presenting the data for a wide age spectrum in COVID-19 indicates an increase of the number of hours spent in bed at night [37]. Likewise, the type of the activity changed during the pandemic; however, the data pertaining directly to older subjects are lacking, indicating the necessity of specific studies in this sense.

15.3.2 Post-COVID-19 Syndrome

The recovery from the acute COVID-19 does not mark full return to health. The sarcopenic, cardiovascular, pulmonary, psychological, and other symptoms may lag into a long recovery phase [38, 39]. Further, the physiologic, psychologic, and social aftermath of the disease, framing the so-called post-COVID-19 syndrome, may further negatively impact the physical activity and adversely influence the performance and quality of the muscle, leading to sarcopenia.

One study demonstrated that 87.4% of patients had at least one symptom extending into the post-COVID-19 phase. Most of these symptoms included dyspnea or fatigue [40]. Only 12.6% of patients were free from any symptom. Of note, a proportion of patients had arthralgias or pain in other parts of the body [40]. The analysis including data from previous coronavirus infections indicates that the postinfection physical function and fitness may be deteriorated as late as 2 years after the disease [41]. These factors may purely mechanistically adversely influence the physical performance and thus promote sarcopenia [42]. The emotional disorder post-COVID-19 has been observed [43]. This may result in an increase of number of people with depressed mood with the negative consequences that abulia may have on physical activity [44]. Another study of Nordic population demonstrated that while over a half of the patients were free from symptoms 1.5 to 6 months post-COVID-19. In some patients, the symptoms, especially dyspnea, tarried, possibly translating to less physical activity [45]. The prolonged bedrest, vasculitis with a potential to baroreceptor damage, and autonomic neuropathy may contribute to the orthostatic hypotension and induce fear of falling, which may in turn again limit physical activity [46, 47].

However, long-term data on sarcopenia incidence in COVID-19 are urgently needed to confirm the importance of this infectious disease on muscle mass physiology.

15.4   Possible Treatments of Sarcopenia in COVID-19

15.4.1 Nutritional Approaches to Sarcopenia in COVID-19

Sarcopenia is characterized by a high catabolism. It is therefore not surprising that malnutrition should be a common condition among older persons with COVID-19 [48]. Along these lines, if left untreated, it is also associated with a higher mortality [49], making the nutritional counselling especially important in older COVID-19 survivors [50]. This should not only include advice to increase calorie intake but also to ensure adequate protein, vitamin, and mineral intakes [51]. Establishing protein requirements and ensuring that the protein supply be divided among all meals and snacks is of paramount importance [52]. In these patients, dietary recommendations should include oral nutritional supplements (ONS), especially when the diet alone would not be sufficient to meet the nutritional requirements posed by the developing sarcopenia [51]. The patient with the acutely developing post-COVID-19 sarcopenia may benefit from an ONS providing at least 400 kcal per day, with 30 g protein or more. Such strategy should be continued for at least 30 days [53]. The strategy should be stepped-up to 600 kcal per day in persons at a particularly high risk of malnutrition [51]. In the post-COVID-19, post-ICU patients, the high intensity ONS should be continued for over 60 days [53].

The link between vitamin D deficiency and COVID-19 has been postulated [54]. Vitamin D deficiency may be of a prognostic importance, especially in the severe COVID-19 cases [55, 56]. However, whether the supplementation of vitamin D might reduce the risk of a negative outcome, including in the sarcopenic patients, remains to be established. Despite that, in some countries, the authorities recommended the vitamin D supplementation as a possible preventive measure in persons with a high risk of COVID-19 [57]. In a pooled analysis of data from 30 interventional studies, vitamin D has been shown to improve, to some extent, muscle strength. The effect has been greater in persons with baseline vitamin D deficiency [58]. These results should be confirmed in future studies that would lead to a better understanding of the prognostic role of low serum vitamin D levels and the effect of vitamin D supplementation in the acute post-COVID-19 sarcopenia.

The COVID-19 in many patients leads to the fatal outcome [59]. The changing gut microbiota have been implicated in the change of the immune response, and thus might in part be associated with a greater morbidity and possibly mortality due to COVID-19. The support of the gut microbiota with probiotics could therefore improve the immunity and help fighting the SARS-CoV-2 infection [60]. The probiotics and prebiotics have been postulated to be beneficial in the frail older persons; however, the conclusive evidence as regards the post-COVID-19 older patients is still to be obtained [61].

15.4.2 Rehabilitation for Sarcopenia in COVID-19

The rehabilitation in the COVID-19 and post-COVID-19 older patients has been earmarked as the especially important therapeutic modality [62]. Recently, a comprehensive approach to the pulmonary rehabilitation in the COVID-19 patients has been proposed [63]. This includes stratified protocols considering the setting and the severity of the pathological involvement. Such approaches may be of special importance as the organ-related consequences of the COVID-19, for instance, respiratory or cardiovascular [64], but also psychological, are far reaching. Respiratory rehabilitation, which in a small study of 6-week duration, has been shown to improve pulmonary function and has indeed been able to influence quality of life and reduce anxiety [65]. The rehabilitation is always a task for a multidisciplinary team. In the case of the acute sarcopenia after COVID-19, the involvement of a multidisciplinary team is crucial to foster awareness, education, and support whenever required [66, 67]. An important aspect of the rehabilitation of the post-COVID-19 patients, as shown based on the data from persons who had been treated in the ICU setting, is to combine its classic forms with other approaches such as dietary intervention, and the instrumental techniques involving the neuromuscular electrical stimulation [68].

There have been a relative paucity of data concerning the physical rehabilitation in the sarcopenic post-COVID-19 persons. A Cochrane Review from September 2020 concluded that most studies are not focusing on the issues of rehabilitation and the efficacy of the physiotherapeutic interventions [69], a finding in-line with earlier reviews [70]. However, some data did emerge, pointing for instance to the tangible beneficiary effects of post-ICU post-COVID-19 daily 30-min multicomponent exercise program comprising resistance, endurance, and balance training [71].

The COVID-19 has been associated with the incident stroke. Therefore, the modalities employed in the general poststroke rehabilitation may be useful in a subset of post-COVID-19 patients [72, 73]. A small case series proposed that in the ICU-treated COVID-19 patients who would develop focal amyotrophy possibly associated with the prone position, electrostimulation should be used early in the treatment [74]. However, whether similar approach might be effective in the acute sarcopenia after the infection should be verified in future studies.

Finally, with the COVID-19 imposed social distancing, older persons experience more loneliness [75, 76]. Therefore, as pointed out by the World Health Organization, the emotional and indeed the practical support of older persons with the daily living tasks is much advised [77]. Also, the cognitive consequences of COVID-19, with possible obvious implications for physical activity and thus sarcopenia, have been pointed to [78]. Therefore, the cognitive training programs may be a valid part of any post-COVID-19 rehabilitation aiming to fight sarcopenia [79, 80].

15.5 Conclusions

COVID-19 currently is a pandemic affecting particularly older people in terms of hospitalization and mortality. Current data suggested that COVID-19 is associated with sarcopenia through several ways, including malnutrition, bedrest, physical inactivity, medications, cytokines storm and many other that we do not actually know. The preliminary data on this condition suggested that COVID-19 is associated with a higher presence of sarcopenia, but future long-term researches are urgently needed to better understand the real role of this acute disease in muscle mass quality and performance.

References

1. Coronaviridae Study Group of the International Committee on Taxonomy of Viruses. The species severe acute respiratory syndrome-related coronavirus: classifying 2019-nCoV and naming it SARS-CoV-2. Nat Microbiol. 2020;5(4):536–44.
2. Dong E, Du H, Gardner L. An interactive web-based dashboard to track COVID-19 in real time. Lancet Infect Dis. 2020;20(5):533–4.
3. Mueller AL, McNamara MS, Sinclair DA. Why does COVID-19 disproportionately affect older people? Aging (Albany NY). 2020;12(10):9959–98.
4. Martinez-Ferran M, de la Guía-Galipienso F, Sanchis-Gomar F, Pareja-Galeano H. Metabolic impacts of confinement during the COVID-19 pandemic due to modified diet and physical activity habits. Nutrients. 2020;12(6):1549.
5. Kirwan R, McCullough D, Butler T, Perez de Heredia F, Davies IG, Stewart C. Sarcopenia during COVID-19 lockdown restrictions: long-term health effects of short-term muscle loss. GeroScience. 2020:1–32.
6. Morley JE, Kalantar-Zadeh K, Anker SD. COVID-19: a major cause of cachexia and sarcopenia? J Cachexia Sarcopenia Muscle. 2020;11(4):863–5.
7. Kilroe SP, Fulford J, Jackman SR, VAN Loon LJC, Wall BT. Temporal muscle-specific disuse atrophy during one week of leg immobilization. Med Sci Sports Exerc. 2020;52:944–54.
8. Fernández-Aranda F, Casas M, Claes L, Bryan DC, Favaro A, Granero R, Gudiol C, Jiménez-Murcia S, Karwautz A, Le Grange D, Menchón JM, Tchanturia K, Treasure J. COVID-19 and implications for eating disorders. Eur Eat Disord Rev. 2020;28(3):239–45.
9. Di Filippo L, De Lorenzo R, D'Amico M, Sofia V, Roveri L, Mele R, Saibene A, Rovere-Querini P, Conte C. COVID-19 is associated with clinically significant weight loss and risk of malnutrition, independent of hospitalisation: a post-hoc analysis of a prospective cohort study. Clin Nutr. 2020;S0261-5614(20):30589–6.
10. Cummings MJ, Baldwin MR, Abrams D, Jacobson SD, Meyer BJ, Balough EM, Aaron JG, Claassen J, Rabbani LE, Hastie J, Hochman BR, Salazar-Schicchi J, Yip NH, Brodie D, O'Donnell MR. Epidemiology, clinical course, and outcomes of critically ill adults with COVID-19 in New York City: a prospective cohort study. Lancet. 2020;395(10239):1763–70.
11. Baqui P, Bica I, Marra V, Ercole A, van der Schaar M. Ethnic and regional variations in hospital mortality from COVID-19 in Brazil: a cross-sectional observational study. Lancet Glob Health. 2020;8(8):e1018–26.
12. Sheshah E, Sabico S, Albakr RM, Sultan AA, Alghamdi KS, Al Madani K, Alotair HA, Al-Daghri NM. Prevalence of diabetes, management and outcomes among Covid-19 adult patients admitted in a specialized tertiary hospital in Riyadh. Saudi Arabia Diabetes Res Clin Pract. 2021;172:108538.

13. Robinson E, Boyland E, Chisholm A, Harrold J, Maloney NG, Marty L, Mead BR, Noonan R, Hardman CA. Obesity, eating behavior and physical activity during COVID-19 lockdown: a study of UK adults. Appetite. 2021;156:104853.
14. Wang PY, Li Y, Wang Q. Sarcopenia: an underlying treatment target during the COVID-19 pandemic. Nutrition. 2021;84:111104.
15. Teshome A, Adane A, Girma B, Mekonnen ZA. The impact of Vitamin D level on COVID-19 infection: systematic review and meta-analysis. Front Public Health. 2021;9:624559. https://doi.org/10.3389/fpubh.2021.624559.
16. Alguwaihes AM, Al-Sofiani ME, Megdad M, Albader SA, Alsari MH, Alelayan A, Alzahrani SA, Sabico S, Al-Daghri NM, Jammah AA. Diabetes and Covid-19 among hospitalized patients in Saudi Arabia: a single-centre retrospective study. Cardiovasc Diabetol. 2020;19:205.
17. Alguwaihes AM, Sabico S, Hasanato R, Al-Sofiani ME, Megdad M, Albader SS, Alsari MH, Alelayan A, Alyusuf EY, Alzahrani SH, Al-Daghri NM, Jammah AA. Severe vitamin D deficiency is not related to SARS-CoV-2 infection but may increase mortality risk in hospitalized adults: a retrospective case-control study in an Arab gulf country. Aging Clin Exp Res. 2021:1–8. https://doi.org/10.1007/s40520-021-01831-0.
18. Bassatne A, Basbous M, Chakhtoura M, Zein OE, Rahme M, Fuleihan GE. The link between COVID-19 and vitamin D (VIVID): a systematic review and meta-analysis. Metabolism. 2021;154753. https://doi.org/10.1016/j.metabol.2021.
19. Xiao D, Li X, Su X, Mu D, Qu Y. Could SARS-CoV-2-induced lung injury be attenuated by vitamin D? Int J Infect Dis. 2021;102:196–202.
20. Ganapathy A, Nieves JW. Nutrition and sarcopenia—what do we know? Nutrients. 2020;12(6):1755.
21. Feyaerts AF, Luyten W. Vitamin C as prophylaxis and adjunctive medical treatment for COVID-19? Nutrition. 2020;79–80:110948.
22. Hunter J, Arentz S, Goldenberg J, Yang G, Beardsley J, Mertz D, Leeder S. Rapid review protocol: zinc for the prevention or treatment of COVID-19 and other coronavirus-related respiratory tract infections. Integr Med Res. 2020;9(3):100457.
23. Bae M, Kim H. Mini-review on the roles of Vitamin C, Vitamin D, and selenium in the immune system against COVID-19. Molecules. 2020;25(22):5346.
24. Hathaway D, Pandav K, Patel M, Riva-Moscoso A, Singh BM, Patel A, Min ZC, Singh-Makkar S, Sana MK, Sanchez-Dopazo R, Desir R, Fahem MMM, Manella S, Rodriguez I, Alvarez A, Abreu R. Omega 3 fatty acids and COVID-19: a comprehensive review. Infect Chemother. 2020;52(4):478–95.
25. Tang CF, Ding H, Jiao RQ, Wu XX, Kong LD. Possibility of magnesium supplementation for supportive treatment in patients with COVID-19. Eur J Pharmacol. 2020;886:173546.
26. Vazquez J, Islam T, Gursky J, Beller J, Correa DJ. Access to care matters: remote health care needs during COVID-19. Telemed J E Health. 2021;27(4):468–71.
27. Welch C, Greig C, Masud T, Wilson D, Jackson TA. COVID-19 and acute sarcopenia. Aging Dis. 2020;11(6):1345–51.
28. Kirwan R, McCullough D, Butler T, Perez de Heredia F, Davies IG, Stewart C. Sarcopenia during COVID-19 lockdown restrictions: long-term health effects of short-term muscle loss. GeroScience. 2020;42:1547–78.
29. Kortebein P, Symons TB, Ferrando A, Paddon-Jones D, Ronsen O, Protas E, et al. Functional impact of 10 days of bed rest in healthy older adults. J Gerontol A Biol Sci Med Sci. 2008;63:1076–81.
30. Kortebein P, Ferrando A, Lombeida J, Wolfe R, Evans WJ. Effect of 10 days of bed rest on skeletal muscle in healthy older adults. JAMA. 2007;297:1772–4.
31. Mayer KP, Thompson Bastin ML, Montgomery-Yates AA, Pastva AM, Dupont-Versteegden EE, Parry SM, et al. Acute skeletal muscle wasting and dysfunction predict physical disability at hospital discharge in patients with critical illness. Crit Care. 2020;24:637.
32. Michel J-P, Maggi S, Ecarnot F. Raising awareness of the needs of older COVID patients after hospital discharge. Aging Clin Exp Res. 2020;32:1595–8.

33. Stam HJ, Stucki G, Bickenbach J. European Academy of Rehabilitation Medicine. Covid-19 and post intensive care syndrome: a call for action. J Rehabil Med. 2020;52:jrm00044.
34. Olsen RH, Krogh-Madsen R, Thomsen C, Booth FW, Pedersen BK. Metabolic responses to reduced daily steps in healthy nonexercising men. JAMA. 2008;299:1261–3.
35. Krogh-Madsen R, Thyfault JP, Broholm C, Mortensen OH, Olsen RH, Mounier R, et al. A 2-wk reduction of ambulatory activity attenuates peripheral insulin sensitivity. J Appl Physiol Bethesda Md 1985. 2010;108:1034–40.
36. Ammar A, Brach M, Trabelsi K, Chtourou H, Boukhris O, Masmoudi L, et al. Effects of COVID-19 home confinement on eating behaviour and physical activity: results of the ECLB-COVID19 international online survey. Nutrients. 2020;12:1583.
37. Di Renzo L, Gualtieri P, Cinelli G, Bigioni G, Soldati L, Attinà A, et al. Psychological aspects and eating habits during COVID-19 home confinement: results of EHLC-COVID-19 Italian online survey. Nutrients. 2020;12:2152.
38. Arnold DT, Hamilton FW, Milne A, Morley AJ, Viner J, Attwood M, et al. Patient outcomes after hospitalisation with COVID-19 and implications for follow-up: results from a prospective UK cohort. Thorax. 2020;76(4):399–401.
39. Halpin SJ, McIvor C, Whyatt G, Adams A, Harvey O, McLean L, et al. Postdischarge symptoms and rehabilitation needs in survivors of COVID-19 infection: a cross-sectional evaluation. J Med Virol. 2021;93:1013–22.
40. Carfi A, Bernabei R, Landi F. Gemelli against COVID-19 post-acute care study group. Persistent symptoms in patients after acute COVID-19. JAMA. 2020;324:603–5.
41. Rooney S, Webster A, Paul L. Systematic review of changes and recovery in physical function and fitness after severe acute respiratory syndrome-related coronavirus infection: implications for COVID-19 rehabilitation. Phys Ther. 2020;100:1717–29.
42. Garrigues E, Janvier P, Kherabi Y, Le Bot A, Hamon A, Gouze H, et al. Post-discharge persistent symptoms and health-related quality of life after hospitalization for COVID-19. J Infect. 2020;81:e4–6.
43. Janiri D, Kotzalidis GD, Giuseppin G, Molinaro M, Modica M, Montanari S, et al. Psychological distress after Covid-19 recovery: reciprocal effects with temperament and emotional dysregulation. An exploratory study of patients over 60 years of age assessed in a post-acute care service. Front Psych. 2020;11:590135.
44. Stanton R, To QG, Khalesi S, Williams SL, Alley SJ, Thwaite TL, et al. Depression, anxiety and stress during COVID-19: associations with changes in physical activity, sleep, tobacco and alcohol use in Australian adults. Int J Environ Res Public Health. 2020;17:4065.
45. Stavem K, Ghanima W, Olsen MK, Gilboe HM, Einvik G. Persistent symptoms 1.5-6 months after COVID-19 in non-hospitalised subjects: a population-based cohort study. Thorax. 2020;76(4):405–7.
46. Morley JE. Editorial: COVID-19—the long road to recovery. J Nutr Health Aging. 2020;24:917–9.
47. Krishnamoorthy Y, Nagarajan R, Saya GK, Menon V. Prevalence of psychological morbidities among general population, healthcare workers and COVID-19 patients amidst the COVID-19 pandemic: a systematic review and meta-analysis. Psychiatry Res. 2020;293:113382.
48. Li T, Zhang Y, Gong C, Wang J, Liu B, Shi L, et al. Prevalence of malnutrition and analysis of related factors in elderly patients with COVID-19 in Wuhan, China. Eur J Clin Nutr. 2020;74:871–5.
49. Hu X, Deng H, Wang Y, Chen L, Gu X, Wang X. Predictive value of the prognostic nutritional index for the severity of coronavirus disease 2019. Nutr Burbank Los Angel Cty Calif. 2020;84:111123.
50. BDA. Critical Care Specialist Group Guidance on management of nutrition and dietetic services during the COVID-19 pandemic [Internet]. https://www.bda.uk.com/resource/critical-care-dietetics-guidance-covid-19.html. Accessed 28 Feb 2021.
51. Cawood AL, Walters ER, Smith TR, Sipaul RH, Stratton RJ. A review of nutrition support guidelines for individuals with or recovering from COVID-19 in the community. Nutrients. 2020;12:3230.

52. Holdoway A. Nutritional management of patients during and after COVID-19 illness. Br J Community Nurs. 2020;25:S6–10.
53. Barazzoni R, Bischoff SC, Breda J, Wickramasinghe K, Krznaric Z, Nitzan D, et al. ESPEN expert statements and practical guidance for nutritional management of individuals with SARS-CoV-2 infection. Clin Nutr Edinb Scotl. 2020;39:1631–8.
54. De Smet D, De Smet K, Herroelen P, Gryspeerdt S, Martens GA. Serum 25(OH)D level on hospital admission associated with COVID-19 stage and mortality. Am J Clin Pathol. 2021;155:381–8.
55. Carpagnano GE, Di Lecce V, Quaranta VN, Zito A, Buonamico E, Capozza E, et al. Vitamin D deficiency as a predictor of poor prognosis in patients with acute respiratory failure due to COVID-19. J Endocrinol Invest. 2020;44(4):765–71.
56. Jain A, Chaurasia R, Sengar NS, Singh M, Mahor S, Narain S. Analysis of vitamin D level among asymptomatic and critically ill COVID-19 patients and its correlation with inflammatory markers. Sci Rep. 2020;10:20191.
57. Vitamin D and clinically extremely vulnerable (CEV) guidance [Internet]. GOV.UK. https://www.gov.uk/government/publications/vitamin-d-for-vulnerable-groups/vitamin-d-and-clinically-extremely-vulnerable-cev-guidance. Accessed 28 Feb 2021.
58. Beaudart C, Buckinx F, Rabenda V, Gillain S, Cavalier E, Slomian J, et al. The effects of vitamin D on skeletal muscle strength, muscle mass, and muscle power: a systematic review and meta-analysis of randomized controlled trials. J Clin Endocrinol Metab. 2014;99:4336–45.
59. Case-fatality rate and characteristics of patients dying in relation to COVID-19 in Italy—PubMed [Internet]. https://pubmed.ncbi.nlm.nih.gov/32203977/. Accessed 28 Feb 2021
60. Patra S, Saxena S, Sahu N, Pradhan B, Roychowdhury A. Systematic network and meta-analysis on the antiviral mechanisms of probiotics: a preventive and treatment strategy to mitigate SARS-CoV-2 infection. Probiot Antimicrob Proteins. 2021; https://doi.org/10.1007/s12602-021-09748-w.
61. Jayanama K, Theou O. Effects of probiotics and prebiotics on frailty and ageing: a narrative review. Curr Clin Pharmacol. 2020;15:183–92.
62. De Biase S, Cook L, Skelton DA, Witham M, Ten Hove R. The COVID-19 rehabilitation pandemic. Age Ageing. 2020;49:696–700.
63. Gautam AP, Arena R, Dixit S, Borghi-Silva A. Pulmonary rehabilitation in COVID-19 pandemic era: The need for a revised approach. Respirol Carlton Vic [Internet]. 2020. https://www.ncbi.nlm.nih.gov/pmc/articles/PMC7536923/. Accessed 28 Feb 2021.
64. Boukhris M, Hillani A, Moroni F, Annabi MS, Addad F, Ribeiro MH, et al. Cardiovascular implications of the COVID-19 pandemic: a global perspective. Can J Cardiol. 2020;36:1068–80.
65. Liu K, Zhang W, Yang Y, Zhang J, Li Y, Chen Y. Respiratory rehabilitation in elderly patients with COVID-19: a randomized controlled study. Complement Ther Clin Pract. 2020;39:101166.
66. Barker-Davies RM, O'Sullivan O, Senaratne KPP, Baker P, Cranley M, Dharm-Datta S, et al. The Stanford hall consensus statement for post-COVID-19 rehabilitation. Br J Sports Med. 2020;54:949–59.
67. Thomas P, Baldwin C, Bissett B, Boden I, Gosselink R, Granger CL, et al. Physiotherapy management for COVID-19 in the acute hospital setting: clinical practice recommendations. J Physiother. 2020;66:73–82.
68. Trethewey SP, Brown N, Gao F, Turner AM. Interventions for the management and prevention of sarcopenia in the critically ill: a systematic review. J Crit Care. 2019;50:287–95.
69. Andrenelli E, Negrini F, De Sire A, Patrini M, Lazzarini SG, Ceravolo MG, et al. Rehabilitation and COVID-19: a rapid living systematic review 2020 by Cochrane rehabilitation field. Update as of September 30th, 2020. Eur J Phys Rehabil Med. 2020;56:846–52.
70. Ceravolo MG, de Sire A, Andrenelli E, Negrini F, Negrini S. Systematic rapid "living" review on rehabilitation needs due to COVID-19: update to march 31st, 2020. Eur J Phys Rehabil Med. 2020;56:347–53.
71. Udina C, Ars J, Morandi A, Vilaró J, Cáceres C, Inzitari M. Rehabilitation in adult post-COVID-19 patients in post-acute care with therapeutic exercise. J Frailty Aging [Internet]. 2021. Accessed 28 Feb 2021. https://doi.org/10.14283/jfa.2021.1.

72. Burridge J, Alt Murphy M, Buurke J, Feys P, Keller T, Klamroth-Marganska V, et al. A systematic review of International clinical guidelines for rehabilitation of people with neurological conditions: what recommendations are made for upper limb assessment? Front Neurol. 2019;10:567.
73. Needham EJ, Chou SH-Y, Coles AJ, Menon DK. Neurological implications of COVID-19 infections. Neurocrit Care. 2020;32:667–71.
74. Nasuelli NA, Pettinaroli R, Godi L, Savoini C, De Marchi F, Mazzini L, et al. Critical illness neuro-myopathy (CINM) and focal amyotrophy in intensive care unit (ICU) patients with SARS-CoV-2: a case series. Neurol Sci. 2021;42:1119–21.
75. Luchetti M, Lee JH, Aschwanden D, Sesker A, Strickhouser JE, Terracciano A, et al. The trajectory of loneliness in response to COVID-19. Am Psychol. 2020;75:897–908.
76. Mukhtar S. Psychological impact of COVID-19 on older adults. Curr Med Res Pract. 2020;10:201–2.
77. Organization WH. Mental health and psychosocial considerations during the COVID-19 outbreak, 18 March 2020. World Health Organization; 2020. https://apps.who.int/iris/handle/10665/331490. Accessed 28 Feb 2021.
78. Alonso-Lana S, Marquié M, Ruiz A, Boada M. Cognitive and neuropsychiatric manifestations of COVID-19 and effects on elderly individuals with dementia. Front Aging Neurosci. 2020;12:588872.
79. Bernini S, Stasolla F, Panzarasa S, Quaglini S, Sinforiani E, Sandrini G, et al. Cognitive telerehabilitation for older adults with neurodegenerative diseases in the COVID-19 era: a perspective study. Front Neurol. 2020;11:623933.
80. Salawu A, Green A, Crooks MG, Brixey N, Ross DH, Sivan M. A proposal for multidisciplinary tele-rehabilitation in the assessment and rehabilitation of COVID-19 survivors. Int J Environ Res Public Health. 2020;17:4890.

Printed in the United States
by Baker & Taylor Publisher Services